# Sepsis

*Editors*

JULIE A. BASTARACHE
ERIC J. SEELEY

# CLINICS IN
# CHEST MEDICINE

www.chestmed.theclinics.com

June 2016 • Volume 37 • Number 2

**ELSEVIER**

1600 John F. Kennedy Boulevard • Suite 1800 • Philadelphia, Pennsylvania, 19103-2899

http://www.theclinics.com

**CLINICS IN CHEST MEDICINE Volume 37, Number 2**
**June 2016 ISSN 0272-5231, ISBN-13: 978-0-323-44611-2**

Editor: Patrick Manley
Developmental Editor: Casey Jackson

*Clinics in Chest Medicine* (ISSN 0272-5231) is published quarterly by Elsevier Inc., 360 Park Avenue South, New York, NY 10010-1710. Months of issue are March, June, September, and December. Periodicals postage paid at New York, NY and additional mailing offices. Subscription prices are $345.00 per year (domestic individuals), $621.00 per year (domestic institutions), $100.00 per year (domestic students/residents), $380.00 per year (Canadian individuals), $771.00 per year (Canadian institutions), $470.00 per year (international individuals), $771.00 per year (international institutions), and $230.00 per year (international and Canadian students/residents). International air speed delivery is included in all Clinics subscription prices. All prices are subject to change without notice. **POSTMASTER:** Send address changes to Clinics in Chest Medicine, Elsevier Health Sciences Division, Subscription Customer Service, 3251 Riverport Lane, Maryland Heights, MO 63043. **Customer Service: Telephone: 1-800-654-2452** (U.S. and Canada); **1-314-447-8871** (outside U.S. and Canada). **Fax: 1-314-447-8029. E-mail: journalscustomerservice-usa@elsevier.com (for print support); journalsonlinesupport-usa@elsevier.com (for online support).**

*Reprints.* For copies of 100 or more of articles in this publication, please contact the Commercial Reprints Department, Elsevier Inc., 360 Park Avenue South, New York, NY 10010-1710. Tel.: 212-633-3874; Fax: 212-633-3820; E-mail: reprints@elsevier.com.

*Clinics in Chest Medicine* is covered in *MEDLINE/PubMed (Index Medicus), Current Contents/Clinical Medicine, EMBASE/ Excerpta Medica, Science Citation Index,* and *ISI/BIOMED.*

# Contributors

## EDITORS

**JULIE A. BASTARACHE, MD**
Assistant Professor of Medicine, Division of Allergy, Pulmonary, and Critical Care Medicine, Department of Medicine, Vanderbilt University School of Medicine, Nashville, Tennessee

**ERIC J. SEELEY, MD, FCCP**
Assistant Professor of Medicine; Director of Interventional Pulmonary Medicine, Division of Pulmonary, Critical Care Medicine and Allergy, Department of Medicine, University of California San Francisco, San Francisco, California

## AUTHORS

**GORDON R. BERNARD, MD**
Melinda Owen Bass Professor of Medicine, Division of Allergy, Pulmonary and Critical Care Medicine, Vanderbilt University Medical Center, Nashville, Tennessee

**KAREN C. CARROLL, MD**
Professor, Division of Medical Microbiology, Department of Pathology, The Johns Hopkins Hospital, The Johns Hopkins University School of Medicine, Baltimore, Maryland

**FABRICE CHRÉTIEN, MD, PhD**
Institut Pasteur - Unité Histopathologie Humaine et Modèles Animaux, Département Infection et Épidémiologie; Sorbonne Paris Cité, Paris Descartes University; Laboratoire de Neuropathologie, Centre Hospitalier Sainte Anne, Paris, France

**JAMES F. COLBERT, MD**
Postdoctoral Fellow, Division of Infectious Diseases, Department of Medicine, University of Colorado School of Medicine, Aurora, Colorado

**ADAM M. DEANE, PhD**
Discipline of Acute Care Medicine, University of Adelaide; Department of Critical Care Services, Royal Adelaide Hospital, Adelaide, Australia

**JOSHUA A. ENGLERT, MD**
Assistant Professor of Internal Medicine, Division of Pulmonary, Allergy, Critical Care, and Sleep Medicine, The Ohio State University Wexner Medical Center, Columbus, Ohio

**KIMBERLY E. FENTON, MD, FAAP**
Clinical Associate Professor of Pediatrics, Stony Brook University School of Medicine, Stony Brook, New York

**OGNJEN GAJIC, MD, MSc, FCCP, FCCM**
Professor of Medicine, Division of Pulmonology and Critical Care Medicine, Mayo Clinic, Rochester, Minnesota

**JEAN P. GELINAS, MD**
Research Fellow, Centre for Heart Lung Innovation, St. Paul's Hospital, University of British Columbia, Vancouver, British Columbia, Canada

**LAURENT GUÉRIN, MD**
Intensive Care Unit, Section Thorax-Vascular Diseases-Abdomen-Metabolism, Hôpital Ambroise Paré, AP-HP, University Hospital Ambroise Paré, Boulogne Billancourt, France; Faculté de Médecine Paris Ile de France Ouest, Université de Versailles Saint Quentin en Yvelines, Versailles, France

**ANDREW M. HARRISON, PhD**
MD-PhD Student, Medical Scientist Training Program, Mayo Clinic, Rochester, Minnesota

**NICHOLAS HEMING, MD, PhD**
General Intensive Care, Assistance Publique
Hopitaux de Paris, Raymond Poincaré
Teaching Hosptal, Garches, France

**DANIEL J. HENNING, MD, MPH**
Acting Instructor of Medicine, Division of
Emergency Medicine, Harborview Medical
Center, University of Washington School of
Medicine, Seattle, Washington

**VITALY HERASEVICH, MD, PhD, MSc,
FCCM**
Associate Professor of Anesthesiology and
Medicine, Department of Anesthesiology,
Mayo Clinic, Rochester, Minnesota

**JORDAN A. KEMPKER, MD, MSc**
Division of Pulmonary, Allergy, Sleep and
Critical Care Medicine, Emory University
School of Medicine, Atlanta, Georgia

**KATHLEEN D. LIU, MD, PhD, MAS**
Division of Nephrology, Department of
Medicine; Division of Critical Care Medicine,
Department of Anesthesia, University of
California San Francisco, San Francisco,
California

**JASON H. MALEY, MD**
Department of Medicine, Perelman School of
Medicine at the University of Pennsylvania,
Philadelphia, Pennsylvania

**GREG S. MARTIN, MD, MSc**
Division of Pulmonary, Allergy, Sleep and
Critical Care Medicine, Emory University
School of Medicine, Atlanta, Georgia

**AURELIEN MAZERAUD**
Institut Pasteur - Unité Histopathologie
Humaine et Modèles Animaux, Département
Infection et Épidémiologie, Paris, France;
Sorbonne Paris Cité, Paris Descartes
University, Paris, France; General Intensive
Care, Assistance Publique Hopitaux de Paris,
Raymond Poincaré Teaching Hosptal,
Garches, France

**MARK E. MIKKELSEN, MD, MSCE**
Department of Medicine, Division of
Pulmonary, Allergy, and Critical Care; Center
for Clinical Epidemiology and Biostatistics,
Perelman School of Medicine at the University
of Pennsylvania, Philadelphia, Pennsylvania

**MARGARET M. PARKER, MD, MCCM**
Professor of Pediatrics, Anesthesia and
Medicine, Stony Brook University School of
Medicine, Stony Brook, New York

**QUENTIN PASCAL, DVM**
Institut Pasteur - Unité Histopathologie
Humaine et Modèles Animaux, Département
Infection et Épidémiologie, Paris, France

**XOSÉ L. PÉREZ, MD**
Intensive Care Medicine, Bellvitge University
Hospital, Barcelona, Spain

**BRIAN W. PICKERING, MB, BCh, MSc,
FFARCSI**
Assistant Professor of Anesthesiology,
Department of Anesthesiology, Mayo Clinic,
Rochester, Minnesota

**MARK P. PLUMMER, MBBS**
Discipline of Acute Care Medicine, University
of Adelaide; Department of Critical Care
Services, Royal Adelaide Hospital, Adelaide,
Australia

**TODD W. RICE, MD, MSc**
Associate Professor of Medicine, Pulmonary
and Critical Care Medicine, Division of Allergy,
Pulmonary, and Critical Care Medicine,
Vanderbilt University Medical Center,
Nashville, Tennessee

**STEFAN RIEDEL, MD, PhD, D(ABMM)**
Associate Professor, Department of Pathology,
Beth Israel Deaconess Medical Center,
Harvard Medical School, Boston,
Massachusetts

**ANGELA J. ROGERS, MD, MPH**
Assistant Professor of Medicine, Division of
Pulmonary and Critical Care Medicine,
Stanford University, Stanford, California

**JAMES A. RUSSELL, MD**
Professor of Medicine, Centre for Heart Lung
Innovation, Division of Critical Care Medicine,
St. Paul's Hospital, University of British
Columbia, Vancouver, British Columbia,
Canada

**ERIC P. SCHMIDT, MD**
Associate Professor, Division of Pulmonary
Sciences and Critical Care Medicine,
Department of Medicine, Denver Health
Medical Center, University of Colorado School
of Medicine, Aurora, Colorado

**ERIC J. SEELEY, MD, FCCP**
Assistant Professor of Medicine; Director of
Interventional Pulmonary Medicine, Division of
Pulmonary, Critical Care Medicine and Allergy,
Department of Medicine, University of
California San Francisco, San Francisco,
California

**MATTHEW W. SEMLER, MD**
Fellow, Division of Allergy, Pulmonary, and
Critical Care Medicine, Vanderbilt University
Medical Center, Nashville, Tennessee

**NATHAN I. SHAPIRO, MD, MPH**
Associate Professor of Emergency
Medicine, Beth Israel Deaconess Medical
Center, Harvard Medical School, Boston,
Massachusetts

**TAREK SHARSHAR, MD, PhD**
Institut Pasteur - Unité Histopathologie
Humaine et Modèles Animaux, Département
Infection et Épidémiologie, Paris, France;
General Intensive Care, Assistance Publique
Hopitaux de Paris, Raymond Poincaré
Teaching Hosptal, Garches, France;
Versailles-Saint Quentin University, Avenue
de Paris, Versailles, France

**TIMOTHY E. SWEENEY, MD, PhD**
Department of Surgery, Institute for Immunity,
Transplantation and Infection, Stanford

University School of Medicine, Stanford,
California

**FRANCK VERDONK**
Institut Pasteur - Unité Histopathologie
Humaine et Modèles Animaux, Département
Infection et Épidémiologie; Sorbonne Paris
Cité, Paris Descartes University, Paris,
France

**ANTOINE VIEILLARD-BARON, MD, PhD**
Intensive Care Unit, Section Thorax-Vascular
Diseases-Abdomen-Metabolism, Hôpital
Ambroise Paré, AP-HP, University Hospital
Ambroise Paré, Boulogne Billancourt, France;
Faculté de Médecine Paris Ile de France Ouest,
Université de Versailles Saint Quentin en
Yvelines, Versailles, France; INSERM U-1018,
CESP, Team 5 (EpReC, Renal and
Cardiovascular Epidemiology), UVSQ, Villejuif,
France

**KEITH R. WALLEY, MD**
Professor of Medicine, Centre for Heart Lung
Innovation, St. Paul's Hospital, University of
British Columbia, Vancouver, British Columbia,
Canada

**PAUL D. WEYKER, MD**
Division of Critical Care, Department of
Anesthesia, Columbia University, New York,
New York

**HECTOR R. WONG, MD**
Division of Critical Care Medicine, Cincinnati
Children's Hospital Medical Center, Cincinnati
Children's Research Foundation; Department
of Pediatrics, University of Cincinnati College
of Medicine, Cincinnati, Ohio

# Contents

**Preface: Sepsis** xv

Julie A. Bastarache and Eric J. Seeley

**The Changing Epidemiology and Definitions of Sepsis** 165

Jordan A. Kempker and Greg S. Martin

This article describes the trends in the incidence of and mortality from sepsis in the United States and globally. The article then discusses the known factors associated with increased risk for developing sepsis and the limitations of the current clinical definition and the clinical correlations of the current epidemiology.

**Therapeutic Targets in Sepsis: Past, Present, and Future** 181

Eric J. Seeley and Gordon R. Bernard

Antibiotics and fluids have been standard treatment for sepsis since World War II. Many molecular mediators of septic shock have since been identified. In models of sepsis, blocking these mediators improved organ injury and decreased mortality. Clinical trials, however, have failed. The absence of new therapies has been vexing to clinicians, clinical researchers, basic scientists, and the pharmaceutical industry. This article examines the evolution of sepsis therapy and theorizes about why so many well-reasoned therapies have not worked in human trials. We review new molecular targets for sepsis and examine trial designs that might lead to successful treatments for sepsis.

**Early Identification and Treatment of Pathogens in Sepsis: Molecular Diagnostics and Antibiotic Choice** 191

Stefan Riedel and Karen C. Carroll

Sepsis and septic shock are serious conditions associated with high morbidity and mortality. Rapid molecular methods for detection of microorganisms and antimicrobial resistance genes from positive blood cultures or whole blood have evolved over the past 10 years. Such diagnostic methods coupled with therapeutic interventional programs are desirable to improve the overall clinical outcome and mortality. This article discusses the usefulness of current molecular test methods for the diagnosis of sepsis and their potential to enhance the success of antimicrobial stewardship programs. Clinicians and laboratories alike must appreciate key factors influencing the appropriate use and potential impact of these methods.

**Risk Stratification and Prognosis in Sepsis: What Have We Learned from Microarrays?** 209

Timothy E. Sweeney and Hector R. Wong

Sepsis mortality rates have decreased in recent years but remain unacceptably high. Risk stratification and prognostication is of particular importance because high-risk patients may benefit from earlier clinical interventions, whereas low-risk patients may benefit from not undergoing unnecessary procedures. Prognostication is currently done mostly via clinical criteria and blood lactate levels. This article summarizes the literature on the complexity of changes at the molecular level for the casual reader.

## Development and Implementation of Sepsis Alert Systems

219

Andrew M. Harrison, Ognjen Gajic, Brian W. Pickering, and Vitaly Herasevich

Development and implementation of sepsis alert systems is challenging, particularly outside the monitored intensive care unit (ICU) setting. Barriers to wider use of sepsis alerts include evolving clinical definitions of sepsis, information overload, and alert fatigue, due to suboptimal alert performance. Outside the ICU, barriers include differences in health care delivery models, charting behaviors, and availability of electronic data. Current evidence does not support routine use of sepsis alert systems in clinical practice. Continuous improvement in the afferent and efferent aspects will help translate theoretic advantages into measurable patient benefit.

## Goal-Directed Resuscitation in Septic Shock: A Critical Analysis

231

Daniel J. Henning and Nathan I. Shapiro

The Early Goal-Directed Therapy versus Standard Care for Sepsis trial by Rivers and colleagues in 2001 suggested that a significant mortality reduction may be realized through goal-directed interventions early in the care of patients with septic shock. However, the recent publication of the Protocol-Based Care for Early Septic Shock (ProCESS), Australasian Resuscitation in Sepsis Evaluation (ARISE), and Protocolised Management in Sepsis (ProMISE) trials did not demonstrate the superiority of early goal-directed therapy over usual care. If usual care includes timely and meticulous care, a protocol may not be needed to realize the continued lowering mortality rates.

## Sepsis Resuscitation: Fluid Choice and Dose

241

Matthew W. Semler and Todd W. Rice

Sepsis is a common and life-threatening inflammatory response to severe infection treated with antibiotics and fluid resuscitation. Despite the central role of intravenous fluid in sepsis management, fundamental questions regarding which fluid and in what amount remain unanswered. Recent advances in understanding the physiologic response to fluid administration, and large clinical studies examining resuscitation strategies, fluid balance after resuscitation, colloid versus crystalloid solutions, and high- versus low-chloride crystalloids, inform the current approach to sepsis fluid management and suggest areas for future research.

## Vasopressors During Sepsis: Selection and Targets

251

Jean P. Gelinas and James A. Russell

Clinicians have greatly improved care for septic shock. Urgent resuscitation using intravenous fluids and vasopressors as well as rapid administration of broad spectrum antibiotics are probably the most basic and universally accepted interventions. Various trials have compared different types of vasopressors, associations of vasopressors and inotropes, and pressure targets. End goal-directed therapy algorithms are now in question because of three recent negative trials. Patients who have a poor response to resuscitation and patients with known severe ventricular dysfunction might merit advanced hemodynamic monitoring. This review examines important vasopressor and septic shock trials.

**Endothelial and Microcirculatory Function and Dysfunction in Sepsis**          263

James F. Colbert and Eric P. Schmidt

The microcirculation is a series of arterioles, capillaries, and venules that performs essential functions of oxygen and nutrient delivery, customized to the unique physiologic needs of the supplied organ. The homeostatic microcirculatory response to infection can become harmful if overactive and/or dysregulated. Pathologic microcirculatory dysfunction can be directly visualized by intravital microscopy or indirectly measured via detection of circulating biomarkers. Although several treatments have been shown to protect the microcirculation during sepsis, they have not improved patient outcomes when applied indiscriminately. Future outcomes-oriented studies are needed to test sepsis therapeutics when personalized to a patient's microcirculatory dysfunction.

**Management of Acute Kidney Injury and Acid-Base Balance in the Septic Patient**          277

Paul D. Weyker, Xosé L. Pérez, and Kathleen D. Liu

Acute kidney injury (AKI) is an abrupt decrease in kidney function that takes place over hours to days. Sepsis is the leading cause of AKI and portends a particularly high morbidity and mortality, although the severity may vary from a transient rise in serum creatinine to end-stage renal disease. With regard to acid-base management in septic AKI, caution should be used with hyperchloremic crystalloid solutions, and dialysis is often used in the setting of severe acidosis. In the future, biomarkers may help clinicians identify AKI earlier and allow for potential interventions before the development of severe AKI.

**Cardiac Function and Dysfunction in Sepsis**          289

Kimberly E. Fenton and Margaret M. Parker

Cardiac function and dysfunction are important in the clinical outcomes of sepsis and septic shock. Cardiac dysfunction is not a single entity, but is a broad spectrum of syndromes that result in biventricular cardiac dysfunction manifested by both systolic and diastolic dysfunction and is influenced by cardiac loading conditions (ie, preload and afterload). Elucidating the underlying pathophysiology has proved to be complex. This article emphasizes the underlying pathophysiology of cardiac dysfunction and explores recent evidence related to diagnosis, including the utility of biomarkers, the role of echocardiography, and management goals and treatment.

**The Use of Ultrasound in Caring for Patients with Sepsis**          299

Laurent Guérin and Antoine Vieillard-Baron

Echocardiography is a noninvasive and accurate tool used in the intensive care unit to assess cardiac function and monitor hemodynamics in shocked patients. During severe sepsis or septic shock, several mechanisms can lead to hemodynamic failure and have to be quickly and precisely diagnosed to propose adequate, personalized, and timely hemodynamic therapy. Echocardiography truly provides intensivists with this diagnostic possibility, whether or not there is fluid responsiveness, cardiac dysfunction, or persistent vasoplegia. Acquiring skills in critical care echocardiography is mandatory in improving management and monitoring of patients with sepsis at the bedside. How critical care echocardiography in managing patients with septic shock improves prognosis remains to be elucidated.

**Dysglycemia and Glucose Control During Sepsis**    309

Mark P. Plummer and Adam M. Deane

Sepsis predisposes to disordered metabolism and dysglycemia; the latter is a broad term that includes hyperglycemia, hypoglycemia, and glycemic variability. Dysglycemia is a marker of illness severity. Large randomized controlled trials have provided considerable insight into the optimal blood glucose targets for critically ill patients with sepsis. However, it may be that the pathophysiologic consequences of dysglycemia are dynamic throughout the course of a septic insult and also altered by premorbid glycemia. This review highlights the relevance of hyperglycemia, hypoglycemia, and glycemic variability in patients with sepsis with an emphasis on a rational approach to management.

**Metabolism, Metabolomics, and Nutritional Support of Patients with Sepsis**    321

Joshua A. Englert and Angela J. Rogers

Sepsis is characterized by profound changes in systemic and cellular metabolism that disrupt normal metabolic homeostasis. These metabolic changes can serve as biomarkers for disease severity. Lactate, a metabolite of anaerobic metabolism, is the most widely used ICU biomarker and it is incorporated into multiple management algorithms. Technological advances now make broader metabolic profiling possible, with early studies identifying metabolic changes associated with sepsis mortality. Finally, given the marked changes in metabolism in sepsis and the association of worse prognosis in patients with severe metabolic derangements, we summarize the seminal trials conducted to optimize nutrition in the ICU.

**Neuroanatomy and Physiology of Brain Dysfunction in Sepsis**    333

Aurelien Mazeraud, Quentin Pascal, Franck Verdonk, Nicholas Heming, Fabrice Chrétien, and Tarek Sharshar

Sepsis-associated encephalopathy (SAE), a complication of sepsis, is often complicated by acute and long-term brain dysfunction. SAE is associated with electroencephalogram pattern changes and abnormal neuroimaging findings. The major processes involved are neuroinflammation, circulatory dysfunction, and excitotoxicity. Neuroinflammation and microcirculatory alterations are diffuse, whereas excitotoxicity might occur in more specific structures involved in the response to stress and the control of vital functions. A dysfunction of the brainstem, amygdala, and hippocampus might account for the increased mortality, psychological disorders, and cognitive impairment. This review summarizes clinical and paraclinical features of SAE and describes its mechanisms at cellular and structural levels.

**Beyond the Golden Hours: Caring for Septic Patients After the Initial Resuscitation**    347

Jean P. Gelinas and Keith R. Walley

Recognition and management of agitation, delirium, and pain are key areas. Reduced use of sedatives is an important measure that must be coupled with increased patient engagement, mobilization, and exercise. Use of low tidal volumes and low mean airway pressures during mechanical ventilation is helpful. A key hemodynamic principle following early aggressive volume resuscitation is subsequent careful assessment to avoid unnecessary additional volume administration and adverse consequences of frank volume overload. Substantial evidence now supports a lower hemoglobin transfusion threshold of 7 g/dL. A rush to initiate enteral or parenteral feeds is not clearly supported by the current evidence.

**Short-term Gains with Long-term Consequences: The Evolving Story of Sepsis Survivorship**          367

Jason H. Maley and Mark E. Mikkelsen

Sepsis is an acute, life-threatening condition that afflicts millions of patients annually. Advances in care and heightened awareness have led to substantial declines in short-term mortality. An expanding body of literature describes the long-term impact of sepsis, revealing long-term cognitive and functional impairments, sustained inflammation and immune dysfunction, increased healthcare resource use, reduced health-related quality of life, and increased mortality. The evidence challenges the notion that sepsis is an acute, transient illness, revealing rather that sepsis is an acute illness with lingering consequences. This article provides a state-of-the-art review of the emerging literature of the long-term consequences of sepsis.

**Index**          381

## PROGRAM OBJECTIVE
The goal of the *Clinics in Chest Medicine* is to provide practitioners with state-of-the-art information that is clinically useful, concise, well referenced, and comprehensive.

## TARGET AUDIENCE
All practicing physicians and healthcare professionals who provide patient care utilizing findings from *Chest Medicine Clinics of North America*.

## LEARNING OBJECTIVES
Upon completion of this activity, participants will be able to:
1. Review the epidemiology and definitions of sepsis.
2. Discuss metabolic and nutritional support for patients with sepsis.
3. Recognize therapeutic targets and management strategies for patients with sepsis.

## ACCREDITATION
The Elsevier Office of Continuing Medical Education (EOCME) is accredited by the Accreditation Council for Continuing Medical Education (ACCME) to provide continuing medical education for physicians.

The EOCME designates this enduring material for a maximum of 15 *AMA PRA Category 1 Credit*(s)™. Physicians should claim only the credit commensurate with the extent of their participation in the activity.

All other health care professionals requesting continuing education credit for this enduring material will be issued a certificate of participation.

## DISCLOSURE OF CONFLICTS OF INTEREST
The EOCME assesses conflict of interest with its instructors, faculty, planners, and other individuals who are in a position to control the content of CME activities. All relevant conflicts of interest that are identified are thoroughly vetted by EOCME for fair balance, scientific objectivity, and patient care recommendations. EOCME is committed to providing its learners with CME activities that promote improvements or quality in healthcare and not a specific proprietary business or a commercial interest.

**The planning committee, staff, authors and editors listed below have identified no financial relationships or relationships to products or devices they or their spouse/life partner have with commercial interest related to the content of this CME activity:**

Fabrice Chrétien, MD, PhD; James F. Colbert, MD; Adam M. Deane, PhD; Joshua A. Englert, MD; Kimberly E. Fenton, MD, FAAP; Anjali Fortna; Jean P. Gelinas, MD; Laurent Guérin, MD; Andrew M. Harrison, PhD; Nicholas Heming, MD, PhD; Jordan A. Kempker, MD, MSc; Kathleen D. Liu, MD, PhD, MAS; Jason H. Maley, MD; Patrick Manley; Greg S. Martin, MD, MSc; Aurelien Mazeraud; Mark E. Mikkelsen, MD, MSCE; Palani Murugesan; Margaret M. Parker, MD, MCCM; Quentin Pascal, DVM; Mark P. Plummer, MBBS; Todd W. Rice, MD, MSc; Angela J. Rogers, MD, MPH; Erin Scheckenbach; Eric P. Schmidt, MD; Matthew W. Semler, MD; Tarek Sharshar, MD, PhD; Franck Verdonk; Antoine Vieillard-Baron, MD, PhD; Keith R. Walley, MD; Paul D. Weyker, MD.

**The planning committee, staff, authors and editors listed below have identified financial relationships or relationships to products or devices they or their spouse/life partner have with commercial interest related to the content of this CME activity:**

**Julie A. Bastarache, MD** has stock ownership in HealthStream, and is a consultant/advisor for Abbott Laboratories.

**Gordon R. Bernard, MD** has research support from AstraZeneca.

**Karen C. Carroll, MD** is on the speakers' bureau for Quidel Corporation.

**Ognjen Gajic, MD, MSc, FCCP, FCCM** has stock ownership in, and receives royalties/patents from, Ambient Clinical Analytics.

**Daniel J. Henning, MD, MPH** has research support from Roche Diagnostics, USA.

**Vitaly Herasevich, MD, PhD, MSc, FCCM** has stock ownership in, and receives royalties/patents from, Ambient Clinical Analytics.

**Brian W. Pickering, MB, BCh, MSc, FFARCSI** is a consultant/advisor for, has stock ownership in, and receives royalties/patents from Ambient Clinical Analytics.

**Stefan Riedel, MD, PhD, D(ABMM)** is on the speakers' bureau for BD, is a consultant/advisor for OpGen, and has research support from BD and Nanosphere, Inc.

**James A. Russell, MD** is a consultant/advisor for Ferring Pharmaceuticals; AKPA; Leading BioSciences, Inc; La Jolla Pharmacuetical Company; Merck & Co., Inc; and Grifols, has stock ownership in Cyon Therapeutics and Leading BioSciences, Inc, has research support from Grifols, and receives roylaties/patents from Cyon Pharmaceuticals.

**Eric J. Seeley, MD, FCCP** is a consultant/advisor for Pulmonx and Cheetah Medical.

**Nathan I. Shapiro, MD, MPH** is a consultant/advisor for Cheetah Medical, and has research support from Cheetah Medical and Thermo Fisher Scientific, Inc.

**Timothy E. Sweeney, MD, PhD** is a consultant/advisor for, with stock ownership in, Multerra Biosciences, LLC, and has research support from Society of University Surgeons and Stanford Medicine.

**Hector R. Wong, MD** has research support from the National Institutes of Health.

## UNAPPROVED/OFF-LABEL USE DISCLOSURE

The EOCME requires CME faculty to disclose to the participants:

1. When products or procedures being discussed are off-label, unlabelled, experimental, and/or investigational (not US Food and Drug Administration [FDA] approved); and
2. Any limitations on the information presented, such as data that are preliminary or that represent ongoing research, interim analyses, and/or unsupported opinions. Faculty may discuss information about pharmaceutical agents that is outside of FDA-approved labelling. This information is intended solely for CME and is not intended to promote off-label use of these medications. If you have any questions, contact the medical affairs department of the manufacturer for the most recent prescribing information.

## TO ENROLL

To enroll in the *Chest Medicine Clinics* Continuing Medical Education program, call customer service at 1-800-654-2452 or sign up online at http://www.theclinics.com/home/cme. The CME program is available to subscribers for an additional annual fee of USD $225.

## METHOD OF PARTICIPATION

In order to claim credit, participants must complete the following:

1. Complete enrolment as indicated above.
2. Read the activity.
3. Complete the CME Test and Evaluation. Participants must achieve a score of 70% on the test. All CME Tests and Evaluations must be completed online.

## CME INQUIRIES/SPECIAL NEEDS

For all CME inquiries or special needs, please contact elsevierCME@elsevier.com.

# CLINICS IN CHEST MEDICINE

**FORTHCOMING ISSUES**

*September 2016*
**Rare and Orphan Lung Diseases**
Robert Kotloff and Francis McCormack, *Editors*

*December 2016*
**Advances in Mechanical Ventilation**
Neil MacIntyre, *Editor*

*March 2017*
**Viral and Atypical Pneumonia**
Charles De La Cruz and Richard Wunderlink, *Editors*

**RECENT ISSUES**

*March 2016*
**Cystic Fibrosis**
Jonathan L. Koff, *Editor*

*December 2015*
**Sarcoidosis**
Robert P. Baughman and Daniel A. Culver, *Editors*

*September 2015*
**Advances and Challenges in Critical Care**
Shyoko Honiden and Jonathan M. Siner, *Editors*

**RELATED INTEREST**

*Critical Care Clinics,* Vol. 32, No. 2 (April 2016)
**Gastrointestinal Issues in Critical Care**
Rahul S. Nanchal and Ram M. Subramanian, *Editors*

**THE CLINICS ARE AVAILABLE ONLINE!**
Access your subscription at:
www.theclinics.com

# Preface
# Sepsis

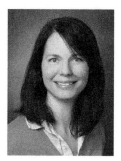 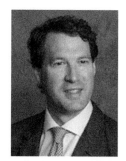

Julie A. Bastarache, MD    Eric J. Seeley, MD, FCCP
*Editors*

The definitions, diagnostics, and demographics of sepsis are changing. However, the development of new targeted therapies or protocolized treatments for sepsis has not kept pace. In fact, no new treatment has been widely adopted since the last installment of *Clinics in Chest Medicine*, Sepsis issue, in 2008. Actually, some treatments that were considered standard of care in 2008, including tight glycemic control and activated protein C, are no longer part of sepsis therapy. We review these new trials and place them in the context of the latest epidemiologic, physiologic, and biologic studies of sepsis.

This issue of *Clinics in Chest Medicine*, Sepsis issue, can be roughly divided into 4 sections. The first focuses on the recently updated definition of sepsis, new epidemiologic studies of sepsis, and a historical overview of attempts at molecular therapeutics for sepsis. In addition, this section addresses the heterogeneity of patients enrolled in trials of new therapies for sepsis, in terms of the source of sepsis, the pathogen involved, and the host immune response to infection. Several articles in this issue of Updates in Sepsis focus on how to classify septic patients with greater sophistication and also explore new targets and trial designs that might improve the quality of sepsis trials.

A second series of articles focuses on the acute resuscitation phase of patients with sepsis and septic shock. Specifically, these articles focus on properly identifying septic patients using molecular tools and the electronic medical record and address treatments critical to the early resuscitation phase. In addition, early physiologic goals

for resuscitation are reviewed in the context of new evidence regarding the golden hours of resuscitation. Furthermore, fluid choice and dose, one of the key enduring therapies of sepsis, is discussed with an eye toward preventing downstream organ injury.

With widespread adoption of early antibiotics and fluids, sepsis mortality is decreasing; however, filling the vascular compartment and supporting injured organs can lead to new physiologic derangements, including severe acidosis, endothelial injury, and volume overload. In the third section of the series, we address how to correctly identify and support organs injured due to the initial septic insult and resuscitation. This includes a review of how the endothelium is injured and the potential role of resuscitation in this injury. We hope that clinical care after the initial resuscitation might be fine tuned, in order to avoid the consequences of postresuscitation volume overload and potential organ injury due to continued unnecessary volume administration.

In the final section of this series, we examine the burden of sepsis survivorship. In particular, we review the metabolic, neurologic, and physical insults that take place during the initial resuscitation, stabilization, and resolution phases of sepsis.

We hope that this series of articles will provide an update for clinicians to hone the current management of patients presenting with sepsis and septic shock. In addition, we hope that epidemiologists, clinical trialists, and basic biologists might view this set of articles as a springboard toward a more informed investigation of sepsis, an

Clin Chest Med 37 (2016) xv–xvi
http://dx.doi.org/10.1016/j.ccm.2016.04.001
0272-5231/16/$ – see front matter © 2016 Published by Elsevier Inc.

enduring disease in need of new targeted protocols and therapies.

Julie A. Bastarache, MD
Vanderbilt University School of Medicine
1161 21st Avenue South
T-1218 MCN
Nashville, TN 37232, USA

Eric J. Seeley, MD, FCCP
400 Parnassus Avenue
5th Floor ACC
San Francisco, CA 94143, USA

E-mail addresses:
julie.bastarache@vanderbilt.edu
(J.A. Bastarache)
eric.seeley@ucsf.edu (E.J. Seeley)

# The Changing Epidemiology and Definitions of Sepsis

 CrossMark

Jordan A. Kempker, MD, MSc*, Greg S. Martin, MD, MSc

## KEYWORDS

- Sepsis • Severe sepsis • Septic shock • Epidemiology

## KEY POINTS

- In the epidemiology of sepsis in the United States, different case definitions have produced varied results, with recent estimates of an average annual age-adjusted incidence between approximately 300 to 1000 sepsis cases per 100,000 persons. Estimates consistently show trends toward an increasing incidence in sepsis with a decreasing case fatality.
- In the United States and globally, respiratory tract infections are consistently the most common source of sepsis although there is more variability in the microbiological distribution of common pathogens.
- Although evidence regarding the epidemiology of sepsis in developing countries is scarce, they seem to have 3-fold to 4-fold increased incidence of mortality from sepsis-related infections.
- Although data for longitudinal risk factors for sepsis are lacking, in the United States this syndrome disproportionately affects the very young and old, males, blacks, and the southeastern states.

## INTRODUCTION

Although the first written description of the sepsis syndrome appears in an Egyptian papyrus circa 1600 BC, the origin of the term sepsis comes from the Ancient Greek word sêpsis, which means putrefaction or the decay of organic matter.[1,2] The Greek word is first encountered in Homer's *Iliad* and was also used in the Hippocratic corpus in the fourth century BC.[2] More than 2000 years passed before humankind first considered the causes and prevention of this syndrome. In the nineteenth century, Hungarian obstetrician Ignaz Semmelweis recognized that physician handwashing drastically decreased the incidence of puerperal sepsis on the maternity ward.[2] Although Semmelweis' theories were rejected during his lifetime, they were later unknowingly validated by Louis Pasteur and Robert Koch, whose works gave birth to the germ theory of infectious diseases[2] (**Fig. 1**). This pivotal achievement paved the way for further developments in defining the spectrum of sepsis syndromes and studying their impact on human life, which is summarized in this article.

The following overview of the modern epidemiology of sepsis begins with discussion of the recent epidemiology of sepsis in the United States (US) and globally, followed by a review of the literature on the associated risk factors for sepsis, and ends with a discussion of the clinical utility of current definitions of sepsis and future directions in the field.

## UNITED STATES TRENDS IN INCIDENCE AND MORTALITY FROM SEPSIS

The epidemiology of sepsis in the US has been primarily based on studies using large, administrative

Disclosure: The authors have nothing to disclose.
Division of Pulmonary, Allergy, Sleep and Critical Care Medicine, Emory University School of Medicine, 615 Michael Street, Suite 205, Atlanta, GA 30322, USA
* Corresponding author.
*E-mail address:* jkempke@emory.edu

Clin Chest Med 37 (2016) 165–179
http://dx.doi.org/10.1016/j.ccm.2016.01.002
0272-5231/16/$ – see front matter © 2016 Elsevier Inc. All rights reserved.

chestmed.theclinics.com

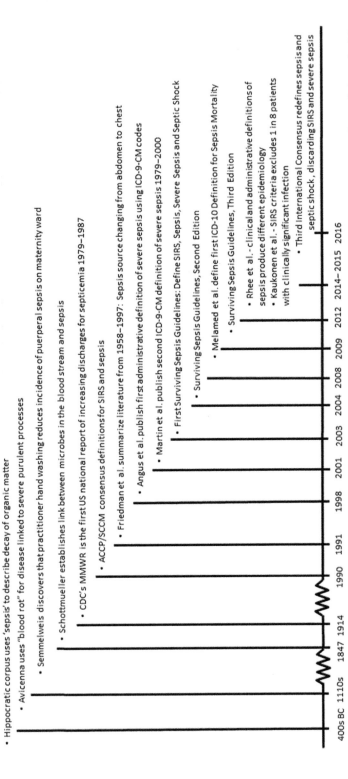

**Fig. 1.** Abbreviated timeline of the conceptual definition of sepsis. 9-CM, Ninth Revision, Clinical Modification; ACCP/SCCM, American College of Chest Physicians and the Society of Critical Care Medicine; CDC, Centers for Disease Control and Prevention; ICD, International Classification of Diseases; MMWR, morbidity and mortality weekly report; SIRS, systemic inflammatory response syndrome.

databases. Therefore, some initial discussion of the administrative definitions used is necessary to understand the observed variability in the estimates. Various investigators have defined sepsis cases using different combinations of diagnostic codes listed on hospital discharge records and using the International Classification of Diseases (ICD), Ninth Revision, Clinical Modification (9-CM) coding scheme. **Table 1** summarizes details of several ICD-9-CM definitions, demonstrating that there is a wide range of the types of coding schemas used to create a case definition of severe sepsis from various infections and associated organ dysfunctions.[3–5] Various attempts have been made to assess the validity of these administrative definitions, which demonstrated the Martin definition to have sensitivity of 17% to 81% and specificity of 88% to 100%, and the Angus definition to have a sensitivity of 47% to 50% and specificity of 92%.[5–7] Although these data support that the administrative definitions are approximating the clinical definitions of severe sepsis, other studies have revealed problems in the accuracy of these administrative definitions. One recent study compared the 2003 to 2012 trends in severe sepsis between various administrative definitions and cases defined with objective clinical data, demonstrating large increases (54%–706%) in rates of severe sepsis based on administrative definitions in the absence of comparable increases in bacteremia and shock based on objective clinical data. This suggests an increase in the use of severe sepsis ICD-9-CM codes on hospital discharge documentation in the absence of objectively proven severe sepsis cases.[8] This increasing use of the sepsis codes on hospital discharges was also demonstrated in an analysis that showed an 11% increase in hospital claims with an infection code and a disproportionately higher 49% increase in hospital claims with a sepsis code from 2003 to 2009.[9] Overall, these data inform us that the epidemiology of sepsis in the US is based on imperfect administrative definitions and these factors must be taken into account when examining the estimates and trends.

Based on the methodology and years evaluated, studies examining hospital discharges to estimate the incidence and case fatality of sepsis have produced various estimates. The first published report to characterize the national epidemiology of sepsis syndromes was a 1990 Morbidity and Mortality Weekly Report from the Centers for Disease Control and Prevention (CDC) that described trends in hospital discharges with ICD-9-CM codes for septicemia.[10] From 1979 through 1987, discharges with septicemia codes increased from 74 to 176 per 100,000 persons while case fatality decreased from 31% to 25%.[10] More than a decade later, several investigators independently produced varied sepsis incidence estimates, trends, and case-fatalities using different datasets and definitions (see **Table 1**). Applying these various definitions to a single national dataset covering 2004 to 2009, the average annual incidence varies widely by definition, ranging from 300 to 1031 per 100,000 persons, yet all with a similar average annual increase of 13% (**Fig. 2**).[11] Examining sepsis mortality indices, this study demonstrated similar patterns of variation. Although case fatality varies up to 2-fold by administrative definition, the case fatality trends are similar with a 4% to 5% decline per year.[12] Additionally, the total incidence of mortality from severe sepsis in the US continued to increase nationally even while the case fatality decreased (numbers not reported).[11] Another study specifically looked at sepsis-related mortality with the CDC's Multiple Causes of Death database from 1999 to 2005 and, using a novel sepsis definition based on ICD-10 coding, again demonstrated a small increases in the incidence of sepsis-related mortality during the study period of 50 to 52 per 100,000.[13] One important note on examining sepsis deaths using the National Vital Statistics Reports is that this report separates out septicemia codes from other infections, notably the combined influenza and pneumonia category, which comprise the largest proportion of sepsis sources in the incidence studies.[14] Within the National Vital Statistics Reports' schema, influenza and pneumonia were the eighth leading cause of death in the US in 2011 at 17 deaths per 100,000, whereas septicemia does not make the top 10 list for reporting.[14]

Some common trends emerge from these reports. Although the case fatality of severe sepsis is decreasing, the national incidence of severe sepsis cases is increasing at a larger rate. This larger increase in incident cases seems to be driving the proportionately smaller increase of total sepsis-related deaths, despite the trend of improving case fatality from sepsis during the same period. Potential reasons for the increasing incidence of severe sepsis may be an aging population, a larger number of people with disease comorbidities, greater improvements in disease-specific mortality from other competing causes of death, growing bacterial drug resistance, and increasing recognition and more frequent and liberal use of sepsis codes on hospital discharges. Reasons for improving case fatality include scientific advances in care, dissemination of effective protocolized treatment and increasing inclusion of sepsis coding for nonsepsis systemic inflammatory response syndrome (SIRS) patients and less severe sepsis patients.

**Table 1**
Comparison of administrative methodologies for epidemiology of sepsis in the United States

| Study Author | Sepsis Spectrum | Patients | ICD | Number of Infection Codes | Number Organ Dysfunction Codes | Geography | Years | Incidence[a] | Average Annual Trend | Case Fatality |
|---|---|---|---|---|---|---|---|---|---|---|
| CDC MMWR[10] | Septicemia | All | 9-CM | 17 | 0 | US | 79-87 | 74-176 | +17% | 25%-31% |
| Angus[3] | Severe sepsis | All | 9-CM | 1286 | 13 | 7 states[b] | 95 | 300 | NA | 29% |
| Martin[5] | Severe Sepsis | All | 9-CM | 6 | 32 | US | 79-00 | 83-240 | +9% | 18%-28% |
| Dombrovskiy[4] | Severe sepsis | ≥18 | 9-CM | 15-17[c] | 29-30[d] | 1 state[e] | 95-02 | 135-208 | +7% | 45%-51% |
| Melamed[13] | Sepsis mortality | All | 10 | 21 | NA | US | 99-05 | 50-52 | +1% | NA |

*Abbreviations:* CDC, Centers for Disease Control and Prevention; MMWR, morbidity and mortality weekly report; NA, not applicable.

[a] Age and gender adjusted incidence per 100,000 population except for Dombrovskiy and Melamed studies, which are crude rate per 100,000 population.

[b] Florida, Maryland, Massachusetts, New York, New Jersey, New York, Virginia, and Washington statewide databases used to generate national estimates.

[c] In October 2002, 995.91 (sepsis) and 995.92 (severe sepsis) were added to ICD-9-CM and the study's definition.

[d] In October 2002, 995.92 (severe sepsis) was added to ICD-9-CM and the study's definition.

[e] New Jersey.

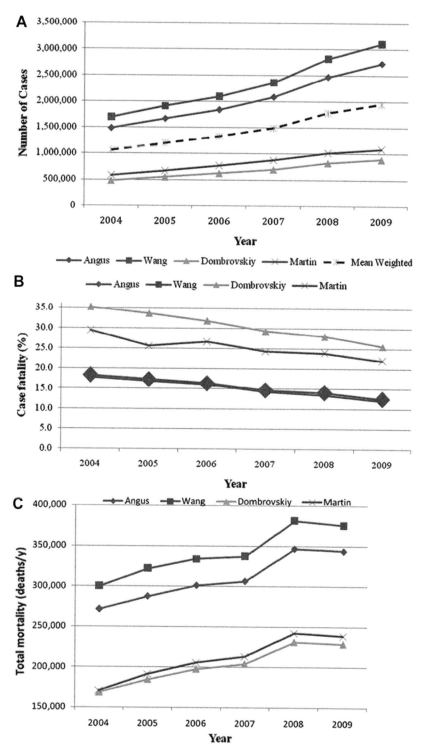

**Fig. 2.** Comparison of epidemiologic trends of severe sepsis in the US between 3 case definitions. (*A*) Number of cases. (*B*) Case fatality (%). (*C*) Total mortality (deaths/y). (*From* Gaieski DF, Edwards JM, Kallan MJ, et al. Benchmarking the incidence and mortality of severe sepsis in the United States. Crit Care Med 2013;41(5):1170; with permission.)

In addition to incidence and mortality trends, the infection sources and causative pathogens for sepsis in the US have changed. From 1979 through 2000 in the US, although the proportions of hospital discharges for severe sepsis with concomitantly documented pathogens increased for all classes of organisms, gram-positive bacterial infections increased the most with an average 26% per year, surpassing gram-negative organisms in 1987 as the predominant class of organism associated with severe sepsis.[5] Furthermore, the proportion of severe sepsis cases with concomitant fungal infections increased 207% during this 22-year period.[5] In 2000, gram-positive organisms accounted for 52% of severe sepsis cases whereas gram-negative and fungal organisms comprised 38% and 5% of cases, respectively.[5] Several reports have demonstrated the respiratory tract to be the most commonly identified (29%–42%) source of infection in US sepsis, followed by either primary bacteremia or genitourinary sources, depending on the study.[3,15–17]

## GLOBAL EPIDEMIOLOGY OF SEPSIS

The studies describing the epidemiology of sepsis outside of the US are summarized in **Table 2** and, in general, use intensive care unit (ICU)-based observational cohort study designs and clinical definitions instead of administrative databases and definitions. In those studies that estimate a population incidence of severe sepsis there is a range from 38 to 110 per 100,000 persons, which is in the lower range of the estimates produced in the US.[3–5,18–27] The case fatality rates of reported severe sepsis range from 22% to 55% and are comparable to those observed in US studies of similar years.[3–5,18–21,23–33] With a few exceptions, the respiratory tract is the most common source of infection, although the pathogen distribution observed just is variable.[20,26,28–30,34–37]

Data regarding the epidemiology of sepsis incidence from developing countries are exceedingly scarce; therefore, to make estimations, this article extrapolates from the World Health Organization (WHO) reports on causes of global mortality. Although the WHO does not individually record sepsis or septicemia as a cause of death, it does report deaths due to lower respiratory tract infections, a leading cause of sepsis. From this data, the WHO Africa Region and countries designated as low-income by the World Bank disproportionately suffer higher mortality rates from lower respiratory infections. More specifically, in 2012, lower respiratory tract infections were the leading cause of death among low-income countries at 91 deaths per 100,000 persons, 3-fold higher than

the rate among high-income countries.[38,39] Additionally, of the WHO geographic regions in 2012, the Africa region suffered the highest mortality rate from lower respiratory tract infections at 116 per 100,000 persons, more than 4-fold higher than the European region at 24 deaths per 100,000 persons (**Fig. 3**).[38,39] Although using deaths due to lower respiratory infection as a surrogate for sepsis-related deaths is imperfect and likely underestimates measures of sepsis epidemiology, it is clear that this is large global problem with a disproportionately heavy burden on developing nations.

## FACTORS ASSOCIATED WITH AN INCREASED INCIDENCE OF SEPSIS

At the time of this article's preparation, there are no longitudinal cohort studies examining prehospital risk factors for the subsequent development of sepsis and the factors associated with sepsis listed below are based on hospital cohorts and cross-sectional administrative data.

Age
- Several studies have demonstrated that older age is a risk factor for sepsis.[3,10,18,21,27,28,40–42]
- The risk for sepsis has a bimodal age distribution, with increased age-adjusted incidences in infants that decrease through childhood and increase again in adulthood with a steep inflection upwards around 50 to 60 years of age.[3,27,41]
- The average annual increases in sepsis incidence interact with age, with greatest increases in older age groups. From 1979 to 2002 in the US, the average annual increase of sepsis incidence was 20% faster in adults older than 65 years old when compared with the younger group.[10,41]

Sex
- Although there is some variation in the distribution of sexes in the prevalence of sepsis, male sex is consistently associated with higher incidence of sepsis.[3,5,15,18,22–27,31,33,37,40,43–45]
- There seems to be interaction between sex and age in the incidence of severe sepsis, such that men have a similar age-adjusted incidence of women 5 years older.[3,5]

Race
- In the US, black race has been associated with an approximately 2-fold increase in the incidence of severe sepsis when compared with whites.[5,15,43,46,47]
- The racial disparity in severe sepsis in the US depends on age with the most occurring

among the 35 to 44 year-old age group.[5,13,16,47]

- The distribution of comorbid illnesses may be different among races. There is some evidence that nonwhites have a higher proportion of diabetes mellitus, human immunodeficiency virus, chronic renal failure, and alcohol abuse; whereas whites more often have pulmonary disease and cancer.[15,16]
- The distribution of pathogens may be different by race. There is some evidence that blacks had higher rates of gram-positive infections and higher rates of invasive pneumococcal disease.[15,16]

Comorbid conditions

- There is some evidence that individuals with a higher number of comorbid illnesses are at higher risks of sepsis.[42]
- Comorbid illnesses that have been associated with sepsis include diabetes mellitus, congestive heart failure, chronic pulmonary disease, immunosuppression, liver disease, cancer, and chronic renal failure.[15,28,33,41,48]
- One study demonstrated that the number of high-risk organ transplantations that the institution performed was associated with a higher sepsis attack rate.[40]

Geography and season

- There is evidence for increased incidences of respiratory infections, streptococcal, and pneumococcal sepsis diagnoses in the winter but not other causes of septicemia.[46,49]
- In the US from 1979 to 1987, septicemia increased the most in the West.[10] In a study of the US from 1979 to 2003, the West had the lowest average annual sepsis rate when compared with the South and the Northeast but was not significantly different from the Midwest.[49]
- A data extraction performed for this article shows the average annual incidence of sepsis-related mortality from 1999 to 2013 by US state, revealing higher incidence of mortality among southeastern states (**Fig. 4**).

## CLINICAL CORRELATIONS AND THE FUTURE OF SEPSIS EPIDEMIOLOGY

The current clinical criteria of sepsis syndromes have a nonlinear history and have recently undergone extensive revisions to improve clinical utility and accuracy (see **Fig. 1**).[50,51] By the time the American College of Chest Physicians and the Society of Critical Care Medicine (ACCP/SCCM) published the first consensus definition of sepsis

syndromes in 1992, it was recognized that there had been a century's worth of proliferation of various terms describing these syndromes, including infection, bacteremia, sepsis, septicemia, septic syndrome, and septic shock.[52] In an effort to "improve [the] ability to make early bedside detection of the disease possible … [and allow] the standardization of research protocols…" the ACCP/SCCM consensus committee: (1) specified the clinical criteria for SIRS, (2) defined sepsis as SIRS in the presence of a known or suspected infection, and (3) identified severe sepsis and septic shock as the potential progression of sepsis to multiple organ dysfunction and death.[52]

The basic structure of the 1992 ACCP/SCCM consensus definitions of SIRS, sepsis, severe sepsis, and septic shock had gone largely unchanged in the 3 editions of the Surviving Sepsis Campaign Guidelines published in 2003, 2008, and 2012.[53–55] While these definitions have demonstrated clinical endurance and been critical to research developments in the field. Nevertheless, there has been a shifting perception that the SIRS definition may be overly sensitive and nonspecific.[50] In 2006, a survey of European ICUs demonstrated the SIRS criteria to be 100% sensitive but only 18% specific for severe infections.[37] Furthermore, in 2012 a prospective observational study in the Netherlands demonstrated that minor variations in the timing and method of capture of SIRS criteria, such as manual versus automated data collection, significantly changed the measured incidences of sepsis syndromes.[56] Furthermore, this study demonstrated that 6% to 17% (depending on the method of SIRS capture) of infected ICU patients did not meet SIRS criteria.[56] More recently, a study of a 14-year survey of all ICUs in New Zealand highlighted the significant potential problems with the clinical definition of sepsis. This study found that the SIRS criteria missed 1 in 8 patients with severe infections and that these missed cases were associated with substantial hospital morbidity and mortality.[57] More specifically, the SIRS-negative sepsis patients still had high rates of organ failure; with 42% having septic shock, 55% requiring mechanical ventilation, and 12% experiencing acute renal failure.[57] Furthermore, when compared with SIRS-positive sepsis patients, the SIRS-negative sepsis patients had a lower but still substantial hospital mortality (16% vs 23%).[57] These data call into question the utility of the SIRS component of the sepsis diagnostic criteria in aiding in timely recognition and treatment of severe infections. It is in this context that the Third International Consensus Sepsis Definitions Task Force

**Table 2**
Summary of studies of the epidemiology of sepsis outside of the United States

| Country | Study Design | Definition | Time Period (mo/y) | Number of Subjects (ICUs) | Attack Rate per 100 ICU Admissions (per 100,000 population/y) | Sources | Organisms | Mortality |
|---|---|---|---|---|---|---|---|---|
| **Europe** | | | | | | | | |
| France[28] | Cohort | Consensus[52] | 1–2/93 | 11,828 (170) | Severe sepsis 6% | Pulmonary 40% Abdomen 32% | Gram-positive 51% Gram-negative 59% | 28-d Severe sepsis 56% |
| Italy[32] | Cohort | Consensus | 4/93–3/94 | 1101 (99) | Severe sepsis 2% | NA | NA | Hospital Severe sepsis 52% |
| England, Wales, and Northern Ireland[18] | Cohort | PROWESS[64] | 95–00 | 56,673 (91) | Severe sepsis 27% (51) | NA | NA | Hospital Severe sepsis 47% |
| England, Wales, and Northern Ireland[24] | Cohort | PROWESS | 12/95–1/05 | 343,860 (172) | Severe sepsis (46–66) | NA | NA | Hospital Severe sepsis 48%–45% |
| 8 countries[45,a] | Cohort | Consensus | 5/97–5/98 | 3946[b] (28) | Severe sepsis 7% | Pulmonary 62% Abdominal 14% | Gram-positive 39% Gram-negative 49% | NA |
| Croatia[34] | Cohort | Consensus | 1/00–12/05 | 5022 (1) | Sepsis 6% | Urinary 54% Pulmonary 14% | Gram-positive 32% Gram-negative 64% | Hospital Sepsis 17% |
| Norway[21] | Cohort | ICD-10 septicemia codes | 1–12/99 | (NA)[c] 700,107 | Severe sepsis (50) | NA | NA | Hospital Severe sepsis 27% |
| Netherlands[22] | 1-day point prevalence | PROWESS | 12/01 | 455 (47) | Severe sepsis 30% (54) | Pulmonary 47% Abdomen 34% | NA | NA |
| France[19] | 2-week point prevalence | Consensus | 11/01 | 3738 (206) | Severe sepsis[d] 15% (95) | NA | NA | 30-day Severe sepsis 35% |
| Slovakia[23] | Cohort | PROWESS | 7/02–12/02 | 1533 (12) | Severe sepsis 8% (80–90) | Pulmonary 55% Abdomen 39% | NA | Hospital Severe Sepsis 51% |
| 24 European Countries[37] | 2-week prevalence | Consensus | 5/02 | 3147 (198) | Sepsis 37% | Pulmonary 68% Abdomen 22% | Gram-positive 40% Gram-negative 38% | Hospital Sepsis 30% |

| Region/Country | Type | Definition | Dates | No. (centers) | Severity/prevalence | Source of infection | Microbiology | Mortality |
|---|---|---|---|---|---|---|---|---|
| Germany[25] | 1-day point prevalence | Consensus 03 | | 3877 (454) | Severe sepsis[d] 11% (76–110) | Pulmonary 63% Abdominal 25% | NA | Hospital Severe sepsis[d] 55% |
| Finland[26] | Cohort | Consensus | 11/04–2/05 | 4500 (24) | Severe sepsis NA (38) | Pulmonary 43% Abdominal 32% | Gram-positive 59% Gram-negative 33% | Hospital Severe sepsis 28% |
| Republic of Macedonia[29] | Cohort | Consensus | 1/08–12/10 | 875 (1) | Severe sepsis 21% | Pulmonary 66% Meningitis 9% | Gram-positive 78% Gram-negative 22% | Hospital Severe sepsis 52% |
| **South America** | | | | | | | | |
| Brazil[33] | Cohort | PROWESS | 5/01–1/02 | 1383 (5) | Severe sepsis 17% | Pulmonary 66% Urinary 6% | NA | 28-day Severe sepsis 47% |
| Colombia[31] | Cohort | Modified IHI definition | 9/07–2/08 | 49,739 (10)[e] | Sepsis 4%[d] | NA | NA | 28-day Severe sepsis 22% |
| **Pacific and Asia** | | | | | | | | |
| Australia and New Zealand[20] | Cohort | Consensus | 5/99–7/99 | 5878 (23) | Severe sepsis 12% (77) | Pulmonary 50% Abdominal 19% | Gram-positive 48% Gram-negative 39% | Hospital Severe sepsis 38% |
| Australia and New Zealand[65] | Cohort | Consensus | 1/00–12/12 | 1,037,115 (171) | 10% | NA | NA | Hospital Severe sepsis 24% |
| South Korea[30] | Cohort | Consensus | 4/05–2/09 | NA (22) | NA | Pulmonary 30% Urinary 26% | Gram-positive 20% Gram-negative 43% | 28-day Severe sepsis 23% |
| South Vietnam[36] | Cohort | Positive blood culture | 6/93–5/94 | 437 (1)13 | Bacteremia 2%[d] | NA | Gram-positive NA Gram-negative 90% | Hospital Bacteremia 6% |
| **Middle East** | — | — | — | — | — | — | — | — |
| Kuwait[35] | Cohort | Positive blood culture | 1/82–6/83 | 3845 (1)13 | Bacteremia 11%[d] | NA | Gram-positive 20% Gram-negative 80% | NA |

Abbreviations: ICU, intensive care unit; IHI, Institute of Healthcare Improvement; NA, not available; PROWESS, Prospective Recombinant Human Activated Protein C Worldwide Evaluation in Severe Sepsis trial.

a Included in the European subsection because it contained mostly European countries: Italy, France, Spain, Germany, Portugal, United Kingdom, Canada, and Israel.
b Total number of subjects who stayed in ICU >24 hours, which was the one strata of the study with data on sepsis density.
c The cohort includes all Norwegian hospitals but an exact number is not supplied.
d Also included severe sepsis and septic shock.
e Total number of hospitals in the study instead of ICUs.

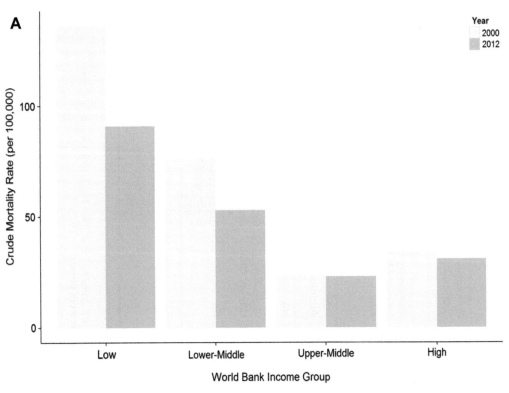

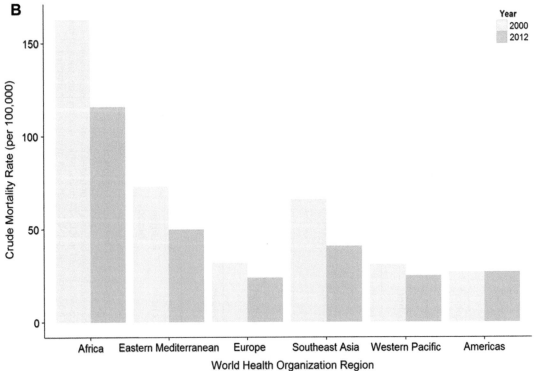

**Fig. 3.** Crude mortality from lower respiratory tract infections. (*A*) World Bank by income group. (*B*) WHO by region. (*Data from* World Health Organization. Global Health Data Repository: Death Rates. Available at: http://apps.who.int/gho/data/node.main.CODRATE?lang=en. Accessed August 12, 2015)

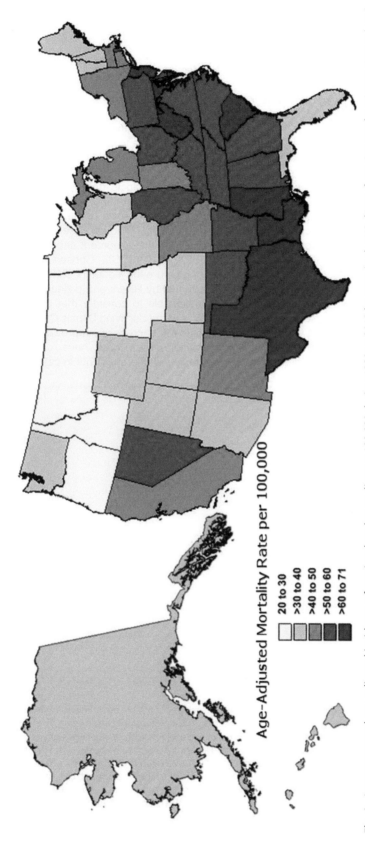

**Fig. 4.** Average annual age-adjusted incidence of sepsis-related mortality per 100,000 during 1999 to 2013 by state in the US. (*Data from* Centers for Disease Control and Prevention, National Center for Health Statistics. Multiple Cause of Death Statistics. Multiple Cause of Death 1999–2013 on CDC WONDER Online Database. Data are from the Multiple Cause of Death Files, 1999–2013, as compiled from data provided by the 57 vital statistics jurisdictions through the Vital Statistics Cooperative Program. 2015. Available at: http://wonder.cdc. gov/mcd-icd10.html. Accessed August 27, 2015.)

**Age-Adjusted Mortality Rate per 100,000**

20 to 30
>30 to 40
>40 to 50
>50 to 60
>60 to 71

proposed new criteria for sepsis syndromes in 2016.[51] In summary

(i) SIRS was respectfully regarded as a useful tool for identification of infection but discarded as criteria for sepsis
(ii) The quick SOFA and SOFA scores were introduced as a screening tool and clinical criteria for sepsis, respectively
(iii) The term *severe sepsis* was discarded and
(iv) septic shock was defined as persistent hypotension necessitating vasopressors with an elevated serum lactate despite volume resuscitation.[51]

The development of these new criteria demonstrate a sophisticated process combining data-driven derivation and validation with expert panel opinion; however, the authors self-reflectively acknowledge that simplicity, outcome prediction, testing burden and pathobiology were all taken into account in the challenging task of deriving clinical criteria for a syndrome of varied inciting etiologies with no gold standard confirmatory diagnostic test.[51,58,59] The initial assessments of

performance demonstrate improved in-hospital mortality prediction of SOFA and quick SOFA over SIRS criteria, with criteria met in 67%, 70% and 55% of decedents with initially suspected infection outside of the ICU setting, respectively.[59] While these new criteria have improved predictive ability, they serve as a cautionary reminder that the necessary reliance on a clinical case definition that is syndromic rather than pathologically defined will likely continue to introduce some misclassification error in epidemiological surveillance.

Despite these issues of case definition, overall the epidemiologic data is encouragingly consistent in demonstrating that, despite the increasing incidence of sepsis cases, there is a decreasing case fatality. Although case fatality was improving before the development and dissemination of the 1992 ACCP/SCCM Consensus definitions and long before the landmark early goal-directed therapy trial by Rivers and colleagues[60] in 2001, it is reasonable to consider that the monumental efforts of the Surviving Sepsis Campaign to disseminate evidence-based improvements in sepsis and critical illness care have contributed to the continued improvements in case fatality.

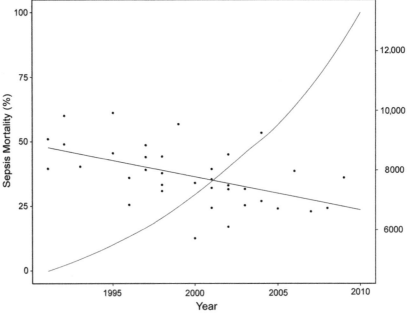

**Fig. 5.** Total sample size required to show a relative risk difference of 10% based on mortality from control arms of randomized controlled trials of severe sepsis and septic shock. The x-axis is publication years. The left-side y-axis is to the reported case fatality of the control arms of trials enrolling subjects with severe sepsis or septic shock, dots are individual trials, blue line is a simple unweighted linear regression of case fatality by year. The right-side y-axis is the total sample size (experimental and control arms) required to show a relative mortality risk difference of 10% with a power of 90% at an alpha of 0.05 for a hypothetical experimental trial with the control arm's mortality rate estimated from the aforementioned regression of that given year. The red line is a simple plot of this total sample size calculated from the control arm's mortality estimated from the blue regression line for each year. (*Data from* supplement of Stevenson EK, Rubenstein AR, Radin GT, et al. Two decades of mortality trends among patients with severe sepsis: a comparative meta-analysis*. Crit Care Med 2014;42(3):625–31.)

The improving case fatality of sepsis also has implications for the future of research into effective sepsis therapies. As the baseline mortality of the standard care of sepsis improves, it becomes increasingly difficult to statistically demonstrate the benefit of newer therapies. As the baseline mortality approaches 25%, sample sizes greater than 10,000 participants are required to show relative risk differences of 10%, thus making future research much more time, cost, and labor intensive (**Fig. 5**). This statistical effect of decreasing case fatality from sepsis helps to contextualize the null findings of the recent trials re-examining the efficacy of early goal-directed therapy when compared with standard care a decade after the original trial.[61–63]

Another inference from the epidemiology of sepsis is that, although the case fatality of sepsis is decreasing, the incidence of sepsis cases continues to increase and drive a smaller but still significant increase in national rates of sepsis-related mortality.[13] Within this context, in addition to improving the treatment of sepsis cases, the next paradigms in curbing the growing problem of sepsis may focus on identifying and treating prehospital risk factors for sepsis. More longitudinal studies are needed to identify high-impact, corrigible prehospital risk factors for sepsis and the highest incidence subpopulations in which to study ambulatory interventions. In addition to exploring these general risk factors, examination of the specific risk factors mediating the racial and gender disparities in the incidence of sepsis is needed to take the next steps toward eliminating these inequalities.

## SUMMARY

In the epidemiology of sepsis in the US, different case definitions have produced varied results. Estimates show trends toward increasing incidence in sepsis and decreasing case fatality. In the US and globally, respiratory tract infections are the most common source of sepsis, although there is more variability in the microbiological distribution of common pathogens. Evidence on the epidemiology of sepsis in developing countries is scarce; however, there is a 3-fold to 4-fold increased incidence of mortality from sepsis-related infections. Although data for longitudinal risk factors for sepsis are lacking, in the US it disproportionately affects the very young and old, males, blacks, and the southeastern states.

## REFERENCES

1. Moss M. Epidemiology of sepsis: race, sex, and chronic alcohol abuse. Clin Infect Dis 2005; 41(Suppl 7):S490–7.

2. Botero JSH, Pérez MCF. The history of sepsis from ancient Egypt to the XIX century. 2012. Available at. http://www.intechopen.com/books/export/citation/EndNote/sepsis-an-ongoing-and-significant-challenge/the-history-of-sepsis-from-ancient-egypt-to-the-xix-century. Accessed August 5, 2015.

3. Angus DC, Linde-Zwirble WT, Lidicker J, et al. Epidemiology of severe sepsis in the United States: analysis of incidence, outcome, and associated costs of care. Crit Care Med 2001;29(7):1303–10.

4. Dombrovskiy VY, Martin AA, Sunderram J, et al. Facing the challenge: decreasing case fatality rates in severe sepsis despite increasing hospitalizations. Crit Care Med 2005;33(11):2555–62.

5. Martin GS, Mannino DM, Eaton S, et al. The epidemiology of sepsis in the United States from 1979 through 2000. N Engl J Med 2003;348(16):1546–54.

6. Whittaker SA, Mikkelsen ME, Gaieski DF, et al. Severe sepsis cohorts derived from claims-based strategies appear to be biased toward a more severely ill patient population. Crit Care Med 2013;41(4):945–53.

7. Iwashyna TJ, Odden A, Rohde J, et al. Identifying patients with severe sepsis using administrative claims: patient-level validation of the angus implementation of the international consensus conference definition of severe sepsis. Med Care 2014;52(6):e39–43.

8. Rhee C, Murphy MV, Li L, et al, Centers for Disease Control and Prevention Epicenters Program. Comparison of trends in sepsis incidence and coding using administrative claims versus objective clinical data. Clin Infect Dis 2014;60(1):88–95.

9. Walkey AJ, Wiener RS. Trends in infection source and mortality among patients with septic shock. Am J Respir Crit Care Med 2014;190(6):709–10.

10. From the Centers for Disease Control. Increase in National Hospital Discharge Survey rates for septicemia–United States, 1979-1987. JAMA 1990;263(7):937–8.

11. Gaieski DF, Edwards JM, Kallan MJ, et al. Benchmarking the incidence and mortality of severe sepsis in the United States. Crit Care Med 2013;41(5):1167–74.

12. Stevenson EK, Rubenstein AR, Radin GT, et al. Two decades of mortality trends among patients with severe sepsis: a comparative meta-analysis*. Crit Care Med 2014;42(3):625–31.

13. Melamed A, Sorvillo FJ. The burden of sepsis-associated mortality in the United States from 1999 to 2005: an analysis of multiple-cause-of-death data. Crit Care 2009;13(1):R28.

14. Heron M. Deaths: Leading Causes for 2011. Department of Health and Human Services-National Vital Statistics Reports; 2015. Available at. http://www.cdc.gov/nchs/data/nvsr/nvsr64/nvsr64_07.pdf). Accessed August 10, 2015.

15. Esper AM, Moss M, Lewis CA, et al. The role of infection and comorbidity: factors that influence disparities in sepsis. Crit Care Med 2006;34(10): 2576–82.

16. Mayr FB, Yende S, Linde-Zwirble WT, et al. Infection rate and acute organ dysfunction risk as explanations for racial differences in severe sepsis. JAMA 2010;303(24):2495–503.

17. Wang HE, Shapiro NI, Angus DC, et al. National estimates of severe sepsis in United States emergency departments. Crit Care Med 2007;35(8):1928–36.

18. Padkin A, Goldfrad C, Brady AR, et al. Epidemiology of severe sepsis occurring in the first 24 hrs in intensive care units in England, Wales, and Northern Ireland. Crit Care Med 2003;31(9):2332–8.

19. Brun-Buisson C, Meshaka P, Pinton P, et al. EPISEPSIS: a reappraisal of the epidemiology and outcome of severe sepsis in French intensive care units. Intensive Care Med 2004;30(4):580–8.

20. Finfer S, Bellomo R, Lipman J, et al. Adult-population incidence of severe sepsis in Australian and New Zealand intensive care units. Intensive Care Med 2004;30(4):589–96.

21. Flaatten H. Epidemiology of sepsis in Norway in 1999. Crit Care 2004;8(4):R180–4.

22. van Gestel A, Bakker J, Veraart CP, et al. Prevalence and incidence of severe sepsis in Dutch intensive care units. Crit Care 2004;8(4):R153–62.

23. Zahorec R, Firment J, Strakova J, et al. Epidemiology of severe sepsis in intensive care units in the Slovak Republic. Infection 2005;33(3):122–8.

24. Harrison DA, Welch CA, Eddleston JM. The epidemiology of severe sepsis in England, Wales and Northern Ireland, 1996 to 2004: secondary analysis of a high quality clinical database, the ICNARC Case Mix Programme Database. Crit Care 2006; 10(2):R42.

25. Engel C, Brunkhorst FM, Bone HG, et al. Epidemiology of sepsis in Germany: results from a national prospective multicenter study. Intensive Care Med 2007;33(4):606–18.

26. Karlsson S, Varpula M, Ruokonen E, et al. Incidence, treatment, and outcome of severe sepsis in ICU-treated adults in Finland: the Finnsepsis study. Intensive Care Med 2007;33(3):435–43.

27. Dombrovskiy VY, Martin AA, Sunderram J, et al. Rapid increase in hospitalization and mortality rates for severe sepsis in the United States: a trend analysis from 1993 to 2003. Crit Care Med 2007;35(5): 1244–50.

28. Brun-Buisson C, Doyon F, Carlet J, et al. Incidence, risk factors, and outcome of severe sepsis and septic shock in adults. A multicenter prospective study in intensive care units. French ICU Group for Severe Sepsis. JAMA 1995;274(12):968–74.

29. Grozdanovski K, Milenkovic Z, Demiri I, et al. Prediction of outcome from community-acquired severe sepsis and septic shock in tertiary-care university hospital in a developing country. Crit Care Res Pract 2012;2012:182324.

30. Park DW, Chun BC, Kim JM, et al. Epidemiological and clinical characteristics of community-acquired severe sepsis and septic shock: a prospective observational study in 12 university hospitals in Korea. J Korean Med Sci 2012;27(11):1308–14.

31. Rodriguez F, Barrera L, De La Rosa G, et al. The epidemiology of sepsis in Colombia: a prospective multicenter cohort study in ten university hospitals. Crit Care Med 2011;39(7):1675–82.

32. Salvo I, de Cian W, Musicco M, et al. The Italian SEPSIS study: preliminary results on the incidence and evolution of SIRS, sepsis, severe sepsis and septic shock. Intensive Care Med 1995;21(Suppl 2):S244–9.

33. Silva E, Pedro Mde A, Sogayar AC, et al. Brazilian Sepsis Epidemiological Study (BASES study). Crit Care 2004;8(4):R251–60.

34. Degoricija V, Sharma M, Legac A, et al. Survival analysis of 314 episodes of sepsis in medical intensive care unit in university hospital: impact of intensive care unit performance and antimicrobial therapy. Croat Med J 2006;47(3):385–97.

35. Elhag KM, Mustafa AK, Sethi SK. Septicaemia in a teaching hospital in Kuwait–I: incidence and aetiology. J Infect 1985;10(1):17–24.

36. Hoa NT, Diep TS, Wain J, et al. Community-acquired septicaemia in southern Viet Nam: the importance of multidrug-resistant Salmonella typhi. Trans R Soc Trop Med Hyg 1998;92(5):503–8.

37. Vincent J-L, Sakr Y, Sprung CL, et al. Sepsis in European intensive care units: results of the SOAP study. Crit Care Med 2006;34(2):344–53.

38. World Health Organization. The top 10 causes of death. Available at: http://www.who.int/mediacentre/factsheets/fs310/en/index1.html. Accessed August 12, 2015.

39. World Health Organization. Global health data repository: death rates. Available at: http://apps.who.int/gho/data/node.main.CODRATE?lang=en. Accessed August 12, 2015.

40. Sands KE, Bates DW, Lanken PN, et al. Epidemiology of sepsis syndrome in 8 academic medical centers. JAMA 1997;278(3):234–40.

41. Martin GS, Mannino DM, Moss M. The effect of age on the development and outcome of adult sepsis. Crit Care Med 2006;34(1):15–21.

42. Banta JE, Joshi KP, Beeson L, et al. Patient and hospital characteristics associated with inpatient severe sepsis mortality in California, 2005-2010. Crit Care Med 2012;40(11):2960–6.

43. Barnato AE, Alexander SL, Linde-Zwirble WT, et al. Racial variation in the incidence, care, and outcomes of severe sepsis: analysis of population, patient, and hospital characteristics. Am J Respir Crit Care Med 2008;177(3):279–84.

44. Rangel-Frausto MS, Pittet D, Costigan M, et al. The natural history of the systemic inflammatory response syndrome (SIRS). A prospective study. JAMA 1995;273(2):117–23.

45. Alberti C, Brun-Buisson C, Burchardi H, et al. Epidemiology of sepsis and infection in ICU patients from an international multicentre cohort study. Intensive Care Med 2002;28(2):108–21.

46. Baine WB, Yu W, Summe JP. The epidemiology of hospitalization of elderly Americans for septicemia or bacteremia in 1991-1998. Application of Medicare claims data. Ann Epidemiol 2001;11(2):118–26.

47. Dombrovskiy VY, Martin AA, Sunderram J, et al. Occurrence and outcomes of sepsis: influence of race. Crit Care Med 2007;35(3):763–8.

48. McBean M, Rajamani S. Increasing rates of hospitalization due to septicemia in the US elderly population, 1986-1997. J Infect Dis 2001;183(4):596–603.

49. Danai PA, Sinha S, Moss M, et al. Seasonal variation in the epidemiology of sepsis. Crit Care Med 2007;35(2):410–5.

50. Vincent JL, Opal SM, Marshall JC, et al. Sepsis definitions: time for change. Lancet 2013;381(9868):774–5.

51. Singer M, Deutschman CS, Seymour CW, et al. The Third International Consensus Definitions for Sepsis and Septic Shock (Sepsis-3). Jama 2016;315(8):801–10.

52. Bone RC, Balk RA, Cerra FB, et al. Definitions for sepsis and organ failure and guidelines for the use of innovative therapies in sepsis. The ACCP/SCCM Consensus Conference Committee. American College of Chest Physicians/Society of Critical Care Medicine. Chest 1992;101(6):1644–55.

53. Dellinger RP, Levy MM, Rhodes A, et al. Surviving Sepsis Campaign: international guidelines for management of severe sepsis and septic shock, 2012. Intensive Care Med 2013;39(2):165–228.

54. Dellinger RP, Levy MM, Carlet JM, et al. Surviving Sepsis Campaign: international guidelines for management of severe sepsis and septic shock: 2008. Crit Care Med 2008;36(1):296–327.

55. Dellinger RP, Carlet JM, Masur H, et al. Surviving Sepsis Campaign guidelines for management of severe sepsis and septic shock. Crit Care Med 2004;32(3):858–73.

56. Klein Klouwenberg PM, Ong DS, Bonten MJ, et al. Classification of sepsis, severe sepsis and septic shock: the impact of minor variations in data capture and definition of SIRS criteria. Intensive Care Med 2012;38(5):811–9.

57. Kaukonen KM, Bailey M, Pilcher D, et al. Systemic inflammatory response syndrome criteria in defining severe sepsis. N Engl J Med 2015;372(17):1629–38.

58. Shankar-Hari M, Phillips GS, Levy ML, et al. Developing a New Definition and Assessing New Clinical Criteria for Septic Shock: For the Third International Consensus Definitions for Sepsis and Septic Shock (Sepsis-3). Jama 2016;315(8):775–87.

59. Seymour CW, Liu VX, Iwashyna TJ, et al. Assessment of Clinical Criteria for Sepsis: For the Third International Consensus Definitions for Sepsis and Septic Shock (Sepsis-3). Jama 2016;315(8):762–74.

60. Rivers E, Nguyen B, Havstad S, et al. Early goal-directed therapy in the treatment of severe sepsis and septic shock. N Engl J Med 2001;345(19):1368–77.

61. Peake SL, Delaney A, Bailey M, et al. Goal-directed resuscitation for patients with early septic shock. N Engl J Med 2014;371(16):1496–506.

62. Yealy DM, Kellum JA, Huang DT, et al. A randomized trial of protocol-based care for early septic shock. N Engl J Med 2014;370(18):1683–93.

63. Mouncey PR, Osborn TM, Power GS, et al. Trial of early, goal-directed resuscitation for septic shock. N Engl J Med 2015;372(14):1301–11.

64. Bernard GR, Vincent JL, Laterre PF, et al. Efficacy and safety of recombinant human activated protein C for severe sepsis. N Engl J Med 2001;344(10):699–709.

65. Kaukonen KM, Bailey M, Suzuki S, et al. Mortality related to severe sepsis and septic shock among critically ill patients in Australia and New Zealand, 2000-2012. JAMA 2014;311(13):1308–16.

# Therapeutic Targets in Sepsis: Past, Present, and Future

Eric J. Seeley, MD, FCCP[a],*, Gordon R. Bernard, MD[b]

## KEYWORDS

- Sepsis • Antibiotics • Treatment • Therapeutic targets

## KEY POINTS

- Antibiotics and fluids have been the therapy of choice for sepsis since shortly after World War II.
- Although goal-directed targets and timing have changed since then, no additional targeted therapy is part of standard practice for sepsis.
- New approaches to translational investigation of targets are needed.
- Several new targets including the endothelium and late mediators of septic organ injury merit thorough investigation.
- Adaptive trial design might help to speed the large clinical trials of new sepsis therapies.

## INTRODUCTION

Long before van Leeuwenhoek peered through his microscope to describe bacteria in 1676, microbial infections have been an enduring cause of human death. Although the evolution of modern germ theory identified and classified many of the pathogens that led to infectious death, it was not until the administration of intravenous fluids, first described during the English cholera epidemic of 1831,[1,2] and the discovery of penicillin, by Flemming in 1928,[3] that the first steps toward modern day management of sepsis were taken.

One striking characteristic of the systemic inflammatory response to infection is that, even after antibiotics kill invading microbes, the host inflammatory response endures and can contribute to organ injury and death.[4] Although many biologically well-informed attempts to limit the inflammatory response have been made in animal models of infection and human clinical trials, severe infection leading to septic organ injury remains a major cause of morbidity and mortality in intensive care units.[5] Furthermore, short of fluids and antibiotics, which have been widely used since the 1950s, no targeted biologic therapy has decreased sepsis mortality and none is currently considered part of standard clinical practice.[6] Significant steps forward in adrenergic pharmacology and organ support have improved mortality. However, mortality and long-term cognitive and physical disability from sepsis remain high and new treatments are needed.

Disclosures: None.
[a] Division of Pulmonary and Critical Care Medicine, Department of Medicine, University of California San Francisco, 400 Parnassus Avenue, 5th Floor ACC, San Francisco, CA 94143, USA; [b] Division of Allergy, Pulmonary and Critical Care Medicine, Vanderbilt University Medical Center, Nashville, TN 37232, USA
* Corresponding author.
E-mail address: eric.seeley@ucsf.edu

Clin Chest Med 37 (2016) 181–189
http://dx.doi.org/10.1016/j.ccm.2016.01.015
0272-5231/16/$ – see front matter © 2016 Elsevier Inc. All rights reserved.

This article reviews the historical evolution of sepsis therapy (**Table 1**) and identifies possible causes for why rational therapies failed in human trials. In addition, this article examines potential future sepsis targets and considers which trial designs might optimize their success (**Box 1, Table 2**).

## EVOLUTION OF SEPSIS THERAPY
### Fluids

Although intravenous fluids did not become a mainstay of sepsis therapy until the early 20th century, the idea of delivering intravenous salt solutions to improve hemodynamics during infection can be traced to the cholera pandemic of 1831.[7] Dr William O'Shaughnessy, a 22 year-old recent medical graduate of Edinburgh University, with a keen interest in medical chemistry, traveled to Sunderland, England, the nidus of the cholera outbreak, to study and treat patients infected with cholera. His observations led him to question the use of bloodletting and emetics, which were the current state of the art therapies for cholera. He studied the blood of patients infected with cholera and found "a material diminution of water in the blood ... and a notable decrease in the soluble salts," which he described in the Lancet in 1832.[1] Instead of bloodletting, O'Shaughnessy argued that trying to restore the original characteristics of healthy blood by delivering a salt solution, could improve the underlying diminution of the "water in blood."

Several months later, during the same cholera epidemic, Dr Thomas Latta drew on the observations of O'Shaughnessy and was the first recorded physician to deliver a warmed salt solution intravenously. He wrote "I have no doubt that it will be found ... to be one of the most powerful, and one of the safest remedies yet used in this ... hopeless state of collapse."[1] Although the intravenous delivery of saline would not become a standard treatment for sepsis until many years later, O'Shaughnessy's initial impressions of the central importance of fluid resuscitation for sepsis endures today.

### Antibiotics

Alexander Flemming's sharp eye first noted that "mold juice" from the fungus *Penicillium chrysogenum* could kill *Staphylococcus* in culture on September 28, 1928.[3] His initial thought was that bacterial susceptibility to "mold juice" might help him to subclassify bacteria. However, eventually, he realized that "mold juice" or the key compounds within it, which he called "penicillin," might be used to treat bacterial infections in humans. Flemming worked hard to produce quantities of penicillin sufficient for in vivo study, but given the difficulty of purifying the compound from mold, he abandoned this pursuit 1940. Fortunately, in the same year, the team of Florey and Chain, working at Oxford, published a paper outlining a method of penicillin purification in quantities sufficient for clinical testing.[3] It then took many additional bright physicians, chemists, mycologists and defense-related funding from both England and the United States during World War II to advance Flemming's antibacterial "mold juice" to a reasonably priced clinical treatment for bacterial infections.[3]

### Supporting Injured Organs

Today, timely administration of broad-spectrum antibiotics and restoration of intravascular fluid volume remain the cornerstones of treatment for sepsis. Even after the delivery of these 2 key therapies, patients frequently develop septic shock, requiring catecholamine vasopressors. Although the advances of fluids, antibiotics, and vasopressors have decreased mortality, a significant portion of patients still progress to develop organ injury. Although artificial organ support, including mechanical ventilation and continuous renal replacement therapy, can maintain organs after they have been injured, unraveling the early molecular events during sepsis held the promise of avoiding organ injury altogether.

**Table 1**
**Major events in the treatment of sepsis**

| Year | Intervention |
| --- | --- |
| 1832 | Intravenous fluids for cholera |
| 1905 | Epinephrine for shock |
| 1928 | Penicillin discovered |
| 1930 | First use of penicillin for infection |
| 1949 | Norepinephrine used for shock |
| 1970s | Steroids used for sepsis |
| 1982 | Polyclonal anti-LPS trial |
| 1991 | Monoclonal anti-LPS trials |
| 1993 | Anti-TNF trials |
| 2001 | Early goal-directed therapy |
| 2014 | ProCESS, ARISE, ProMISe |

*Abbreviations:* ARISE, Australasian Resuscitation in Sepsis Evaluation; LPS, lipopolysaccharide; ProCess, Protocolized Care for Early Septic Shock; ProMISe, Protocolised Management in Sepsis; TNF, tumor necrosis factor.

## THE GOLDEN AGE OF CYTOKINES

The mid to late 20th century was marked by great steps forward in understanding the molecular underpinnings of the host inflammatory response. However, the origins of identifying tumor necrosis factor (TNF) date back as far as 1893, when Coley[8] first described the necrolytic effect of inoculating erysipelas into patients with malignant tumors.[9] Attempts were even made to treat cancer patients systemically with bacterial broth; however, not surprisingly, the side effects were too extreme. Nearly 80 years later, Williamson and colleagues[10] reported "An endotoxin-induced serum factor that causes necrosis of tumors"; this factor was tumor necrosis factor. A separate string of investigations into the metabolic wasting common to cancer and chronic infection led to the identification of cachectin,[11,12] a soluble factor that led to the suppression of the enzyme lipoprotein lipase in both cancer and infection. Shortly thereafter, it was appreciated that macrophages, a sentinel of early infection, are a key source of cachectin and rapidly increase the production of cachectin after lipopolysaccharide (LPS) stimulation.[13] The tools of modern molecular biology then revealed that cachectin and TNF were, in fact, the same molecule.[14] This surprised many, given the divergent starting points of inquiry. However, these converging scientific paths underscore the central role of TNF in orchestrating the host response to infection and chronic illness.

Tracey, Beutler, Lowry and Cerami, in an amazing string of papers published in *Science*, the *Proceedings of the National Academy of Science*, and the *Journal of Experimental Medicine* dissected the causal pathway of LPS in leading to TNF production and then systemic shock.[14–17] They showed that the exogenous administration of recombinant human TNF, in levels that are achieved during infection, caused hypotension, metabolic acidosis, hemoconcentration, and death in mice. The same group went on to show that anti-TNF antibodies, given before a lethal dose of *Escherichia coli*, could stave off the development of septic shock in baboons.[15] Last, this group showed that TNF blockade, through passive immunization, could also decrease the downstream inflammatory mediators of interleukin (IL)-1β and IL-6.[16]

This molecular dissection of the inflammatory cascade, from LPS to TNF and shock, led to great optimism that blocking this pathway could halt the inflammatory response that lingered after antibiotics killed the inciting bacteria. Synchronous improvements in scalable monoclonal antibody production allowed for the production of clinical grade blocking antibodies to LPS and TNF. In animal models, these antibodies lead to a dramatic improvement in outcomes, including improved survival.[15] In step with these research advancements, pharmaceutical companies raced to test antibodies in human sepsis, because there was a large unmet clinical need for a common and highly morbid disease.

## HUMAN SEPSIS TRIALS: FROM OPTIMISM TO DISAPPOINTMENT
### Blocking Lipopolysaccharide and Tumor Necrosis Factor

Biopharmaceutical money poured into sepsis research and trials. The first large-scale trial of anti-LPS antibodies was published in 1991 in the *New England Journal of Medicine*.[18] With great excitement, it seemed that administration of the anti-LPS HA-1A antibody (or centoxin) in patients with gram-negative sepsis improved survival.[18] Subsequent trials, however, did not show a mortality benefit, and the HA-1A antibody was not approved by the US Food and Drug Administration.[19] The 1990s saw no fewer than 11 large randomized controlled trials (RCTs) of anti-TNF therapy in sepsis.[20] The trials used 2 approaches. First, a TNF receptor, namely, immunoglobulin G1 fusion protein (TNFR:Fc), which was well-vetted in large animal models; and second, a monoclonal antibody against TNF. The soluble TNF receptor sepsis study group published the results of a 141-person dose escalation trial in septic patients treated with TNFR:Fc. The primary end point was 28-day mortality. Patients treated with the higher doses of the TNF receptor fusion protein had a higher mortality than the placebo group.[21] The trial of an anti-TNF monoclonal antibody showed a trend toward improved mortality at day 3; however, this benefit was not durable out to 28 days.[22] Several subsequent trials of blocking cytokines suggested no benefit for gram-negative sepsis and possible harm in gram-positive sepsis, and distinguishing between the 2 infectious agents proved impossible at the time of treatment. This initial excitement for blocking cytokines in sepsis rapidly turned to disappointment as a result of these trials.

### Why Did These Therapies Fail?

In the wake of these trials, the enthusiastic balloon of pharmaceutical funding for sepsis popped, and a shadow has been cast on private funding for sepsis research and trials. Some have even said, "Sepsis is where big pharma goes to die." However, for practitioners and clinical researchers, sepsis remains a growing problem with a large unmet need for targeted therapies. A lingering question has remained after all of these trials: why did these therapies, which were well-vetted in mouse and larger animal models of sepsis, fail in humans? We would submit 4 main theories. First, there was unqualified exuberance on behalf of biopharmaceutical companies owing to the very large unmet clinical need for sepsis. Thus, these companies may have raced into human trials prematurely. Second, the animal models in which these therapies were tested did not adequately recapitulate human sepsis. For example, for pragmatic reasons, common mouse models of sepsis include single-dose administration of LPS or single-dose administration of large bacterial innoculations. The mice included in these experiments are often 8 to 12 weeks old and they are not treated with antibiotics or fluids. In contrast, human sepsis frequently occurs in older adults who are treated with antibiotics, fluids, catecholamines, and mechanical organ support. This topic has recently been reviewed thoroughly.[23] Third, the delivery of cytokine-blocking antibodies may have been attempted long after peak serum levels of inflammatory cytokines had passed. And last, there is likely redundancy to the immune response. Thus, blocking a single cytokine may not halt the injurious inflammatory response. This supposition is based on the key evolutionary role that host–pathogen defense has played over the course of primate evolution.[4] This characteristic of the immune response may be central to the failure of biopharmaceutical-funded attempts at blocking a single cytokine, because other inflammatory mediators continue the injurious inflammatory response. Future attempts at therapeutic interventions for sepsis may want to take into account each of these possible explanations.

## QUANTITATIVE RESUSCITATION REEXAMINED

During the unraveling of biologically targeted therapies for human sepsis, several emergency department and critical care physicians sought to optimize resuscitation by putting into place hemodynamic targets or "goals" by which to optimize oxygen delivery through fluids, red blood cell transfusion, and ionotropic/vasopressor support. The most notable of these studies was the Trial of Early Goal Directed Therapy (EGDT) by Rivers and colleagues,[24] published in the New England Journal of Medicine in 2000. The trial set in motion a major paradigm shift in the care of septic patients. Many centers "adopted" EGDT; however, strict adherence to the protocol was low.[25] The bundled resuscitation plan set goals for hematocrit

that were above standard practice, and the protocol required an expensive and invasive continuous central venous oximeter to guide hemodynamics. Multiple implementation studies showed benefit to this new protocol.[26] However, many physicians questioned the usefulness of several components of the protocol, especially the hemoglobin goal, the central venous oxygen goal, and the use dobutamine to boost cardiac output.

Three large, multicenter, multinational trials named Protocolized Care for Early Septic Shock (ProCESS), Australasian Resuscitation in Sepsis Evaluation (ARISE) and Protocolised Management in Sepsis (ProMISe) were recently published and answered several of these lingering questions.[27–29] The take-home points are that central venous oximetry to target oxygen delivery, CVP targeted resuscitation, and transfusion goals of a hemoglobin of greater than 10 were not superior to "Rivers light" and "usual care."[27] Usual care was not fully defined, but included central venous cannulation in approximately 50% of patients, predominately for vasopressor administration. Thus "usual care" should become standard practice, but it is not entirely clear what "usual care" is, short of rapid administration of antibiotics, fluids as needed for shock, and vasopressor support. Thus, in some ways this is a remarkable return to Dr Latta's 1832 conclusion that fluids remain "one of the most powerful … remedies for this hopeless state of collapse," which we have come to know as septic shock.

## FUTURE TARGETS
### Healing the Injured Epithelium

It is clear that the early cytokine storm is not a viable molecular target for sepsis therapy and that a rigorously protocolized resuscitation strategy is not better than "usual care," which was largely based on EGDT as described by Rivers and colleagues.[24] So what targets hold potential for sepsis therapies in the future (see **Table 2**) and how future sepsis trials might be designed to optimize finding a measurable benefit in an age of decreasing sepsis mortality (see **Box 1**)?

Two promising targets include the endothelium and late molecular mediators of septic organ injury. Endothelial injury during sepsis leads to increased endothelial permeability and the release of usually sequestered subendothelial coagulation factors. Furthermore, injury to the endothelium in discrete organs, such as the lung and kidneys, may be responsible for septic organ injury. Therapy directed at the endothelium is appealing. One approach would be targeting

## Table 2
## Emerging therapeutic targets in Sepsis

| Biological Target | Function/Target |
|---|---|
| **Endothelium** | |
| Angiopoietin-1 (Ang1) | Blocks VE-cadherin internalization[30] |
| Slit2N | Stabilizes VE-cadherin at tight junctions[30] |
| Sphingosine 1-phosphate (S1P) | Increases junctional targeting of VE-cadherin[30] |
| **Late mediators of inflammation** | |
| Histones | Leads to endothelial injury and cardiomyopathy[32,52] |
| Pentraxin 3 (PTX3) | Binds histones and decreases their toxicity[36] |
| HMGB1 | Leads to endothelial barrier dysfunction[38,53] |
| **Immune tolerance/autophagy** | |
| Anthracyclines | Autophagy in the lung[43] |

*Abbreviation:* VE, vascular endothelial.

tight junctions, including angiopoietin-1 and Slit2N.[30] Both of these molecules alter endothelial cell permeability in mouse models of sepsis. The endothelial glycocalyx is another potential target. The biology of these targets and potential approaches to therapy are thoroughly reviewed In another article in this series (See, Colbert JF, Schmidt EP. Endothelial and Microcirculatory Function and Dysfunction in Sepsis).

### Late Mediators of Septic Organ Injury

Targeting early mediators of septic inflammation, including TNF and IL-1B, may not have worked because these mediators may have already reached peak concentrations by the time septic patients arrive in the emergency department. The transcriptional programs of innate and adaptive immune cells and key target tissues have likely been activated by the time a blocking antibody or small molecule can be delivered. Another approach to therapy would be to identify and target late mediators of septic organ injury. These mediators could potentially be measured in the serum at the time of admission and then blocked based on the level of elevation and risk–benefit profile of the treatment.

Histones, which are usually sequestered in eukaryotic cell nuclei and function to package

DNA, have been shown to mediate late endothelial and cardiac injury. Using a selective screening method, Esmon and colleagues[31] found that histones, and in particular histones H3 and H4, were late mediators or sepsis-induced endothelial injury. This group found that injection of purified histones led to cellular injury, inflammation, and death in mice. Treating mice with a monoclonal antibody against histone H4 could improve survival during cecal ligation and puncture (CLP)- and LPS-induced injury in mice. Subsequent studies of human serum samples suggest that histones contribute to cardiac and endothelial injury during the clinical syndrome of sepsis,[32,33] and some support the use of a synthetic histone mimic as therapy.[34]

In addition to antihistone antibodies, another method of decreasing the toxicity of histones is by the administration of pentraxin 3 (PTX3), which is a naturally occurring pattern recognition molecule. PTX3 is produced by cells of the innate and adaptive immune system as well as in other organs and increases in the serum during sepsis.[35] Hamakubo and colleagues[36] found that PTX3 binds histones and a truncated N-terminal fragment of the protein can rescue mice from histone induced inflammatory injury as well improve organ injury during LPS- and CLP-induced sepsis. This is a good example of a host-protective naturally occurring protein that was isolated, truncated, and then used as therapy.

Another potential late mediator of septic organ injury is the cytokine-like protein high mobility group B-1 (HMGB1).[37] Much like histones, HMGB1 is principally a nuclear protein where it acts as a DNA chaperone protein. However, it is released from cells during injury or infection and accumulates in the serum of septic animals and humans.[38,39] Importantly, the measured increase in HMGB1 is delayed compared with the traditional early inflammatory cytokines, including TNF and IL1B. HMGB1 can be measured in the serum of infected mice for more than 30 days and seems to remain increased in humans for an even longer duration during sepsis. Administration of HMGB1 to mice leads to hepatic and renal injury as well as endothelial barrier dysfunction. Blocking the actions of HMGB1, either with a monoclonal antibody or small interfering RNA, can improve survival even in mouse models of existing septic organ injury.[37,39–42] These therapies await assessment in clinical trials of human sepsis.

### Large-Scale Screens of Compounds Safe for Human Use

Another approach to finding new potential therapies for sepsis is through large-scale screens of medications currently approved as safe for use in humans. This repurposing of existing medications obviates the need for extensive dose finding and toxicity studies. However, the approach may also decrease the potential upside profits for biopharmaceutical companies if the repurposed therapy is already off patent. An example of this approach was used by Moita and colleagues,[43] who used a large-scale screen of 2320 compounds to identify new molecules that decreased inflammatory cytokine production in THP-1 cells, a human monocyte cell line, in response to E coli challenge. Moita and colleagues found that members of the anthracycline chemotherapeutic family, including epirubicin, doxorubicin, and daunorubicin, were among the most potent suppressors of inflammatory cytokines. The authors used an antibiotic-treated CLP model to show that epirubicin improved sepsis outcomes in CLP, even when delivered 24 hours after the induction of septic peritonitis. The authors then went on to show that the beneficial effects of epirubicin were through its induction of authophagy in the lungs, which protected this vulnerable organ bed from TNF-driven necroptosis. This path of inquiry, screening known human-safe compounds on human cell lines and then testing them in a model of antibiotic-treated murine sepsis, may facilitate the clinical application of repurposed pharmaceuticals. However, for molecules that are not patentable for sepsis, funding for phase II/III trials may require government support.

## OPTIMIZING TRIAL DESIGN

Large collaborative research networks, analogous to the ARDS Clinical Trials Network research

---

| Box 1 |
| :--- |
| **Innovative trial designs in sepsis** |
| *Adaptive trial design* |
| Adaptive randomization |
| Adaptive group sequential design |
| Flexible sample size reestimation design |
| Adaptive dose finding |
| Biomarker-adaptive design |
| Adaptive treatment switching |
| Adaptive hypothesis design |
| *Time to event design* |
| Time to acute kidney injury |
| Time to acute respiratory distress syndrome |
| Time to intubation |
| Time to resolution of shock |

---

collaborative, will be essential for developing future therapies in sepsis. Although the remarkable reduction in sepsis mortality over the last 10 to 20 years has been universally celebrated, powering clinical trials for 28-day mortality will require several thousands of patients to be powered to show mortality benefits, especially if small, that is, absolute mortality reductions of less than 10%. This would require either a very large network of enrolling centers (which may increase the risk of regional differences in care) or would require trials that take too long. We present several innovative alternatives to traditional RCTs that might improve trial speed and help optimize the likelihood of identifying beneficial therapies.

### Reducing Heterogeneity

It has been widely recognized that 1 limitation to sepsis trial design has been patient heterogeneity. This stems from inherent differences in sepsis pathogenesis depending on key bacterial factors. There are key differences in site of infection (pneumonia vs urinary tract infection) and virulence factors of infecting pathogens (gram-positive vs gram-negative organisms) and both of these factors contribute to wide variation in host response based on the existing host barrier defense and immune reserve. The same infecting organisms may cause some hosts to become hypoinflammatory, whereas others become hyperinflammatory. Enrollment based on the systemic inflammatory response syndrome criteria with evidence of organ injury or fluid unresponsive hypotension have helped to cast a broad net on the heterogeneous population of patients with sepsis.[44] However, the inclusion of so many heterogeneous patients may in fact mask a potentially beneficial therapy. Well-executed attempts to find transcriptional or cytokine profiles that might discriminate patients into clearer mortality risk categories or temporal categories have not been successful.[45,46] A reasonable attempt to try to study a less heterogeneous group of patients might be to use some combination of site of infection and a biomarker. For example, patients with pneumonia and sepsis who have an elevation in IL-6 greater than some cutoff value could be preferentially enrolled in trials. The downside of this approach is that trials will require more time for enrollment if they are powered for mortality and, in some cases, may become infeasible owing to small numbers of patients.

### Innovative Trial Designs

The prevailing paradigm for phase II and III RCTs in sepsis has been to use 28-day mortality as a primary endpoint. Powering clinical trials for this endpoint will require many patients, for example, the recent ProCESS trial enrolled a total of 1341 patients into 3 different groups[27] and the recent trial of a Toll-like receptor-4 antagonist enrolled 1961 patients.[47] This is a time-intensive and expensive way to test new therapeutic targets in sepsis. Are there new trial designs that might provide for dynamic yet statistically robust adjustments of either power size or trial endpoints?

Several new study designs that might limit the expense and enhance a possible treatment effect have been described. For example, many experts have suggested that adaptive trial designs,[48,49] which have been leveraged to study new oncotherapeutics, could improve the time and expense required to test new therapies for sepsis (see **Box 1**). A full statistical explanation for adaptive trial design is beyond the scope of this article; however, adaptive trials attempt to provide more flexibility in terms of power and effect size compared with traditional RCTs in which power and effective size must be calculated based on previous data. This type of trial design might be especially relevant for sepsis, because mortality seems to be decreasing over time.[27,50,51]

## SUMMARY

The long-standing evolutionary interplay between humans and microbes has likely been calibrated to stave off minor mucosal invasions. However, the focal point of this evolutionary process, small-scale recurrent infections, may have hardwired a poorly calibrated systemic inflammatory response when infections become systemic. Early administration of antibiotics can kill the invading microbes; however, the inflammatory response lingers and often leads to collateral organ injury. As these organ injuries accumulate, mortality increases. Fluids and pressors can support the early hemodynamic collapse, but therapies targeting either the inflammatory response or the end-organ damage have failed. Future attempts at molecular therapies in sepsis might be aided by rigorous testing in "more relevant" animal models of sepsis; however, cost and complexity may limit this approach. Future clinical trials that focus on late mediators of sepsis, such as HMGB1 and histones, might benefit from adaptive trial designs and attempts to limit patient heterogeneity to contains costs and enhance trial efficiency.

## REFERENCES

1. Baskett TF. William O'Shaughnessy, Thomas Latta and the origins of intravenous saline. Resuscitation 2002;55(3):231–4.
2. Awad S, Allison SP, Lobo DN. The history of 0.9% saline. Clin Nutr 2008;27:179–88.
3. Ligon BL. Penicillin: its discovery and early development. Semin Pediatr Infect Dis 2004;15(1):52–7.
4. Seeley EJ, Matthay MA, Wolters PJ. Inflection points in sepsis biology: from local defense to systemic organ injury. Am J Physiol Lung Cell Mol Physiol 2012;303:L355–63.
5. Martin GS, Mannino DM, Eaton S, et al. The epidemiology of sepsis in the United States from 1979 through 2000. N Engl J Med 2003;348(16):1–9.
6. Dellinger RP, Levy MM, Rhodes A, et al, Surviving Sepsis Campaign Guidelines Committee including the Pediatric Subgroup. Surviving sepsis campaign: international guidelines for management of severe sepsis and septic shock: 2012. Crit Care Med 2013;41:580–637.
7. Daly WJ, DuPont HL. The controversial and short-lived early use of rehydration therapy for cholera. Clin Infect Dis 2008;47:1315–9.
8. Coley WB. The treatment of inoperable sarcoma by bacterial toxins (the mixed toxins of the Streptococcus erysipelas and the Bacillus prodigiosus). Proc R Soc Med 1910;3:1–48.
9. Wiemann B, Starnes CO. Coley's toxins, tumor necrosis factor and cancer research: a historical perspective. Pharmacol Ther 1994;64(3):529–64.
10. Carswell EA, Old LJ, Kassel RL, et al. An endotoxin-induced serum factor that causes necrosis of tumors. Proc Natl Acad Sci U S A 1975;72:3666–70.
11. Kawakami M, Pekala PH, Lane MD, et al. Lipoprotein lipase suppression in 3T3-L1 cells by an endotoxin-induced mediator from exudate cells. Proc Natl Acad Sci U S A 1982;79:912–6.
12. Rouzer CA, Cerami A. Hypertriglyceridemia associated with Trypanosoma brucei brucei infection in rabbits: role of defective triglyceride removal. Mol Biochem Parasitol 1980;2:31–8.
13. Beutler B, Mahoney J, Le Trang N, et al. Purification of cachectin, a lipoprotein lipase-suppressing hormone secreted by endotoxin-induced RAW 264.7 cells. J Exp Med 1985;161:984–95.
14. Beutler B, Cerami A. Cachectin and tumour necrosis factor as two sides of the same biological coin. Nature 1986;320:584–8.
15. Tracey KJ, Fong Y, Hesse DG, et al. Anti-cachectin/TNF monoclonal antibodies prevent septic shock during lethal bacteraemia. Nature 1987;330:662–4.
16. Fong Y, Tracey KJ, Moldawer LL, et al. Antibodies to cachectin/tumor necrosis factor reduce interleukin 1 beta and interleukin 6 appearance during lethal bacteremia. J Exp Med 1989;170:1627–33.
17. Beutler B, Greenwald D, Hulmes JD, et al. Identity of tumour necrosis factor and the macrophage-secreted factor cachectin. Nature 1985;316:552–4.
18. Ziegler EJ, Fisher CJ, Sprung CL, et al. Treatment of gram-negative bacteremia and septic shock with

HA-1A human monoclonal antibody against endo-toxin. A randomized, double-blind, placebo-controlled trial. The HA-1A Sepsis Study Group. N Engl J Med 1991;324:429–36.

19. McCloskey RV, Straube RC, Sanders C, et al. Treatment of septic shock with human monoclonal antibody HA-1A. A randomized, double-blind, placebo-controlled trial. CHESS Trial Study Group. Ann Intern Med 1994;121:1–5.

20. Reinhart K, Karzai W. Anti-tumor necrosis factor therapy in sepsis: update on clinical trials and lessons learned. Crit Care Med 2001;29:S121–5.

21. Fisher CJ, Agosti JM, Opal SM, et al. Treatment of septic shock with the tumor necrosis factor receptor:Fc fusion protein. The Soluble TNF Receptor Sepsis Study Group. N Engl J Med 1996;334:1697–702.

22. Abraham E, Wunderink R, Silverman H, et al. Efficacy and safety of monoclonal antibody to human tumor necrosis factor alpha in patients with sepsis syndrome. A randomized, controlled, double-blind, multicenter clinical trial. TNF-alpha MAb Sepsis Study Group. JAMA 1995;273:934–41.

23. Fink MP. Animal models of sepsis. Virulence 2014;5:143–53.

24. Rivers EE, Nguyen BB, Havstad SS, et al. Early goal-directed therapy in the treatment of severe sepsis and septic shock. N Engl J Med 2001;345:1368–77.

25. Kalil AC, Sun J. Why are clinicians not embracing the results from pivotal clinical trials in severe sepsis? A Bayesian analysis. PLoS One 2008;3:e2291.

26. Castellanos-Ortega A, Suberviola B, García-Astudillo LA, et al. Impact of the Surviving Sepsis Campaign protocols on hospital length of stay and mortality in septic shock patients: results of a three-year follow-up quasi-experimental study. Crit Care Med 2010;38:1036–43.

27. ProCESS Investigators, Yealy DM, Kellum JA, et al. A randomized trial of protocol-based care for early septic shock. N Engl J Med 2014;370:1683–93.

28. Mouncey PR, Osborn TM, Power GS, et al. ProMISe Trial Investigators. Trial of early, goal-directed resuscitation for septic shock. N Engl J Med 2015;372:1301–11.

29. ARISE Investigators, ANZICS Clinical Trials Group, Peake SL, et al. Goal-directed resuscitation for patients with early septic shock. N Engl J Med 2014;371:1496–506.

30. Goldenberg NM, Steinberg BE, Slutsky AS, et al. Broken barriers: a new take on sepsis pathogenesis. Sci Translational Med 2011;3:88ps25.

31. Xu J, Zhang X, Pelayo R, et al. Extracellular histones are major mediators of death in sepsis. Nat Med 2009;15:1318–21.

32. Kalbitz M, Grailer JJ, Fattahi F, et al. Role of extracellular histones in the cardiomyopathy of sepsis. FASEB J 2015;29:2185–93.

33. Alhamdi Y, Abrams ST, Cheng Z, et al. Circulating histones are major mediators of cardiac injury in patients with sepsis. Crit Care Med 2015;43(10):2094–103.

34. Nicodeme E, Jeffrey KL, Schaefer U, et al. Suppression of inflammation by a synthetic histone mimic. Nature 2011;468:1119–23.

35. Mauri T, Bellani G, Patroniti N, et al. Persisting high levels of plasma pentraxin 3 over the first days after severe sepsis and septic shock onset are associated with mortality. Intensive Care Med 2010;36:621–9.

36. Daigo K, Nakakido M, Ohashi R, et al. Protective effect of the long pentraxin PTX3 against histone-mediated endothelial cell cytotoxicity in sepsis. Sci Signal 2014;7:ra88.

37. Wang H, Bloom O, Zhang M, et al. HMG-1 as a late mediator of endotoxin lethality in mice. Science 1999;285:248–51.

38. Angus DC, Yang L, Kong L, et al. GenIMS Investigators. Circulating high-mobility group box 1 (HMGB1) concentrations are elevated in both uncomplicated pneumonia and pneumonia with severe sepsis. Crit Care Med 2007;35:1061–7.

39. Wang H, Liao H, Ochani M, et al. Cholinergic agonists inhibit HMGB1 release and improve survival in experimental sepsis. Nat Med 2004;10:1216–21.

40. Ye C, Choi J-G, Abraham S, et al. Human macrophage and dendritic cell-specific silencing of high-mobility group protein B1 ameliorates sepsis in a humanized mouse model. Proc Natl Acad Sci U S A 2012;109:21052–7.

41. Yang H, Ochani M, Li J, et al. Reversing established sepsis with antagonists of endogenous high-mobility group box 1. Proc Natl Acad Sci U S A 2004;101:296–301.

42. Saeed RW. Cholinergic stimulation blocks endothelial cell activation and leukocyte recruitment during inflammation. J Exp Med 2005;201:1113–23.

43. Figueiredo N, Chora A, Raquel H, et al. Anthracyclines induce DNA damage response-mediated protection against severe sepsis. Immunity 2013;39:874–84.

44. Bone RC, Balk RA, Cerra FB, et al. Definitions for sepsis and organ failure and guidelines for the use of innovative therapies in sepsis. The ACCP/SCCM Consensus Conference Committee. American College of Chest Physicians/Society of critical care Medicine. Chest 1992;101:1644–55.

45. Wong HR, Lindsell CJ, Pettilä V, et al. A multibiomarker-based outcome risk stratification model for adult septic shock. Crit Care Med 2014;42:781–9.

46. Bozza FA, Salluh JI, Japiassu AM, et al. Cytokine profiles as markers of disease severity in sepsis: a multiplex analysis. Crit Care 2007;11:R49.

47. Opal SM, Laterre P-F, Francois B, et al. Effect of eritoran, an antagonist of MD2-TLR4, on mortality in patients with severe sepsis: the ACCESS randomized trial. JAMA 2013;309:1154–62.

48. Chow S-C. Adaptive clinical trial design. Annu Rev Med 2014;65:405–15.

49. Maharaj R. Vasopressors and the search for the optimal trial design. Contemp Clin Trials 2011;32:924–30.

50. Kaukonen K-M, Bailey M, Suzuki S, et al. Mortality related to severe sepsis and septic shock among critically ill patients in Australia and New Zealand, 2000-2012. JAMA 2014;311:1308–16.

51. Stevenson EK, Rubenstein AR, Radin GT, et al. Two decades of mortality trends among patients with severe sepsis: a comparative meta-analysis. Crit Care Med 2014;42:625–31.

52. Ekaney ML, Otto GP, Sossdorf M, et al. Impact of plasma histones in human sepsis and their contribution to cellular injury and inflammation. Crit Care 2014;18:543.

53. Qin S. Role of HMGB1 in apoptosis-mediated sepsis lethality. J Exp Med 2006;203:1637–42.

# Early Identification and Treatment of Pathogens in Sepsis
## Molecular Diagnostics and Antibiotic Choice

Stefan Riedel, MD, PhD, D(ABMM)[a],*, Karen C. Carroll, MD[b]

## KEYWORDS

- Sepsis • Bacteremia • Nucleic acid amplification • Microarrays • Antimicrobial stewardship
- Patient outcomes • Resistance markers

## KEY POINTS

- Sepsis and septic shock are significant medical problems, with high mortality rates and are the 10th leading cause of death in the United States.
- Although blood cultures are considered the gold standard, emerging molecular diagnostic methods are providing rapid identification for key organisms and antimicrobial resistance markers from positive blood cultures.
- Assays that provide detection and identification of bacteria directly from whole-blood are in development, and are not yet able to replace existing culture amplification-dependent methods.
- Rapid diagnostic methods can significantly reduce the time to identification of organisms and resistance genes and have the greatest impact on improving time to optimal therapy and patient outcomes when coupled with an antimicrobial stewardship program.

## INTRODUCTION

Sepsis, severe sepsis, and septic shock are stages of increasing severity of the systemic host response to bloodstream infections.[1,2] Since the 1980s, the epidemiologic burden of sepsis in the United States and other developed countries has steadily increased. Despite significant improvements in medical care and the development of newer and more broad-spectrum antibiotics for treatment, sepsis still accounts for significant morbidity and mortality in the United States, and is considered among the top 10 leading causes of death.[3] In 2013, the Agency for Healthcare Research and Quality published data from the Healthcare Cost and Utilization Project, indicating that sepsis was among the top 4 conditions associated with the highest cost to hospitals in the United States.[4,5] Aside from the high mortality rate and economic burden during the acute phase of the illness, sepsis and severe sepsis have

Disclosure Statements: Within the past year or currently, S. Riedel has received research support from the following companies that make products for the detection of bacteremia: Nanosphere, Inc, BD Diagnostics, Inc. Dr S. Riedel is also a member of the scientific advisory board of OpGen, Inc. Within the past year or currently, K.C. Carroll has received research support from the following companies that make products for the detection of bacteremia: Abbott Diagnostics, Inc, Gen Mark, Inc, Accelerate, Inc and BD Diagnostics Inc.
[a] Department of Pathology, Harvard Medical School, Beth Israel Deaconess Medical Center, 330 Brookline Avenue, Boston, MA 02215, USA; [b] Division of Medical Microbiology, Department of Pathology, The Johns Hopkins Hospital, The Johns Hopkins University School of Medicine, 600 North Wolfe Street, Meyer B1-193, Baltimore, MD 21287, USA
* Corresponding author.
*E-mail address:* sriedel@bidmc.harvard.edu

chestmed.theclinics.com

associated indirect costs, such as health care expenditures after hospital discharge and nontrivial productivity loss among sepsis survivors (eg, work absenteeism, early retirement, and overall increased morbidity and mortality).[6] In addition, several other studies described an increased risk of death lasting up to 5 years after survival of 1 episode of sepsis, although many of the mechanisms of the increased morbidity and mortality years after surviving sepsis remain unclear to date. All stages of sepsis combined pose a significant financial and humanistic burden, not only to the individual patients but also to society as a whole.

Despite the technical improvements of continuous monitoring blood culture systems, the value of blood cultures for confirming the clinical suspicion of sepsis has been shown to be suboptimal. The diagnostic limitations and uncertainties of blood cultures related to a low sensitivity (ie, positivity rate), prolonged time to pathogen detection and turn-around-times (TAT) of results, and frequent contamination of blood cultures by patients' skin microbiota during blood culture procurement, are often compensated by the liberal use of broad-spectrum antimicrobial therapy.[2] However, considering rising antimicrobial resistance rates and the emergence of novel antimicrobial resistance types (eg, carbapenem-resistant *Enterobacteriaceae*), it is important to exercise a judicial approach to the use of broad-spectrum antimicrobial therapy. The major role of antimicrobial stewardship programs (ASPs) is to optimize the overall utilization, selection, and dosing of antimicrobial agents to minimize adverse events and prevent the emergence of antimicrobial resistance in the health care setting. During the past decade, development of rapid, often molecular, detection methods for both pathogens and antimicrobial resistance markers has seen a significant upsurge. The implementation of such rapid diagnostic technologies in the clinical microbiology laboratory is critical not only for the confirmatory diagnosis of sepsis, but also for support of ASPs. This article provides an update and assessment of recent improvements in pathogen and antimicrobial resistance detection in sepsis, focusing primarily on diagnostic molecular technologies.

# MOLECULAR METHODS FOR DETECTION OF BACTEREMIA

Tremendous progress has been made over the last 2 decades in the development of diagnostic assays to speed up the detection of bacteria and yeast in blood. The initial wave of these assays involved testing positive blood culture bottles at the time of positivity with molecular methods that determine both the identity of a pathogen or pathogens and associated resistance markers. The second wave, direct from whole blood testing, has been ushered in by the T2 Biosystems *Candida* assay (described in more detail elsewhere in this article), the first such assay to obtain US Food and Drug Administration (FDA) approval; **Table 1** summarizes the assays discussed in this review. Several other assays are in development or have progressed to the clinical trial stage. This section of the review discusses the existing molecular platforms and their performance characteristics. The next section discusses the impact of these methods on antimicrobial stewardship activities and patient outcomes where available.

# NONAMPLIFIED, GROWTH-DEPENDENT METHODS

Rapid pathogen detection is of pivotal importance for the diagnosis of sepsis, and a variety of molecular techniques have been developed over time for the detection of specific pathogens. However, many of these technologies still require an initial growth of the pathogen(s) in blood culture bottles. Fluorescence in situ hybridization (FISH) technologies were among the earliest developed and most studied techniques for the detection of pathogens from positive blood cultures.[2,7] These technologies are typically pathogen specific, and allow for the detection of only a small number (1–3) of organisms per test. Broad-based methods on the other hand detect various pathogens from positive blood culture bottles without nucleic acid amplification; these multiplex, automated methods allow for the identification of genus, species, and specific resistance determinants for the most common organisms implicated in bloodstream infections.

## *Pathogen-Specific Methods*

Peptide nucleic acid PNA-(FISH) technology (AdvanDx, Woburn, MA) is probably the most studied commercially available technology suitable for the detection of pathogens from positive blood cultures.[7,8] The first technology to be commercially available for rapid organism detection, it is now, becoming rapidly surpassed by other molecular detection methods. PNA FISH technology uses fluorescein-labeled probes that target pathogen-specific 16S rRNA of bacteria or 26S rRNA of yeast. FDA-approved PNA FISH probes are available for the following common pathogens implicated in BSIs: *Staphylococcus aureus* and coagulase-negative staphylococci (CoNS); *Enterococcus faecalis* and other *Enterococcus* spp.; *Escherichia*

**Table 1**
Summary of molecular assays for detection of bacteremia

| Assay | Manufacturer | Principle | Pathogens Detected | Resistance Markers | Sensitivity (%) | Specificity (%) | References | TAT (h) | FDA or CE Approved |
|---|---|---|---|---|---|---|---|---|---|
| Nonamplified growth-dependent assays | | | | | | | | | |
| PNA FISH | AdvanDx, USA | Fluorescence-based hybridization with PNA probes | *Staphylococcus aureus* (green)/CoNS (red) | *mecA* (*mecAXpressFISH*) | 94–100 | 87–100 | 9–12 | 1.5–3 | CE/FDA |
| PNA FISH: GNR Traffic Light assay | | | *Enterococcus faecalis* (green)/other enterococci (red) *Escherichia coli* (green)/*Klebsiella pneumoniae* (yellow)/*Pseudomonas aeruginosa* (red) | | | | | | |
| PNA FISH: yeast traffic light assay | | | *Candida albicans* and *Candida parapsilosis* (green)/*Candida tropicalis* (yellow)/*Candida glabrata* and *Candida krusei* (red) | | | | | | |
| *QuickFISH* | | | *S aureus* (green)/CoNS (red) | None | 98–100 | 89–100 | 13–16 | 0.5 | |
| Verigene BC-GP | Nanosphere, Inc, USA | Gold nanoparticle technology | *S aureus, S epidermidis; S lugdunensis, S anginosus* group, *Streptococcus agalactiae, Streptococcus pyogenes, Enterococcus faecalis, Enterococcus faecium, Listeria* spp., *Staphylococcus* spp., *Streptococcus* spp., *Micrococcus* spp. (only approved outside USA). | *mecA, vanA, vanB* | 92–100 | 95–100 | 19–21 | 2.5 | CE/FDA |
| Verigene BC-GN | | Gold nanoparticle technology | *Escherichia coli, Klebsiella pneumoniae, Klebsiella oxytoca, Pseudomonas aeruginosa, Serratia marcescens, Acinetobacter* spp., *Proteus* spp., *Citrobacter* spp., *Enterobacter* spp. | *KPC, NDM, CTX-M, VIM, IMP, OXA* | 89–100 | 93–100 | 22–24 | 2.5 | CE/FDA |

(continued on next page)

**Table 1**
*(continued)*

| Assay | Manufacturer | Principle | Pathogens Detected | Resistance Markers | Sensitivity (%) | Specificity (%) | References | TAT (h) | FDA or CE Approved |
|---|---|---|---|---|---|---|---|---|---|
| *Amplified methods, growth required* | | | | | | | | | |
| *Pathogen specific real-time PCR methods* | | | | | | | | | |
| Staph SR | BD GeneOhm, USA | Real-time PCR | *S aureus* (MRSA/MSSA) | *mecA* | 94–99 | 96.5 | 25,26 | 2.5–3 | CE/FDA |
| Xpert MRSA/SA | Cepheid, USA | Real-time PCR | *S aureus* (MRSA/MSSA) | *mecA* | 98.1–99.6 | 99.5 | 25,26 | 1 | CE/FDA |
| *Broad Based Technologies* | | | | | | | | | |
| Prove-It Sepsis | MobiDiag, Finland | Multiplex PCR plus microarray | 50 different pathogens | *mecA* | 95–99 | 98 | 28,29 | 3 | CE |
| FilmArray BC-ID | BioFire, Inc, USA | Multiplex, nested real-time PCR | *Staphylococcus aureus, Streptococcus agalactiae, Streptococcus pneumoniae, Streptococcus pyogenes, Enterococcus* spp., *Listeria monocytogenes, Neisseria meningitidis, Haemophilus influenzae, Acinetobacter baumanii, Pseudomonas aeruginosa, Escherichia coli, Klebsiella pneumoniae, Klebsiella oxytoca, Enterobacter cloacae, Serratia marcescens, Proteus* spp., *Candida albicans, Candida glabrata, Candida krusei, Candida tropicalis, Candida parapsilosis* | *mecA vanA/B* KPC | 88–100 | 99–100 | 30–35 | 1 | CE/FDA |
| *Broad-based direct from whole blood* | | | | | | | | | |
| SeptiFast | Roche, Germany | Multiplex real-time PCR | 25 different pathogens | *mecA* | 68–75 | 86–92 | 41,42 | 3–30 | CE |

| Test | Manufacturer | Method | Pathogens detected | Resistance markers | Sensitivity | Specificity | References | Turnaround (h) | Approval |
|---|---|---|---|---|---|---|---|---|---|
| SepsiTest | Molzym, Germany | Broad-range PCT followed by sequencing | >300 different pathogens | None | 87 | 85.5 | 43 | 8–12 | CE |
| Vyoo Assay | SIRS-Lab, Germany | Multiplex PCR with gel electrophoreses | 40 different pathogens (including gram-positive, gram-negative, yeast, and *Aspergillus fumigatus*) | *mecA, vanA, vanB, vanC, bla$_{SHV}$* | 60 | 75 | 44 | 8 | CE |
| MagicPlex Sepsis Test | Seegene, Korea | Multiplex real-time PCR | 73 gram-positive organisms (including *Staphylococcus* spp., *Streptococcus* spp., *Enterococcus* spp.), *Acinetobacter baumanii, Pseudomonas aeruginosa, Escherichia coli, Klebsiella oxytoca, Enterobacter cloacae, Enterobacter aerogenes, Serratia marcescens, Proteus mirabilis, Salmonella* ser. *Typhi, Bacteroides fragilis, Stenotrophomonas maltophilia, Candida albicans, Candida glabrata, Candida krusei, Candida tropicalis, Candida parapsilosis, Aspergillus fumigatus* | *mecA, vanA, vanB* | 62–65 | 92–96 | 27,45,46 | 3–4 | CE |
| T2 *Candida* magnetic resonance assay | T2 Biosystems Lexington MA | Magnetic resonance assay | 5 *Candida* spp. reported as 3 independent results: *C albicans/C tropicalis C glabrata/C krusei*, and *C parapsilosis* | None | 88–94 | 98.9–99.9 | 47,48 | 3–5 | FDA |
| IRIDICA BAC BSI | Abbott Molecular, Carlsbad, CA | PCR coupled with electrospray ionization mass spectrometry | Theoretically up to hundreds of organisms | *mecA, vanA, vanB, bla$_{KPC}$* | 83–91 | 94–99 | 49–53 | 8 | Neither |

*Abbreviations:* CE, Confirmité Européenne; FDA, Food and Drug Administration; PCR, polymerase chain reaction; PNA, peptide nucleic acid.

*Adapted from* Riedel S, Carroll KC. Laboratory detection of sepsis: biomarkers and molecular approaches. Clin Lab Med 2013;33(3):413–37; with permission.

*coli, Klebsiella pneumoniae*, and *Pseudomonas aeruginosa*; *Candida albicans, Candida parapsilosis, Candida tropicalis, Candida glabrata*, and *Candida krusei*.[8–12] These PNA FISH assays typically differentiate between 2 and 5 different key pathogens in a blood culture broth by using 2 or 3 different fluorescent dyes. In the *S aureus*/CoNS assay, *S aureus* appears green, and CoNS appears red; for the Yeast-Traffic Light assay, *C albicans*/ *C parapsilosis* appear green, *C tropicalis* is yellow, and *C glabrata/C krusei* appear red. Although all PNA FISH probes have been approved for use with all commercially available continuous monitoring blood culture systems, not all assays have been subject to thorough evaluation using all continuous monitoring blood culture systems. Based on studies published to date, sensitivities and specificities for these 4 assays range from 94% to 100% and 87% to 100%, respectively.[9–12] The original version of the PNA FISH assay required approximately 10 minutes of hands-on time and 90 minutes of incubation time to results reporting. Recently, a more rapid version of the assay, *Quick*FISH, providing results within 30 minutes with less than 5 minutes of hands-on time has been introduced. This improved TAT has been very attractive to both laboratories and clinicians, and all the assays for all the mentioned organisms except the yeast have been cleared by the FDA. In a recent multicenter study, investigating 722 positive blood cultures from the BacT/ALERT systems, the *Quick*FISH assay had a sensitivity of 99.5% for reporting *S aureus* and 98.8% for CoNS, with a combined specificity of 89.5%.[13] In another study, using 173 positive blood cultures from the BACTEC system, sensitivity and specificity for detection of *S aureus* was 100%, and for CoNS 98.5% and 100%, respectively.[14] Another study compared the Candida *Quick*FISH blood culture assay against conventional laboratory methods.[15] In this study, the investigators describe an overall agreement of 99.3% between the *Quick*FISH and conventional methods for 3 major *Candida* species (*C albicans, C glabrata*, and *C parapsilosis*). The overall sensitivity was 99.7%, and the specificity was 98.0%.[15] Studies investigating the economic and antimicrobial stewardship impact of the PNA FISH and *Quick*FISH technology have been published and will be discussed in a subsequent section in this review. Last, the addition of the *mecAXpress*FISH assay (AdvanDx), which is designed for use in conjunction with the *Staphylococcus Quick*FISH assay, allows for the detection of methicillin-resistant *S aureus* (MRSA). In a multicenter study by Salimnia and colleagues,[16] the authors reported a 99.1% sensitivity and 99.6% specificity for detection of

methicillin resistance in *S aureus* by this assay. The authors furthermore demonstrated that the *mecAXpress*FISH assay showed high reproducibility among 6 operators over 5 days of testing, with a 98.9% level of agreement.[16] The authors concluded that this assay would require very little effort for implementation among laboratories that already use any of the currently available *S aureus* PNA FISH tests, and that it has the potential of leading to further improvements of patient outcomes and antibiotic utilization, when applied immediately after the *Staphylococcus Quick*FISH test.[16]

### Broad-Based Methods

The Verigene Blood Culture Nucleic Acid Test (Nanosphere, Northbrook, IL) is a nonamplified, qualitative, multiplex assay that uses gold nanoparticle technology for the detection of bacterial pathogens directly from positive blood culture bottles.[2,17] This system consists of a Verigene bench-top Processor SP and a Verigene Reader.[17] Additional components are the extraction tray, utility tray, and the test cartridge, which are inserted into the Processor SP. After vortexing a sample from a patient's positive blood culture bottle, 350 μL of blood are inoculated into the sample well of the extraction tray; from that point forward, the remaining testing process is automated. Using a magnetic bead-based procedure, bacterial DNA is extracted, fragmented, and denatured in the extraction tray and transferred subsequently by pipette tips to the self-contained test cartridge. Pathogen-specific capture probes are already immobilized on a glass slide. If target DNA is present in the sample, the extracted nucleic acids within the sample hybridize to complimentary sequence-specific capture oligonucleotides that are arranged on the glass slide. A second set of mediator DNA oligonucleotides, which are conjugated to gold nanoparticles, contains complementary sequences to the target DNA and hybridizes with the target DNA present in the sample forming a sandwich. In the final step, elemental silver is deposited onto the gold nanoparticle through a catalytic process, resulting in an amplified signal facilitating the detection of the bound nucleic acids. At the end of the test cycle, the glass slide in its holder is removed and placed into the compartment of the Verigene Reader. Inside the reader, the presence of hybridized probes is determined using optical array scanning technology, and results are reported as detected or not detected for all targets present on the slide. The TAT from positive blood culture to pathogen identification is approximately 2.5 hours. There are 2 FDA-approved panels available for the Verigene system: the Gram-positive Blood Culture (BC-GP) and the Gram-negative Blood Culture (BC-GN) nucleic acid test.[18] The targets for the Verigene BC-GP and the Verigene BC-GN panels are summarized in **Table 1**. Both panels have been evaluated for performance and accuracy in detection of the target organisms using all of the commercially available continuous monitoring blood culture detection systems.[19–23] In these studies, the sensitivity and specificity for the BC-GP assay were 92.6% to 100% and 95.4% to 100%, respectively[19–21]; the sensitivity for the BC-GN assay was found to be 89% to 100%, and the specificity 93% to 100%.[22,23] Although both Verigene assays demonstrated overall high levels of sensitivity, specificity, and accuracy (≥95% accuracy for BC-GP; 85%–100% for BC-GN) for monomicrobial BSIs, a significant difference in performance was identified for polymicrobial blood cultures. Samuel and colleagues[21] reported a 94% concordance of the BC-GP assay compared with traditional blood culture organism identification for monomicrobial blood cultures, but a 76% concordance for polymicrobial blood cultures. Similar differences were reported by other investigators.[20] Likewise the detection of resistance markers performed better for monomicrobial blood cultures than for polymicrobial blood cultures. In the study by Samuel and colleagues,[21] the BC-GP panel detected 93% of resistance markers (vanA/B and mecA) in positive blood cultures with S aureus, S epidermidis, Enterococcus faecium, and/or E faecalis. The level of concordance for monomicrobial blood cultures was 97%, compared with 84% for polymicrobial blood cultures.[21] Although both assays have difficulties detecting all organisms in polymicrobial blood culture samples, it is also important to recognize that the assay does not link the resistance marker to the detected organisms in polymicrobial samples; this issue is of particular importance for the detection of mecA in samples containing both S aureus and CoNS. Although several studies described similar problems with polymicrobial blood cultures, it should be recognized that true polymicrobial sepsis is thought to be uncommon, estimated to occur in only 5% of all sepsis episodes,[24] although in the authors' own institution the rates are somewhat higher (10%; Karen Carroll, personal communication, 2015). Nonetheless, careful judgment is warranted when interpreting results of the Verigene panels from blood culture samples containing multiple organisms. To date, only a few studies have been performed analyzing the impact of utilization of the Verigene system with respect to antimicrobial stewardship, patients' clinical outcomes, and cost effectiveness; these studies are discussed in a subsequent section of this review.

## AMPLIFIED METHODS: GROWTH REQUIRED
### Pathogen-Specific Real-time Methods

There are numerous nucleic amplification assays that identify S aureus in blood culture bottles positive for gram-positive cocci in clusters. All of them also detect the mecA gene for the distinction between methicillin-susceptible S aureus and MRSA.

The BD GeneOhm StaphSR assay (BD Diagnostics, Sparks, MD) is a real-time polymerase chain reaction (PCR) assay that uses molecular beacon technology to amplify 2 targets—a proprietary species-specific target for S aureus identification and SCCmec for the detection of MRSA.[25] The assay is performed on the SmartCycler instrument (Cepheid, Sunnyvale, CA, USA) and requires manual extraction. One instrument can test 16 samples. This assay takes approximately 2.5 hours to perform and reports results as positive for MRSA, positive for S aureus, or negative.

The latest version of the Xpert MRSA/SA blood culture assay (Cepheid) uses proprietary primers and probes to target spa (identifies S aureus), mecA (detection of methicillin resistance), and the SCCmec-orfX junction in a multiplex real-time PCR assay.[25,26] All 3 genes must be amplified for a call of MRSA.[25] Methicillin-sensitive S aureus is defined as the presence of spa alone or in conjunction with SCCmec (but not mecA), or the presence of spa and mecA but the absence of SCCmec-orfX.[25] If spa is not detected then the results are interpreted as negative for S aureus despite the presence of the other genes.[26] The first step involves transferring a 50-μL aliquot of the positive blood culture bottle into an elution reagent vial; after vortexing it for 10 seconds, the entire contents of the vial are inoculated into the test cartridge. The test cartridge is then sealed and inserted into a GeneXpert instrument. These instruments are modular and are available in platforms that contain 1, 2, 4, 16, 28, and 80 individual units.[25] Time to results is about 75 minutes, including sample preparation.

A recent multicenter study (8 sites) compared the current version of the BD GeneOhm StaphSR assay with the Xpert MRSA/SA assay on positive blood culture bottles from the 3 major manufacturers following the manufacturers' recommendations.[26] Both systems were compared with phenotypic methods of identification and cefoxitin disk diffusion for detection of methicillin resistance.[26] A total of 795 blood culture bottles containing gram-positive cocci in clusters were evaluated.[26] The sensitivity and specificity for the

GeneOhm Staph SR and the Xpert MRSA/SA for the detection of *S aureus* compared with routine methods were 99.2% and 96.5%, and 99.6% and 99.5%, respectively.[26] There was greater variability between the 2 assays for the detection of MRSA. The GeneOhm Staph SR missed 6 cultures that contained MRSA for an overall sensitivity of 94.3% whereas the GeneXpert missed 2, for a sensitivity of 98.1%.[26] The Xpert assay had greater specificity 99.5% compared with the GeneOhm assay (96.5%), which demonstrated 15 false positives.[26]

### Broad-based Technologies

The Prove-It Sepsis (Mobidiag, Helsinki, Finland) is not available in the United States but was launched in Europe in 2013. The initial assay used front-end multiplex PCR followed by detection of amplified products in a proprietary tube that contains the microarray at the bottom of the vial.[2,27,28] Subsequently, the assay has been modified into a strip format (StripArray), which consists of 8 successive reaction vials with a chip microarray on the bottom. The test menu now includes 60 bacterial targets and *vanA, vanB* resistance markers in addition to *mecA* and also includes 8 of the most clinically relevant *Candida* spp., namely *C albicans, Candida dubliniensis, C glabrata, C parapsilosis, C tropicalis, Candida guilliermondii, Candida lusitaniae,* and *C krusei*.[29] The array also includes a pan-yeast probe that can detect but not differentiate among 6 other yeasts (5 *Candida* spp. and *Saccharomyces cerevisiae*). Total assay time takes 3.5 hours. In a study performed on spiked BacT/Alert SA standard blood culture bottles, using 69 different clinical isolates representing 8 *Candida* spp., there was 100% concordance by the microarray analysis with the original identification.[29] An additional evaluation of 62 samples containing yeast DNA was also performed. The array identified yeast species in 93.5% of the samples.[29] Two of the missed samples were not contained in the database and the 2 others were not identified by conventional methods.[29] All of the negative cultures and positive bacterial samples yielded a negative yeast result.[29]

The FilmArray Blood Culture Identification (BioFire Diagnostics, Inc Salt Lake City UT) assay consists of a self-contained pouch that stores reagents for sample extraction and purification and nested multiplex PCR. The pouch is inoculated with 200 μL of positive blood culture broth on one end and is hydrated on the opposite end with buffer before placement in the FilmArray instrument. The assay has primers and probes that detect members of the family *Enterobacteriaceae*, 3 Gram-positive and 1 Gram-negative genera, 5 Gram-positive species, 9 Gram-negative species and 5 *Candida* spp. (24 agents in total). In addition, the *mecA* (*S aureus*), *vanA/vanB* (enterococci), and bla$_{KPC}$ genes (*Enterobacteriaceae*) are also detected. Hands-on time is 2 minutes and results are available within 1 hour.

There have been several publications from single institution studies on the performance of this assay and 1 very large multicenter study.[30–35] Among these studies conducted at 13 institutions, the pouch identified 87% to 92% of all pathogens routinely recovered in positive blood cultures. The results of these studies, which are quite variable in their study designs, indicate that the overall accuracy for detection of the genera and species in the panel compared with conventional methods ranged from 94% to 100%.[30–35] The performance for accurately detecting resistance markers ranged from 80.4% to 100%. In 1 study, the FilmArray had difficulty in detecting *mecA* among coagulase-negative staphylococci accounting for the low sensitivity.[35] This was either not observed or not reported in the other studies.[30–34]

Also, like the Verigene assay, in mixed cultures containing *S aureus* and CoNS, correct assignment of a *mecA* gene positive result to the particular species cannot occur. In all of the studies, detection of *mecA* in *S aureus* ranged from 98% to 100%. The FilmArray assay can distinguish *Klebsiella oxytoca* from *Raoultella ornithinolytica*, whereas phenotypic methods cannot. One of the major limitations of this assay, similar to the Verigene assays, is the inability to detect all organisms in polymicrobial cultures.[30–35] Also of note, in the study by Ward and colleagues,[35] a significant number of false-positive results for *P aeruginosa* were observed. It was determined, and the manufacturer, bioMérieux, has confirmed, that this is owing to contamination of the BacTAlert standard anaerobic blood culture bottles with nucleic acid from nonviable organisms.[36] In May 2014, BioFire released an advisory note regarding the possibility of detecting false positive results for *P aeruginosa* and *Enterococcus* spp. when testing bioMérieux BacTAlert standard anaerobic bottles.[37]

## BROAD-BASED TECHNOLOGIES DIRECTLY FROM WHOLE BLOOD

The greatest impact on patient outcomes is likely to occur with assays that offer direct from whole blood testing. There are many challenges to detecting organisms directly from whole blood. The first of these is sensitivity. Often patients with bacteremia will have less than 1 colony forming unit per milliliter (CFU/mL) of bacteria in blood.[27,38] Detecting such low quantities of organisms is challenging even in the era of ultrasensitive nucleic acid amplification techniques. In addition, the repertoire of organisms that can cause bacteremia continues to expand as opportunistic organisms cause serious disease in extremely immunocompromised patients. Clinical specificity is challenged by the possibility of detecting the nucleic acid of dead organisms, random nucleic acid that appears in blood transiently, and also reagent contamination from environmental organisms.[27,36,39] When comparing such assays to conventional blood culture methods, the optimum "gold standard" is unclear. Although these are obstacles, great progress is being made and some of these methods hold promise for detecting noncultivatable or difficult to cultivate pathogens that continue to allude current blood culture methods.

Several assays that detect pathogens in whole blood have been available outside the United States for a number of years. **Table 1** lists the features of these assays and several reviews describe their performance in more detail.[2,27,40]

The LightCycler Septi*FAST* test (Roche Diagnostics, Mannheim Germany) is a 6- to 8-hour assay that detects up to 25 pathogens and *mecA* from whole blood in an assay combining multiplex real-time PCR using dual-fluorescence energy transfer probes (FRET) and melt curve analysis for pathogen differentiation.[2] This assay detects 10 bacteria to species level, several others to the genus level, 5 *Candida* spp., and *Aspergillus fumigatus*, and it has been evaluated extensively in the literature in adult and pediatric patients including 2 recent metaanalyses of its performance.[21,27,41,42] Only the results of the metaanalyses are summarized herein. The systematic review and metaanalysis by Chang and colleagues[41] included 34 primary studies through October 2012. These 34 studies collectively evaluated 6012 patients (8438 episodes), 22.8% of which were confirmed bacterial or fungal infections.[41] Of note, few of the studies were blinded and a wide range of reference standards were applied—some clinical and laboratory, others laboratory based alone. With these shortcomings in mind, the pooled sensitivity was 75% (95% CI, 65%–83%) and the pooled specificity was 92% (95% CI, 90%–95%).[41] The analyses examined the overall positive and negative likelihood ratios (high and moderate, respectively), performance for bacteria and fungi independently, and subgroup analyses examining bacteremic and fungemic patients in studies that had similar settings (such as patients in the intensive care unit [ICU]) and reference methods. The authors concluded that the Septi*FAST* assay is of high "rule-in" value for early detection of septic patients, and in patients with low probability of sepsis, the test may be of value in excluding bacteremia and fungemia.[41]

In the study by Dark and colleagues,[42] the authors likewise found significant heterogeneity and variable quality among the 41 diagnostic accuracy studies evaluated in their analyses. The authors of this metaanalysis used blood culture as the reference standard and included any clinical diagnostic accuracy study that compared Septi*FAST* to the reference method through April 2014.[42] In total, 7727 patients, representing a wide range of age and settings, contributed 10,493 episodes of suspected sepsis in which the median prevalence of blood culture positivity was 17%.[42] Similar to the results of the Chang study, the combined results for sensitivity and specificity, 68% (95% CI, 63%-73%) and 86% (95% CI, 84%-89%), respectively, showed better specificity.[42] The authors concluded that positive results are likely to be of greater diagnostic utility than negative results when compared with blood cultures.[42] Because the upper CI for both sensitivity and specificity did not reach 90% in this pooled analysis, standard blood cultures will still be required to detect false negatives in patients with suspected sepsis and, at least in some settings, even accounting for the superior sensitivity of molecular methods; "false positives" may lead to erroneous diagnoses.[42]

The SepsiTest (Molzym GmbH, Bremen, Germany) uses broad range primers targeting 16S rDNA of bacteria and 18S rDNA of fungi in a real-time PCR assay. The amplicons are sequenced to yield definitive identification of a total of 345 bacteria and fungi. Two 1-mL samples are suggested for testing in duplicate. The manufacturer provides an additional kit called Add-On10 that accommodates up to 10 mL of blood to enhance sensitivity. The assay requires at least 8 hours to complete. In the prospective, multicenter study by Wellinghausen and colleagues,[43] 342 blood samples from 187 patients, mostly adults, were evaluated. Compared with reference blood cultures, the overall diagnostic sensitivity and specificity of the PCR in this study were 87.0% and 85.8%, respectively, and the concordance between the SepsiTest and blood cultures was 86%.[43] There were 7 samples that grew bacteria that were not detected by PCR and 41 samples that were PCR positive but negative by blood cultures. Among the latter group, 12 of the patients were believed to have true bacteremia and in 11 cases, the same species were detected in other body sites. The majority of the remaining samples were obtained from patients who had received antibiotics.[43] Although the performance characteristics of the assay in this study are encouraging, the assay is labor intensive. The practicality of this in a routine clinical laboratory setting is questionable.

Another 8 hours platform, also manufactured in Germany, is the VYOO assay (SIRS-LAB GmbH, Jena, Germany), which combines 16S rRNA gene multiplex PCR with highly specific melting point analysis to identify 34 of the most common bacterial species and 6 fungal species causing bloodstream infections. In addition, 5 resistance markers are also detected: mecA, vanA, vanB, and variants of $bla_{SHV}$ and $bla_{CTX}$, extended spectrum β-lactamase genes.[44] This assay accommodates 5 mL of ethylenediaminetetraacetic acid (EDTA) whole blood.

In the study by Bloos and colleagues,[44] 336 blood samples collected from 245 adult ICU patients were collected for PCR simultaneously with standard blood cultures (311 pairs). The concordance between the PCR assay and standard blood cultures was 72.7%; 67 samples were positive by PCR but negative by standard cultures and 18 were positive by blood cultures that were negative by PCR.[44] Seven of the 18 "false-negative" PCR tests were pathogens not included in the VYOO assay. Two independent arbitrators reviewed the charts of patient with positive PCR results and concluded that 94% of the PCR results yielded clinically meaningful results (ie, not suggestive of contamination), including detection of 12 pathogens that were not treated by initial empiric therapy.[44] In this study, owing to staff limitations, the time for PCR results was 24.2 hours (not the 8 hours possible by the technology) compared with 68.8 hours for standard blood cultures. The overall sensitivity of 60% and specificity of 75% emphasizes the fact that this assay will remain an adjunct to standard blood cultures in a similar fashion to the other assays described.

Seegene (Seoul, Korea) has developed an assay (MagicPlex Sepsis Test) that screens for up to 90 pathogens and 3 resistance markers and definitively identifies 21 bacterial species and 6 fungal species.[27] After DNA extraction from 1 mL of fresh whole blood (EDTA), the first conventional PCR creates an amplicon bank. Real-time PCR using the Magicplex Screening kit screens for the presence of bacteria and fungi. Species identification is then performed on the screen positive samples using the Magicplex ID1-ID-9 real-time detection kit.[45] The assay requires about 7 hours to perform including the DNA extraction step. There are 2 studies that have evaluated the MagicPlex assay. In the study by Carrara and colleagues,[45] the authors compared the Magicplex Sepsis Test to standard blood cultures on 267 patients from an ICU, the emergency department, and a hematology unit. Clinical data were also included in the analysis. The agreement between standard blood cultures and the PCR assay was 73%. Of the 63 positive specimens considered true BSI by clinical assessment, 23 were positive by PCR and standard methods, 18 by PCR only, and 22 by blood cultures only.[45] There was a high rate of contamination by both PCR and standard blood cultures making it difficult to interpret the results that were positive by 1 method alone. The authors concluded that the Magicplex assay shows high specificity overall (92%) but lacks sensitivity (65%) and they recommended technical improvements to the assay.[45]

In the Ljungstrom study, 375 patients who had 383 episodes of sepsis were analyzed by blood cultures, the Magicplex assay performed on whole blood and the Prove-it microarray based assay on positive blood culture bottles.[46] The sensitivity of the Magicplex assay adjudicated by clinical data was 62%, a value similar to the Carrara study.[45,46] In the study by Ljungstrom and colleagues,[46] the specificity was 96% and the concordance with blood cultures was only moderate (kappa 0.50). Also of note in this study was the initial invalid rate of 12% for the Magicplex assay. However, this study was not able to accurately measure the turnaround times because of the variability in the times of the assay performances.[46]

Although such assays, such as SeptiFAST and others have been available in Europe, until recently there has not been an FDA-cleared assay available in the Unites States. Two systems, one that is FDA-cleared and currently available for detection of Candida species in blood and a second more broad-based technology that is in clinical trials in the Unites States are discussed.

### T2 Candida Magnetic Resonance Assay

The T2Dx instrument (T2 Biosystems, Lexington, MA) lyses the Candida cells by standard mechanical bead beating, amplifies the DNA using a proprietary thermostable polymerase and primers targeting the intervening transcribed spacer2 (ITS2) region within the Candida ribosomal operon, and detects the amplification products by hybridization to supermagnetic nanoparticles that are detected by magnetic resonance.[47] The assay has an internal control and requires positive and negative external controls. Whole blood from patients suspected of having candidemia is collected into $K_2$EDTA plastic blood collection vacutainers.[47] The T2 Candida clinical assay detects 5 yeasts reported as 3 independent results. *C albicans/C tropicalis, C glabrata/C krusei,* and *C parapsilosis* in 3 to 5 hours. This reporting arrangement is designed to assist with determining optimum treatment. Preclinical testing revealed a limit of detection for each of these species in whole blood between 1 and 3 CFU/mL. In the clinical trial, performed at 12 centers, 300 contrived samples representing 250 whole blood samples from patients spiked with known concentrations of the 5 targeted *Candida* species and 50 uninoculated whole blood samples were tested as negative controls. In addition, for the prospective arm of the study, 1501 patients were enrolled who had blood cultures drawn concurrently for standard of care testing and the T2MR Candida assay.[48] For the contrived samples, the overall sensitivity was 91% with a range of 88.1% for *C krusei/C glabrata* to 94.2% for *C albicans/C tropicalis*.[48] The specificity results were overall 99.4% with a range of 98.9% (*C albicans/C tropicalis*) to 99.9% (*C krusei/C glabrata*).[48] In the prospective arm of this study, there were only 4 patients who had concomitantly positive T2MR and standard of care blood culture results. There were 31 discordant results, 29 of which were detected only by the T2MR assay and 2 that were T2MR negative but grew *Candida* species in blood cultures. In 5 of these 29 cases, the same *Candida* species grew from other clinical samples and in 6 cases the patients were on antifungal therapy at the time of blood draw. The mean time for completion of standard blood cultures to species level identification in this study was 129.9 ± 26.3 hours and for the T2MR the mean time to species identification was 4.4 ± 1 hours (*P*<.001).[48] Although the negative predictive value of 99.4% may allow for cessation of empiric antifungal therapy for the organisms detected by the assay, it remains to be determined whether this will actually occur among populations at risk for invasive fungal disease beyond *Candida* species. The company is pursuing expanding its menu beyond detection of *Candida* species to include bacterial pathogens.

### IRIDICA BAC-BSI Assay

This commercial assay (IRIDICA BAC-BSI Assay, Ibis Biosciences, Abbott Molecular, Carlsbad, CA), which has undergone numerous iterations, uses broad range multiplex PCR coupled with electrospray ionization mass spectrometry.[49–53] Electrospray ionization mass spectrometry measures the mass of the A, G, C, and T composition of the PCR amplicons.[49] Comparing the base composition of the detected organisms with those of organisms in the database, bacteria and *Candida* species in whole blood can be identified with high accuracy in about 6 to 8 hours. The assay requires 5 mL of whole blood.[53] The current BAC-BSI assay, which is in clinical trials at the time of this publication, definitively detects 48 bacterial pathogens, 5 yeast (*C albicans, C dubliniensis, C glabrata, C parapsilosis,* and *C tropicalis*), and 4 resistance markers *vanA, vanB, mecA,* and *bla_{KPC}*, but it has the capacity to detect many more species. A preliminary study by Bacconi and colleagues[53] describes optimization of the assay in the presence of high levels of human DNA. In the clinical phase of the study, 331 prospectively obtained patient samples (5 mL) were tested by conventional cultures (2 sets each consisting of 1 BD Bactec Plus aerobic/F bottle and 1 BD Bactec anaerobic/F bottle; BD Diagnostics).[53] The BAC-BSI detected 35 positives compared with 18 by standard methods. Fifteen samples were positive by both methods for an overall accuracy compared with standard culture positives of 94% (15/16). Overall, the sensitivity and specificity were 83% and 94%, respectively. Repeat testing of a second whole blood sample improved the sensitivity and specificity to 91% and 99%, respectively.[53]

In Rapid Diagnosis of Infections in the Critically Ill (RADICAL), an observational study performed in 9 ICUs in 6 European countries, the PCR-ESI MS assay was used to test 616 whole blood samples, 185 respiratory samples, and 110 sterile fluid and tissue samples from 529 patients.[54] Only the results for the bloodstream infections are presented herein. PCR-ESI MS detected a pathogen in 228 cases (37%) compared with 68 (11%) using culture. In 13 cases, culture was positive and PCR-ESI MS was negative, and both were negative in 384 cases. Clinical analysis performed by independent investigators suggested that altered treatment would have potentially occurred as a result of the 6-hour availability, enhanced sensitivity, and high negative predictive value (97.5%) of the PCR-ESI MS.[54]

Although the broad spectrum nature of this assay is the best among the platforms described to date, the footprint of this assay and the costs are likely to make implementation of this assay possible for only the largest reference laboratories.

## POTENTIAL ECONOMIC IMPACT OF RAPID MOLECULAR DIAGNOSTIC METHODS AND BENEFITS FOR ANTIMICROBIAL STEWARDSHIP PROGRAMS

Sepsis has been identified as the 10th leading cause of death in the United States, and the overall humanistic and economic burden is extremely high and growing.[2,3,6] The time interval to appropriate/optimal antimicrobial therapy has been recently described as one of the most important factors influencing clinical outcomes and mortality rates in sepsis patients. When considering the goal to shorten the time of empiric, broad-spectrum antimicrobial therapy toward optimal therapy, one must also recognize the globally rising rates of antimicrobial resistance. Infections involving organisms with resistance to various antimicrobial agents have been shown to increase hospital length of stay (LOS), health care costs, and mortality.[55,56] Furthermore, the connection between "unrestricted" broad-spectrum antimicrobial use and the subsequent development of antimicrobial resistance has now been widely accepted. ASPs have been developed as a form of multidisciplinary interventions to allow for selection of the most optimal antimicrobial agent, dosage, and length of therapy to treat an infection.[8] Decreasing the time to appropriate/optimal antimicrobial therapy has been shown to decrease (unnecessary) antimicrobial exposure and can result in cost avoidance.[8,55,56] As stated, the use of blood cultures and routine laboratory methods for organism identification to confirm the clinical suspicion/diagnosis of sepsis has been shown to be suboptimal.[24] Furthermore, studies demonstrated that only 5% to 15% of blood cultures drawn for any reason, and approximately 50% to 60% of the blood cultures collected from patients with clinical signs of septic shock gave positive results using current, continuously monitoring blood culture systems.[57,58] In this review, we presented data on various rapid molecular pathogen detection methods and their performance; although the majority of the methods described in this review demonstrate an acceptable performance and accuracy for implementation in everyday clinical use and can decrease the TAT for reporting results for organism identification and limited AST (ie, presence of predetermined, important genetic resistance markers), only a few studies have been published to date that evaluate the impact of these methods on clinical outcomes, mortality, and costs of health care. The timeline summarized in **Fig. 1** illustrates the potential impact on improving TAT for organism ID by these various detection methods.

One of the first studies investigating the impact of rapid diagnostic tests in conjunction with an ASP on earlier appropriate antimicrobial therapy, patient outcomes, and hospital costs was published by Forrest and colleagues,[59] using the PNA FISH S aureus/CoNS on blood cultures with gram-positive cocci in clusters from ICU patients

with suspected sepsis. PNA FISH results for 139 blood cultures were reported in real time to an ASP for assessment of continued need for vancomycin therapy. The investigators in this study compared the results with a control group of 84 blood cultures with gram-positive cocci in clusters from patients with presumed sepsis for whom PNA FISH was not used. In this study, there was a significant decrease in medium length of hospital stay (approximately 2 days per sepsis episode), a trend toward reduced vancomycin use (approximately 5% decrease), and a decrease in associated hospital cost (approximately $4000 per patient).[59] Subsequently, other studies reported similar data for the PNA FISH S aureus/CoNS and the E faecium/Enterococcus spp. probes.[60,61] Similarly, a study investigating the role of PNA FISH Candida probes demonstrated significant cost savings, mainly attributed to a decreased use of echinocandins.[62] Subsequently, Holtzman and colleagues[63] published results from their study demonstrating the absence of a benefit of the PNA FISH assay(s) with respect to LOS and antimicrobial use without implementation of active notification and antimicrobial stewardship interventions. Few studies investigated the impact of real-time PCR assays in conjunction with an ASP on patient outcomes, antimicrobial use, and cost of patient care. Bauer and colleagues[64] published data from a single-center study, investigating the impact of the Xpert MRSA/SA assay on patient outcomes and associated cost for patients with blood cultures positive for gram-positive cocci in clusters. The investigators reported an overall decrease in hospital LOS by 6.2 days with an associated cost saving of approximately $ 21,000. Finally, only a few studies using broad-based multiplexed platforms for the assessment of impact on antimicrobial stewardship, LOS, and clinical outcome have been performed to date.[34,65–69] Sango and colleagues[66] investigated the impact of Verigene BC-GP platform combined with ASP interventions on patients with enterococcal sepsis. The results of this study, comparing the Verigene BC-GP assay with conventional laboratory methods, demonstrated a decrease in time to effective antimicrobial therapy, together with a decrease in LOS (average, 21.7 days). Bork and colleagues[68] performed a "theoretic antibiotic therapy comparison" study after validation of the Verigene BC-GN assay; in this study, assuming that 100% of the AST/ASP recommendations would be followed by clinicians, the investigators described a statistically significantly shorter time ($P<.01$) from detection of positive blood cultures to effective and/or optimal antimicrobial therapy. The authors

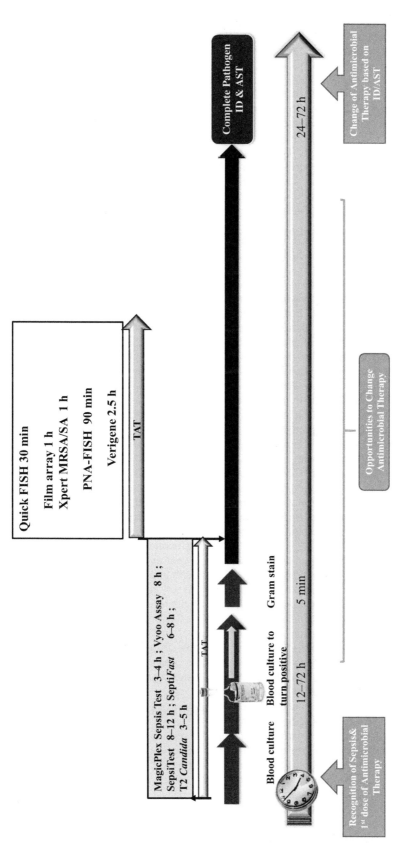

**Fig. 1.** Turnaround time for conventional blood culture results and impact of rapid diagnostic methods. AST, antimicrobial susceptibility testing; ID, organism identification; MRSA, methicillin-resistant *Staphylococcus aureus*; MSSA, methicillin-sensitive *Staphylococcus aureus*; PNA FISH, Peptide nucleic acid fluorescence in-situ hybridization; SA, *S aureus*; TAT, turn-around-time.

therefore concluded, that the use of this assay could potentially decrease to both effective and optimal antimicrobial therapy and significantly improve clinical outcomes in sepsis patients.[68] When reviewing the existing evidence all together, a few limitations must be mentioned here; 2 of these studies[70,71] were retrospective in design, 3 studies[34,67,68] did not specifically investigate the impact of the rapid molecular test method on cost savings per patient, 1 one study was based on a computer-modelling approach to test interventions.[72] Furthermore, all clinical studies were limited by their relatively small sample sizes and absence of a comprehensive assessment of mortality.

To our knowledge, at the time of writing this review only one prospective, randomized controlled trial evaluating clinical outcomes associated with use of a rapid multiplex PCR method for the detection of bacteria, fungi, and resistance genes directly from positive blood cultures has been published.[70] In this study, Banerjee and colleagues[70] investigated the usefulness of a rapid multiplex PCR method (FilmArray Blood Culture Identification; BioFire Diagnostics, Inc) in conjunction with an ASP, compared with the use of rapid multiplex PCR without ASP, and their standard approach to organism ID and AST. In this study, both intervention groups, when compared with the control group, showed a significant decreased use of broad-spectrum antibiotics, less treatment of contaminant organisms, and much shorter time to deescalation of antimicrobials used for treatment. However, the authors did not identify any statistically significant differences in LOS, mortality, or associated cost for treatment.[70]

Finally, 1 study has been published to date investigating the economic impact of a rapid diagnostic method for use on whole blood samples. This study by Bilir and colleagues[72] is a decision tree modeling analysis for the impact of the T2-Candida assay compared with the use of blood culture alone for diagnosis of fungemia in sepsis patients. This study is a computer-based modeling analysis of the economic impact (cost savings and LOS) of the T2 Candida assay over a 1-year period in a hypothetical hospital patient care setting assuming rates of candidemia, approach to intervention, and time to positivity and time to intervention for positive blood cultures based on historical data. In this study, the authors conclude that a hospital could realize a significant cost savings, decreased LOS, and potentially lower mortality rates, when using the T2 Candida assay.[72] At this point, additional, more comprehensive, and preferably prospective studies are necessary to provide more evidence

and a better understanding of the true impact of rapid molecular tests on clinical patient outcomes, mortality, LOS, and cost savings.

## SUMMARY

The use of direct detection and identification methods for pathogens from positive blood cultures or whole blood is a promising approach to improve clinical outcomes in sepsis patients, specifically when these methods are combined with ASPs.[71] The number of commercially available molecular test methods for the diagnosis of sepsis has increased rapidly over the past 10 years. Despite their excellent performance for identification of key pathogens and resistance genes from positive blood cultures, none of these methods by itself has shown sufficient diagnostic accuracy, sensitivity, and/or specificity to fully replace the use of blood cultures and other standard laboratory methods for identification of all organisms potentially implicated as causes of sepsis. Caution must be exercised specifically when considering the performance of these methods for polymicrobial blood cultures. To date, various studies have demonstrated that the rapid molecular tests clearly result in improvements of TAT for identifying key pathogens and resistance genes from positive blood cultures, with the potential for a significant impact on time to optimal antimicrobial therapy, clinical outcomes, and patient mortality. Although these molecular technologies for organism and resistance gene identification, are more expensive to the laboratory when compared with the current conventional methods for ID and AST, there is emerging evidence that the cost for such technologies could be offset by cost savings and cost avoidance in other areas of health care through improvements in clinical care, implementation of earlier, optimal antimicrobial therapy, and decreased ICU LOS and/or overall hospital LOS. Currently ongoing as well as future prospective clinical trials will hopefully provide the evidence to support broader implementation of rapid molecular diagnostic methods in a variety of health care settings.

## REFERENCES

1. Hotchkiss RS, Karl IE. The pathophysiology and treatment of sepsis. N Engl J Med 2003;348(2): 138–50.
2. Riedel S, Carroll KC. Laboratory detection of sepsis: biomarkers and molecular approaches. Clin Lab Med 2013;33:413–37.
3. Chalupka AN, Talmor D. The economics of sepsis. Crit Care Clin 2012;28:57–76.

4. Sutton JP, Friedman B. Trends in septicemia hospitalizations and readmissions in selected HCUP States, 2005 and 2010. H-CUP, Healthcare Cost and Utilization Report; Statistical Brief 161, September 2013. Agency for Healthcare Research and Quality. Available at: www.hcup-us.ahrq.gov/reports/statbriefs/sb161.pdf. Accessed September 18, 2015.

5. Lagu T, Rothberg MB, Nathanson BH, et al. The relationship between hospital spending and mortality in patients with sepsis. Arch Intern Med 2011;171(4):292–9.

6. Tiru B, DiNino EK, Orenstein A, et al. The economic and humanistic burden of severe sepsis. Pharmacoeconomics 2015;33(9):925–37.

7. Stender H, Fiandaca M, Hyldig-Nielsen JJ, et al. PNA for rapid microbiology. J Microbiol Methods 2002;48(1):1–17.

8. Avdic E, Carroll KC. The role of the microbiology laboratory in antimicrobial stewardship programs. Infect Dis Clin North Am 2014;28:215–35.

9. Hensley DM, Tapia R, Encina Y. An evaluation of the AdvanDx Staphylococcus aureus/CNS PNA FISH assay. Clin Lab Sci 2009;22(1):30–3.

10. Della-Latta P, Salimnia H, Painter T, et al. Identification of Escherichia coli, Klebsiella pneumoniae, and Pseudomonas aeruginosa in blood cultures: a multicenter performance evaluation of a three-color peptide nucleic acid fluorescence in situ hybridization assay. J Clin Microbiol 2011;49(6):2259–61.

11. Morgan MA, Marlowe E, Novak-Weekly S, et al. A 1.5 hour procedure for identification of Enterococcus species directly from blood cultures. J Vis Exp 2011;48 [pii:2616].

12. Hall L, Le Febre KM, Deml SM, et al. Evaluation of the Yeast Traffic Light PNA FISH probes for identification of Candida species from positive blood cultures. J Clin Microbiol 2012;50(4):1446–8.

13. Deck MK, Anderson ES, Buckner RJ, et al. Multicenter evaluation of the Staphylococcus QuickFISH method for simultaneous identification of Staphylococcus aureus and coagulase-negative staphylococci directly from blood culture bottles in less than 30 minutes. J Clin Microbiol 2012;50(6):1994–8.

14. Carretto E, Bardaro M, Russello G, et al. Comparison of the Staphylococcus QuickFISH BC test with the tube coagulase test performed on positive blood cultures for evaluation and application in a clinical routine setting. J Clin Microbiol 2013;51(1):131–5.

15. Abdelhamed AM, Zhang SX, Watkins T, et al. Multicenter evaluation of Candida QuickFISH BC for identification of Candida species directly from blood culture bottles. J Clin Microbiol 2015;53(5):1672–6.

16. Salimnia H, Fairfax MR, Lephart P, et al. An international, prospective, multicenter evaluation of the combination of the AdvanDx Staphylococcus QuickFISH BC with mecA XpressFISH for detection of methicillin-resistant Staphylococcus aureus isolates from positive blood cultures. J Clin Microbiol 2014;52(11):3928–32.

17. Nanosphere. Instrumentation 2015. Available at: www.nanosphere.us/products/instrumentation. Accessed September 18, 2015.

18. Nanosphere. Products 2015. Available at: www.nanosphere.us/products/bloodstream-infection-tests. Accessed September 18, 2015.

19. Beal SG, Ciurca J, Smith G, et al. Evaluation of the Nanosphere Verigene gram-positive blood culture assay with the VersaTREK blood culture system and assessment of possible impact on selected patients. J Clin Microbiol 2013;51(12):3988–92.

20. Wojewoda C, Sercia L, Navas M, et al. Evaluation of the Verigene Gram-positive blood culture nucleic acid test for rapid detection of bacteria and resistance determinants. J Clin Microbiol 2013;51(7):2072–6.

21. Samuel LP, Tibbetts RJ, Agotesku A, et al. Evaluation of a microarray-based assay for rapid identification of Gram-positive organisms and resistance markers in positive blood cultures. J Clin Microbiol 2013;51(4):1188–92.

22. Hill JT, Tran KD, Barton KL, et al. Evaluation of the Nanosphere Verigene BC-GN assay for direct identification of gram-negative bacilli and antibiotic resistance markers from positive blood cultures and potential impact for more rapid antibiotic interventions. J Clin Microbiol 2014;52(10):3805–7.

23. Dodemont M, De mendocena R, Nonhoff C, et al. Performance of the Verigene Gram-negative blood culture assay for rapid detection of bacteria and resistance determinants. J Clin Microbiol 2014;52(8):3085–7.

24. Martin GS, Mannino DM, Eaton S, et al. The epidemiology of sepsis in the United States from 1979 through 2000. N Engl J Med 2003;348(16):1546–54.

25. Pence MA, TeKippe EM, Burnham CA. Diagnostic assays for identification of microorganisms and antimicrobial resistance determinants directly from positive blood culture broth. Clin Lab Med 2013;33:651–84.

26. Buchan BW, Allen S, Burnham CAD, et al. Comparison of the next-generation Xpert MRSA/SA BC assay and the GeneOhm StaphSR assay to routine culture for identification of Staphylococcus aureus and methicillin-resistant S. aureus in positive-blood-culture broths. J Clin Microbiol 2015;53:804–9.

27. Loonen AJM, Wolffs PFG, Bruggeman CA, et al. Developments for improved diagnosis of bacterial bloodstream infections. Eur J Clin Microbiol 2014;33:1687–702.

28. Tissari P, Zumla A, Tarkka E, et al. Accurate and rapid identification of bacterial species from positive blood cultures with a DNA-based microarray

platform: an observational study. Lancet 2010;375: 224–30.

29. Aittakorpi A, Kuusela P, Koukila-Kähkölä P, et al. Accurate ad rapid identification of *Candida* spp. frequently associated with fungemia by using PCR and the microarray-based Prove-it sepsis assay. J Clin Microbiol 2012;50:3635–40.

30. Blaschke AJ, Heyrend C, Byington CL, et al. Rapid identification of pathogens from positive blood cultures by multiplex polymerase chain reaction using the FilmArray system. Diagn Microbiol Infect Dis 2012;74:349–55.

31. Altun O, Almuhayawi M, Ullberg M, et al. Clinical evaluation of the FilmArray blood culture identification panel in identification of bacteria and yeasts from positive blood culture bottles. J Clin Microbiol 2013;51:4130–6.

32. Kanack KJ, Salimnia H, Schreckenberger P, et al. Clinical evaluation of a multiplex PCR blood culture identification panel for simultaneous detection of bacteria, yeast and select antimicrobial resistance genes. Abstract presented at the 53rd Intersci Conf Antimicrob Agents Chemother, abstract D-104. Denver, CO, September 10–13, 2013.

33. Bhatti MM, Boonlayangoor S, Beavis KG, et al. Evaluation of the FilmArray and Verigene Systems for rapid identification of positive blood cultures. J Clin Microbiol 2014;52:3433–6.

34. Southern TR, vanSchooneveld TC, Bannister DL, et al. Implementation and performance of the BioFire FilmArray® blood culture identification panel with antimicrobial treatment recommendations for bloodstream infections at a Midwestern academic tertiary hospital. Diagn Microbiol Infect Dis 2015;81:96–101.

35. Ward C, Stocker K, Begum J, et al. Performance of the Verigene (Nanosphere) and FilmArray (BioFire) molecular assays for identification of causative organisms in bacterial bloodstream infections. Eur J Clin Microbiol Infect Dis 2015;34:487–96.

36. Aellen S, Que YA, Guignard B, et al. Detection of live and antibiotic-killed bacteria by quantitative real-time PCR of specific fragments of rRNA. Antimicrob Agents Chemother 2006;50:1913–20.

37. BioFire Diagnostics LLC. Advisory notice. 2014. Available at: ftp://ftp.bmgrp.at/Austria/BioFire-BCID-Lit/Manuals-Beipacktexte/rfit-prt-0224_fa_bcid_ce_ivd_reag_doc_en.pdf. Accessed December 10, 2015.

38. Jonsson B, Nyberg A, Henning C. Theoretical aspects of detection of bacteraemia as a function of volume of blood cultured. APMIS 1993;101:595–601.

39. Birch L, Dawson CE, Cornett JH, et al. A comparison of nucleic acid amplification techniques for the assessment of bacterial viability. Lett Appl Microbiol 2001;33:296–301.

40. Skvarc M, Stubljar D, Rogina P, et al. Non-culture-based methods to diagnose bloodstream infection: does it work? Eur J Microbiol Immunol 2013;2:97–104.

41. Chang SS, Hsieh WH, Liu TS, et al. Multiplex PCR system for rapid detection of pathogens is patients with presumed sepsis—a systematic review and meta-analysis. PLoS One 2013;8:1–10.

42. Dark P, Blackwood B, Gates S, et al. Accuracy of LightCycler® SeptiFast for the detection and identification of pathogens in blood of patients with suspected sepsis: a systematic review and meta-analysis. Intensive Care Med 2015;41:21–33.

43. Wellinghausen N, Kochem A-J, Disqué C, et al. Diagnosis of bacteremia in whole-blood samples by use of a commercial universal 16SrRNA gene-based PCR and sequence analysis. J Clin Microbiol 2009;47:2759–65.

44. Bloos F, Sachse S, Kortgen A, et al. Evaluation of a polymerase chain reaction assay for pathogen detection in septic patients under routine condition: an observational study. PLoS One 2012;7:e46003.

45. Carrara L, Navarro F, Turbau M, et al. Molecular diagnosis of bloodstream infections with a new dual-priming oligonucleotide-based multiplex PCR assay. J Med Microbiol 2013;62:1673–9.

46. Ljungstrom L, Enroth H, Claesson BEB, et al. Clinical evaluation of commercial nucleic acid amplification tests in patients with suspected sepsis. BMC Infect Dis 2015;15:199–209.

47. Neely LA, Audeh M, Phung NA, et al. T2 Magnetic resonance enables nanoparticle-mediated rapid detection of candidemia in whole blood. Sci Transl Med 2013;5:182ra54.

48. Mylonakis E, Clancy CJ, Ostrosky-Zeichner L, et al. T2 Magnetic resonance assay for the rapid diagnosis of candidemia in whole blood: a clinical trial. Clin Infect Dis 2015;60:892–9.

49. Ecker DJ, Sampath R, Massire C, et al. Ibis T5000: a universal biosensor approach for microbiology. Nat Rev Microbiol 2008;6(7):553–8.

50. Ecker DJ, Sampath R, Li H, et al. New technology for rapid molecular diagnosis of bloodstream infections. Expert Rev Mol Diagn 2010;10:399–415.

51. Kaleta EJ, Clark AE, Johnson DR, et al. Use of PCR coupled with electrospray ionization mass spectrometry for rapid identification of bacterial and yeast bloodstream pathogens from blood culture bottles. J Clin Microbiol 2011;49:345–53.

52. Laffler TG, Cummins LL, McClain CM, et al. Enhanced diagnostic yields of bacteremia and candidemia in blood specimens by PCR/electrospray ionization mass spectrometry. J Clin Microbiol 2013;51:3535–41.

53. Bacconi A, Richmond GA, Baroldi MA, et al. Improved sensitivity for molecular detection of bacterial and *Candida* infections in blood. J Clin Microbiol 2014;52:3164–74.

54. Vincent JL, Brealey D, Libert N, et al. Rapid diagnosis of infection in the critically ill, a multicenter study of molecular detection in bloodstream

infections, pneumonia, and sterile site infections. Crit Care Med 2015;43:2283–91.

55. Camins BC, King MD, Wells JB, et al. Impact of an antimicrobial utilization program on antimicrobial use at a large teaching hospital: a randomized controlled trial. Infect Control Hosp Epidemiol 2009;30:931–8.

56. Nowak MA, Nelson RE, Breidenbach JL, et al. Clinical and economic outcomes of a prospective antimicrobial stewardship program. Am J Health Syst Pharm 2012;69:1500–8.

57. Murray PR, Masur H. Current approaches to the diagnosis of bacterial and fungal bloodstream infections for the ICU. Crit Care Med 2012;40(12): 3277–82.

58. Previsdomini M, Gini M, Cerutti B, et al. Predictors of positive blood cultures in critically ill patients: a retrospective evaluation. Croat Med J 2012;53(1): 30–9.

59. Forrest GN, Mehta S, Weekes E, et al. Impact of in situ hybridization testing on coagulase-negative staphylococci positive blood cultures. J Antimicrob Chemother 2006;58:154–8.

60. Ly T, Gulia J, Pyrgos V, et al. Impact upon clinical outcomes of translation of PNA FISH-generated laboratory data from the clinical microbiology bench to bedside in real time. Ther Clin Risk Manag 2008; 4(3):637–40.

61. Forrest GN, Roghmann MC, Toombs LS, et al. Peptide nucleic acid fluorescent in situ hybridization for hospital-acquired enterococcal bacteremia: delivering earlier effective antimicrobial therapy. Antimicrob Agents Chemother 2008;52(10):3558–63.

62. Forrest GN, Mankes K, Jabra-Rizk MA, et al. Peptide nucleic acid fluorescence in situ hybridization-based identification of Candida albicans and its impact on mortality and antifungal costs. J Clin Microbiol 2006;44(9):3381–3.

63. Holtzman C, Whitney D, Barlam T, et al. Assessment of impact of peptide nucleic acid fluorescence in situ hybridization for rapid identification of coagulase-negative staphylococci in the absence of antimicrobial stewardship intervention. J Clin Microbiol 2011;49(4):1581–2.

64. Bauer KA, West JE, Balada-Llasat JM, et al. An antimicrobial stewardship program's impact with rapid polymerase chain reaction methicillin-resistant *Staphylococcus aureus/S. aureus* blood culture test in patients with *S. aureus* bacteremia. Clin Infect Dis 2010;51(9):1074–80.

65. Alby K, Daniels LM, Weber DJ, et al. Development of a treatment algorithm for streptococci and enterococci from positive blood cultures identified with the Verigene Gram-positive blood culture assay. J Clin Microbiol 2013;51(11):3869–971.

66. Sango A, McCarter YS, Johnson D, et al. Stewardship approach for optimizing antimicrobial therapy through use of a rapid microarray assay on blood cultures positive for *Enterococcus* species. J Clin Microbiol 2013;51(12):4008–11.

67. Beal SG, Thomas C, Dhiman N, et al. Antibiotic utilization improvement with the Nanosphere Verigene Gram-positive blood culture assay. Proc (Bayl Univ Med Cent) 2015;28(2):139–43.

68. Bork JT, Leekha S, Heil EL, et al. Rapid testing using the Verigene gram-negative blood culture nucleic acid test in combination with antimicrobial stewardship intervention against gram-negative bacteremia. Antimicrob Agents Chemother 2015;59(3):1588–95.

69. Ledeboer NA, Lopansri BK, Dhiman N, et al. Identification of gram-negative bacteria and genetic resistance determinants from positive blood culture broths by use of the Verigene gram-negative blood culture multiplex microarray-based molecular assay. J Clin Microbiol 2015;53(8):2460–72.

70. Banerjee R, Teng CB, Cunningham SA, et al. Randomized trial of rapid multiplex polymerase chain reaction-based blood culture identification and susceptibility testing. Clin Infect Dis 2015;61: 1071–80.

71. Harbarth S, Nobre V, Pittet D. Does antibiotic selection impact patient outcome? Clin Infect Dis 2007; 44:87–93.

72. Bilir SP, Ferrufino CP, Pfaller MA, et al. The economic impact of rapid Candida species identification by T2Candida among high risk patients. Future Microbiol 2015;10(7):1133–44.

# Risk Stratification and Prognosis in Sepsis
## What Have We Learned from Microarrays?

Timothy E. Sweeney, MD, PhD[a], Hector R. Wong, MD[b,c],*

## KEYWORDS

- Sepsis • Prognostics • Gene expression • Microarray • Biomarker

## KEY POINTS

- Whole-genome expression studies are a useful tool in making sense of the complex and heterogeneous changes that occur in sepsis.
- Prognosis of sepsis at admission is becoming more feasible, with recent validation of some stratification markers such as the pediatric sepsis biomarker risk model (PERSEVERE).
- Splitting patients into subgroups (endotypes) based on gene expression markers may be a way to identify more homogeneous populations of patients with sepsis.
- Better biomarkers may provide for prognostic and phenotypic enrichment strategies in future therapeutic trials.
- Both time and illness severity must be controlled for in future studies of sepsis.

## INTRODUCTION

Sepsis kills more than 750,000 people in the United States annually.[1] Mortality rates have decreased in recent years as a result of clinical process improvements such as adherence to resuscitation protocols and timely administration of antibiotics[2] but remain unacceptably high. Risk stratification and prognostication in sepsis is of particular importance because high-risk patients may benefit from earlier clinical interventions, whereas low-risk patients may benefit from not undergoing unnecessary procedures. Prognostication in sepsis is currently done mostly via clinical criteria (eg, organ dysfunction and/or presence of shock) and blood lactate levels. Although useful, these approaches may not adequately reflect the diversity of clinical presentations seen. In addition, the lack of biomarkers to adequately quantify the heterogeneity of patients with sepsis may have contributed to the numerous failed drug trials in sepsis.[3] Better risk stratification could lead to successful clinical trials through predictive enrichment and prognostic enrichment.[4] Eventually, such biomarkers could personalize treatment based on where a patient resides on the spectrum of inflammation or whether specific organs are failing.

T.E. Sweeney is funded by a Stanford Child Health Research Institute Young Investigator Award (through the Institute for Immunity, Transplantation and Infection), the Society for University Surgeons, and the Stanford Department of Surgery. H.R. Wong is funded by the National Institutes of Health (R01GM099773, R01GM096994, and R01GM108025).

Disclosures: T.E. Sweeney is a scientific advisor to Multerra Biosciences and is a party to a provisional patent filed on the 11-gene sepsis diagnostic.

[a] Department of Surgery, Institute for Immunity, Transplantation and Infection, Stanford University School of Medicine, Stanford, CA, USA; [b] Division of Critical Care Medicine, Cincinnati Children's Hospital Medical Center, Cincinnati Children's Research Foundation, 3333 Burnet Avenue, MLC2005, Cincinnati, OH 45229, USA; [c] Department of Pediatrics, University of Cincinnati College of Medicine, Cincinnati, OH, USA
* Corresponding author. Division of Critical Care Medicine, Cincinnati Children's Hospital Medical Center, 3333 Burnet Avenue, MLC2005, Cincinnati, OH 45229.
E-mail address: hector.wong@cchmc.org

Clin Chest Med 37 (2016) 209–218
http://dx.doi.org/10.1016/j.ccm.2016.01.003

There are multiple approaches to discovering and developing biomarkers. One such approach leverages the high throughput capabilities of transcriptomics in which thousands of genes can be simultaneously measured. These data-driven, systematic studies are particularly amenable to highly complex syndromes such as sepsis because so many changes are occurring at once. Sepsis induces profound changes in the peripheral blood transcriptome, with 70% to 80% of all genes undergoing significant changes in expression.[5,6] To understand and make sense of these changes thus requires a comprehensive view of the transcriptome. As a result, dozens of whole-genome expression studies in clinical human sepsis have now been completed. These studies mostly belong in 3 broad, often overlapping, categories: (1) studies of sepsis at onset; (2) longitudinal studies of sepsis, and (3) studies of organ-specific outcomes in sepsis.

The complexity of changes at the molecular level has made interpreting individual studies difficult for the casual reader; therefore, the authors have summarized the literature. These areas were not reviewed: (1) animal studies of sepsis, (2) studies of critical illness (ie, traumatic injuries) without sepsis, (3) studies that only sampled later time-points in sepsis (more than 48 hours after onset), (4) studies of acute infection only without sepsis, and (5) studies of sepsis that only examined small numbers of genes (ie, studies not using highly parallel technologies). The focus was on synthesizing both validated clinical findings and recurring themes across studies of whole blood or sorted leukocytes evaluating gene expression in sepsis.

## PROGNOSTICATION OF MORTALITY AT ADMISSION: GENE EXPRESSION AT THE ONSET OF SEPSIS

The first microarray study in clinical sepsis was published in 2004; the principle findings were that two-thirds of all genes assayed were differentially expressed, and that septic inflammation was distinctly different from the inflammation that underlies other critical illness.[7] Since that time, both findings have been confirmed my much larger studies with more advanced technologies.[5,6,8,9] Having found that septic inflammation can be distinguished from nonseptic inflammation, the next question was whether subtypes of sepsis both known (ie, survivors and nonsurvivors) and unknown (ie, new classifications based on gene expression patterns) could be discovered in gene expression data. Pachot and colleagues[10] established that, within a cohort, gene expression

patterns in early sepsis could divide survivors from nonsurvivors; however, these results were likely over fit (a common failing in high-dimensional data) because the gene expression pattern that distinguished survivors from nonsurvivors has not been independently validated.

Several other studies have also examined how gene expression in early sepsis differs between eventual survivors and nonsurvivors. Reproduced findings in nonsurvivors include an early decrease in adaptive immunity compared with innate immunity,[11–13] disrupted cell cycle control genes,[12,14,15] increases in protease and metal-ion regulation pathways,[12,14] and increased expression of innate inflammatory cytokines such as interleukin (IL)-1, IL-6, and IL-18 (**Table 1**).[11,12,16] On the other hand, two studies reported either no or very few genes significantly differently regulated between eventual survivors and nonsurvivors at sepsis onset.[5,17]

Another way to stratify patients in a supervised fashion is to examine illness severity instead of the binary outcome of mortality. Although such studies might not be immediately clinically actionable (because a gene expression model to predict a clinical score is made redundant by that clinical score), they might provide pathophysiologic insights or potential markers for risk stratification. Results have been mixed. One group reported that subjects with worse outcomes show a greater degree of change in their gene expression profiles,[18] whereas another reported that among subjects with septic shock more genes were differentially regulated in the lower-severity group than in the higher-severity group (as measured by the simplified acute physiology score).[19] A more targeted approach is to study correlation coefficients between severity scores and gene expression.[20] Almansa and colleagues[12] found modest but significant correlation (mostly absolute Spearman rho<0.5) between the expression levels of 55 genes and sequential organ failure assessment scores (SOFAs) of subjects with sepsis; however, no model of severity was constructed. Such widely divergent results in the study of sepsis severity and mortality are likely explained both by differences in underlying biology between different cohorts and strong confounding from technical and informatics approaches, sampling time, and study design.

More important than qualitative differences in the transcriptome of survivors is a testable clinical model. Here the hypothesis is that a set of genes with a trained predictive model could give a probability of mortality at the time of admission. The pediatric sepsis biomarker risk model (PERSEVERE) is probably the best-validated

**Table 1**
Validated findings of changes in nonsurvivors or higher-mortality subgroups in sepsis

| | Wong et al,[14] 2007 | Parnell et al,[15] 2011 | Dolinay et al,[16] 2012 | Parnell et al,[13] 2013 | Severino et al,[17] 2014 | Tsalik et al,[11] 2014 | Almansa et al,[12] 2015 | Scicluna et al,[5] 2015 |
|---|---|---|---|---|---|---|---|---|
| Suppressed adaptive immune genes | — | — | — | Greater immune suppression integer, decreased lymphocytes | — | Decreased MHC I and MHC II genes | T-cell response genes negatively correlated with SOFA | — |
| Disrupted cell cycle control | — | Increased cyclins and CDKs in higher mortality group | — | — | — | — | Cell cycle control genes correlate with SOFA | — |
| Increased neutrophil-specific proteases | Increased metallothionein, granzyme B | — | — | — | — | Increased metallothioneins and MMP8 or MMP9 | Increased ELANE, MPO, MMP8, CTSG with increased SOFA | — |
| Increased inflammatory cytokines | Increased IL8 gene and protein levels | — | Increased IL18 gene and protein levels | — | — | Increased IL1R2, IL18R1, IL18RAP | Increased IL1R2, IL18R1 with increased SOFA | — |
| Other | — | — | — | — | No significant difference shown, trend toward mitochondrial dysfunction | — | — | Only 3 genes significantly different in nonsurvivors (BCL2L15, NNMT, PRTN) |

Reference is always survivors; thus the direction of change refers to the changes in nonsurvivors.
*Abbreviations:* CDK, cyclin-dependent kinase; SOFA, sequential organ failure assessment score.

biomarker set to estimate the probability of mortality at the time of admission.[21,22] The PERSEVERE model is a decision tree that incorporates the plasma levels of the protein products of 5 genes (initially identified via microarray but subsequently tested with targeted assays) plus patient age. It can accurately predict mortality (area under the curve [AUC] 0.81) in septic children at admission with a high level of sensitivity, and its level is correlated with severity.[21] PERSEVERE also added significant classification power to the pediatric risk of mortality (PRISM) score, with a net reclassification index greater than 0.9. A second model has been developed for adults that includes 4 out of 5 of the same protein products, plus age, lactate level, and presence of chronic disease. This model outperforms the acute physiology and chronic health evaluation (APACHE) II at predicting mortality, with an AUC of 0.76.[23] These sepsis severity models are based on protein assays and should be translatable to clinically actionable predictions of disease severity.

## THE IMPORTANCE OF TIME IN STUDIES OF ACUTE CRITICAL ILLNESS

Several studies have shown the importance of time since illness onset in interpreting the underlying genomic response. The host response to sepsis changes significantly even within the first 24 to 48 hours. In fact, the set of genes differentially expressed in sepsis changes by 20% to 50% within a 24-hour period.[19,24] Ongoing nonlinear changes have been confirmed in the following 5 to 7 days. Similar nonlinear changes in host gene expression have been found as late as a year after traumatic injuries and burn injuries.[6] Two main approaches have thus been taken in longitudinal studies of sepsis. One is to compare cases and controls at matched time points in short enough time windows such that the underlying response approaches linearity.[8,9] The other is to use advanced nonlinear functions to model the underlying changes.[25,26] Both have been leveraged to make use of several longitudinal studies of sepsis.

## FINDINGS FROM LONGITUDINAL STUDIES: PREDICTING HOSPITAL-ACQUIRED SEPSIS

Several studies have not focused on prognosis within sepsis but instead on risk of sepsis in hospitalized subjects. Here the hypothesis is that a set of genes can predict infections earlier than clinical diagnosis. There are several other studies that focus on diagnostic gene sets at the time of diagnosis; however, pure diagnosis is outside the scope of this article. A summary of these studies is found in **Table 2**.

Cobb and colleagues[25] discovered and validated a principal components model of an 85-gene set called the riboleukogram that they used to predict eventual ventilator-associated pneumonia (VAP) in critically ill subjects.[26] In principal component space, the paths for subjects with eventual VAP and those without were significantly different several days before VAP diagnosis.

Johnson and colleagues[8] examined time-matched intensive care unit (ICU) subjects with systemic inflammatory response syndrome (SIRS) who eventually developed infections and showed that 12, 36, and even 60 hours before eventual diagnosis of sepsis, compared with never-infected subjects, preseptic subjects showed upregulation of innate inflammatory networks and pattern recognition receptor pathways. That group did not build models for prognosis.

Yan and colleagues[27] studied subjects with severe burns to predict which subjects would go on to have multiple episodes of infection. They showed that a 14-probe (10-gene) signature could improve on a regression model for multiple infections built from only clinical parameters, suggesting the added utility of genomic markers in clinical medicine.

Sweeney and colleagues[9] performed a meta-analysis of gene expression in 9 cohorts of subjects with noninfectious SIRS versus sepsis and discovered a diagnostic 11-gene set. They validated this 11-gene set in multiple independent public sepsis gene expression datasets. They further found that the 11-gene set was prognostic of sepsis in both discovery and validation in longitudinal trauma subject cohorts 2 to 5 days before onset of sepsis, raising the possibility of earlier diagnosis than is currently clinically possible.

Prognosis of sepsis in the hospitalized patient could potentially reduce both morbidity and mortality; however, its applications are not yet fully understood. Daily testing for monitoring of prognostic gene sets seems both costly and disruptive; more probable is an integrated model of a clinical score that triggers a gene expression test. Further work is necessary before clinical implementation of any of the sepsis-prognostic models.

## IMMUNE PARALYSIS IN SEPSIS: AN UPDATED VIEW

The impaired adaptive immune response in sepsis has been previously referred to as a compensatory anti-inflammatory response syndrome (CARS), also known as immune paralysis. Hypothesis-driven mechanistic studies of immune paralysis in

**Table 2**
Findings in the studies examining prediction of onset of sepsis in hospitalized subjects

| | Johnson et al,[8] 2007 | McDunn et al,[26] 2008 & Cobb et al,[25] 2009 | Yan et al,[27] 2015 | Sweeney et al,[9] 2015 |
|---|---|---|---|---|
| Clinical setting | Prediction of sepsis compared with ICU subjects with noninfectious SIRS | Prediction of VAP in ICU subjects | Prediction of multiple infections in burn subjects | Prediction of sepsis compared with noninfectious SIRS in multicohort analysis |
| Activated inflammatory pathways | KEGG pathways activated: TLR signaling, MAPK signaling, IL-22 signaling, IL-1 signaling | Enriched defense response GO codes; enriched neutrophil activation genes | Multiple pathways, including interleukin and JAK or STAT signaling | Convergence on IL-6 and JUN signaling in IPA |
| Changes in T-cell signaling | Increased Th1 differentiation | — | Impaired T-cell signaling | Trend toward T-reg enrichment |
| Other findings | Increased apoptosis-associated genes | Enriched GO codes for metal ion binding, protein binding, and ATP binding | Enriched epigenetic modulation genes | Signature may be present in band neutrophils |
| Prognostic gene set | None | 85-gene set; see article | Up: THBS1, ARHGEF7; Down: MDFIC, CCND2, OSBPL8, DCAF7, TMEM50B, GOLGA8A or B, SMARCA4, WHSC1L1 | Up: CEACAM1, ZDHHC19, C9orf95, GNA15, BATF, C3AR1 Down: KIAA1370, TGFBI, MTCH1, RPGRIP1, HLA-DPB1 |

*Abbreviations:* GO, gene ontology; ICU, intensive care unit; IPA, ingenuity pathway analysis; MAPK, mitogen-activated protein kinase; SIRS, systemic inflammatory response syndrome; TLR, toll-like receptor; T-reg, regulatory T cell; VAP, ventilator-associated pneumonia.

sepsis have been invaluable in establishing some key events. However, computational analysis of transcriptomic studies has allowed significant advances in understanding the multiple nonlinear changes that occur in the different portions of the immune system. Severe immune dysregulation is present not only in sepsis but also in other severe critical illness, such as the response to traumatic injury. The Glue Grant, a multicenter, longitudinal study of trauma and burn subjects, performed microarray gene expression profiling on both whole blood and sorted-cells of these subjects. Their findings have, in particular, driven and confirmed 2 major paradigm shifts in the understanding of immune paralysis.

Xiao and colleagues[28] showed that adaptive immune gene modules were rapidly and persistently depressed in trauma subjects (and to a greater degree in subjects with complicated ICU course). This showed that, instead of being an adaptive response to critical inflammation, immune paralysis is induced simultaneously with SIRS.

Desai and colleagues[20] looked at the same subjects over their entire hospital stays, and divided them into 5 ordered groups depending on multiorgan dysfunction scores and long-term outcomes. They showed that gene expression modules for adaptive immunity (among others) became more dysregulated over time in subjects with worse outcomes. In particular, the expression of genes associated with antigen-presenting cells fell in correlation with worsening outcomes.

A new characterization of immune dysregulation in chronic critical illness has been proposed in response to this and other studies: the persistent inflammation-immunosuppression catabolism syndrome (PICS).[29] PICS describes the state of ongoing immune dysregulation in chronically critically ill patients. Notably, the group that described PICS was able to validate it with a mix of clinical and microarray data from the Glue Grant database.[30] In particular, they showed that T-cells from subjects with complications late in their course showed gene expression patterns consistent with regulatory T cell (T-reg)-induced suppression, whereas the neutrophils and monocytes from the same subjects still showed persistent activation of innate immune inflammation.

Interestingly, a separate group has used totally separate methods to come to similar conclusions. Pena and colleagues[31] studied the transcriptomes from monocytes with endotoxin tolerance (induced with a 2-hit endotoxin exposure) for a conserved set of endotoxin tolerance genes similar to M2 polarization. They then used RNA sequencing in a validation cohort to show that the endotoxin tolerance signature is more enriched in subjects with more severe sepsis at admission (more organ failure) than in less-complicated cases.[32] They further showed that their endotoxin tolerance module can be found in several independent sepsis datasets. This confirms that the immune paralysis or tolerance seen in late critical illness is also present in early severe sepsis and may contribute to the worse outcomes of high-risk patients.

## MARKERS OF ORGAN-SPECIFIC OUTCOMES IN PERIPHERAL BLOOD

Of particular interest in stratifying patients with sepsis is the notion of predicting specific organ dysfunctions because such predictions might be more clinically actionable than simply stratifying a patient to a higher-mortality group. Predicting lung injury could allow for early low-tidal volume ventilation, for instance, or predicting kidney injury could lead to avoidance of further nephrotoxicity. The hypothesis is that leukocytes (or the sorted cell type being profiled) carry gene expression patterns that are specific for a distant site of injury (ie, the failing organ system being studied). Circulating cells are, in some sense, a step removed from the organ (unlike in studies of systemic inflammation in which circulating cells are generally thought to be the mediators of the effect). However, peripheral blood (or sorted cell) gene expression may still reveal patterns of inflammation that are specific to a failing organ or organ system.

Several studies have examined the transcriptomic whole blood response in lung injury or acute respiratory distress syndrome (ARDS) in sepsis.[16,33–35] The gene sets found to be differentially expressed in ARDS are not highly overlapping in any of the studies. Interestingly, the genes found to be increased in ARDS are often genes associated with more severe sepsis or septic shock in other studies (eg, MMP8, RETN, IL1B, IL18, OLFM4). The most likely explanation for this is that the lung injury signal is strongly confounded by worse systemic inflammation in patients with lung injury. It is also possible, however, that the higher severity of sepsis in other studies also included some degree of lung injury.

Similar results were found in relation to septic shock–associated acute kidney injury (AKI), with MMP8, IL1R2, OLFM4, and other genes previously associated with severity increased in subjects with AKI.[36] However, all subjects were children with septic shock, which removes at least some confounding from clinical severity.

Not all genes associated with specific organ failure have been shown to be associated with sepsis severity. However, they were also not reproduced between studies. In general, the effects of any organ-specific pattern of gene expression may be small compared with the profound changes in systemic inflammation in severe sepsis. Coupled with generally small sample sizes in the studies done so far, the only firm conclusions are that more studies are necessary, and that controlling for severity with advanced informatics approaches will likely be necessary.

## UNSUPERVISED LEARNING OF SEPSIS SUBTYPES

Another approach to risk stratification is to discovery novel subtypes of gene expression (endotypes) in sepsis. The hypothesis is that clinicians may be clinically grouping all patients of a class together (eg, all those with septic shock) although, potentially, there are really 2 or more subtypes (eg, a group with severe endothelial cell dysfunction, another with mitochondrial dysfunction) within that class that may help stratify patients (**Fig. 1**). All such unsupervised clustering studies are highly dependent on clustering method, validation metric, and interpretation; nevertheless, they can yield valuable insights in high-dimensional datasets that are not easily classified by human intuition alone.

Maslove and colleagues[37] performed unsupervised clustering on 365 sepsis-related genes from 2 microarray studies of neutrophils in clinical sepsis. They identified 2 main clusters of septic subjects. Interestingly, they found that the 2 subgroups stratified subjects with severe sepsis but that subjects with septic shock were evenly distributed, suggesting that shock may be less associated with underlying changes in the transcriptome than other kinds of organ dysfunction.

Wynn and colleagues[38] used 2955 probes to cluster the gene expression profiles of neonates with sepsis. They found that early day of life (<3 days) was distinct from late day of life episodes of sepsis at the molecular level. This points to the utility of unsupervised transcriptomic clustering to discover important clinical differences in sepsis.

Wong and colleagues[39] used 6934 genes to cluster children with septic shock only. They identified 3 clusters of subjects (A–C). They found that group A had more deaths and organ failures, and group B had older children and more children receiving corticosteroids. Interestingly, the group was able to reduce the number of classifying genes to 100 and has tested them in independent subjects using visual gene expression mosaics. Here they found that matched subjects in group A, but not group B, carried a significant increased risk of mortality when receiving adjunctive corticosteroids. This type of theranostic approach

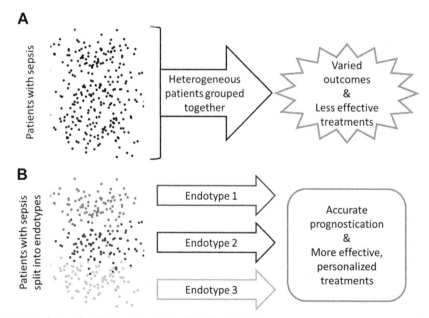

**Fig. 1.** Discovery and use of endotypes in sepsis. (*A*) All subjects in a heterogeneous cohort of septic subjects are treated similarly, reducing the signal-to-noise ratio and rendering prognostic and therapeutic differences less effective. (*B*) The same cohort is split into multiple (here 3, arbitrarily) subgroups based on transcriptomic biomarkers. Each group is treated with a therapy best suited to it and prognostic predictions are more accurate.

illustrates the potential power of identifying new endotypes in sepsis.

## CAVEATS IN GENE EXPRESSION PROFILING: CONSIDERATIONS FOR FUTURE STUDIES

As with all omics (massively parallel) technologies, transcriptomic profiling via microarrays often leads to significant rates of both type I and type II errors. The number of samples is often far less than the number of variables measured; therefore, studies often report false positives. However, the expense of running these studies often leads to publications underpowered to find true effects. Independent validation and/or meta-analysis (either by simple vote counting of study replications, or by true random-effects or Bayesian models) are absolutely required before clinical application.

Many of the studies of sepsis and critical illness focus (appropriately) on whole blood because systemic inflammation is likely largely mediated by circulating leukocytes. However, a gene expression profile of whole blood is a profile of the mixtures of individual cell types present. Thus, differential gene expression can be caused both by actual changes in expression within a cell type and by changes in cell type ratios because each cell type has different background patterns of gene expression. For simple clinical tools, this may not matter because a biomarker must be primarily reliably reproducible, not grounded in pathophysiology. However, for interpretation of pathophysiology, prediction of therapies, and further research directions, cell-type-specific gene expression (either via direct measurement or via bioinformatic deconvolution analysis[40]) will become important. Several studies have thus focused solely on gene expression profiling of peripheral blood mononuclear cells or further-sorted subsets. These studies often have significantly different findings from whole-blood studies, in which signals are dominated by neutrophils, because these are the largest blood cell compartments during acute inflammation. Both approaches offer important insight into sepsis pathophysiology.

Finally, the application of gene expression biomarkers in sepsis has a unique challenge: clinical time. In critical illness, hours count. Accurate gene expression quantitation takes time. Although some technologies are in development to reduce the time required for gene expression quantitation to an hour or less, a standard multiplex polymerase chain reaction still takes 3 to 4 hours. Technologies that can measure more than a handful of genes at once often take much longer. Some

gene expression biomarkers have been converted to protein assays; the rest will require careful optimization before clinical translation.

## WHAT IS LEARNED SO FAR AND FUTURE DIRECTIONS

Despite the caveats, genome-wide expression profiling has yielded some tools that are rapidly approaching clinical deployment, and it has led to several remarkable, reproducible insights into sepsis pathophysiology. Risk stratification via biomarker sets such as PERSEVERE initially discovered in microarray studies have been validated in the research setting to better predict mortality than other clinical scoring systems (eg, PRISM and APACHE II). Further, these models have been reduced to protein assays, making their eventual translation to clinical practice easier.

The understanding of the pathophysiology of severe sepsis has been greatly advanced by transcriptomic studies. Parallel immune dysregulations—overactive innate inflammation and collapse of adaptive immunity—are now known to coexist in sepsis. SIRS seems to be driven largely by activated and immature neutrophils, as evidenced by repeated findings of both increased typical proinflammatory cytokines (IL-1, IL-6, IL-18) and related networks, as well as increased neutrophil proteinase and secretory genes (*MMP8*, *RETN*). Immune paralysis, shown to be activated along with SIRS, is evidenced by both acute and chronic downregulation of adaptive immune genes, possibly by increases in the T-reg compartment. However, immune paralysis is not limited to adaptive immunity because a signature of endotoxin tolerance initially derived in monocyte in vitro has been shown in multiple studies of septic whole blood. Furthermore, because clinical improvements have decreased mortality in the initial acute phases in sepsis, the chronic stage of PICS seems to gaining more relevance. Immune dysregulation in sepsis has been definitively linked to worse outcomes and greater severity (although the causal mechanisms are unknown). Future immunomodulatory therapies for sepsis will likely need to take the new understanding of immune dysregulation into account to succeed.

Stratification of risk for specific types of organ failure is an important area of study in which more research is needed. Whereas many types of omics technologies (eg, metabolomics, lipidomics, proteomics) can potentially find leaked circulating molecules of interest from the target organ in whole blood,[41] transcriptomics has a somewhat greater challenge. Most gene expression signal in the whole blood comes from leukocytes and will thus primarily show patterns of systemic inflammation. Still, decoding this signal (ie, searching for the organ-specific needle in the transcriptomic haystack) could potentially allow for a single diagnostic to yield multiple dimensions of risk stratification, with obvious clinical benefit.

## SUMMARY

Sepsis is a complex, heterogeneous clinical syndrome. At its most basic, better risk stratification can help determine level of care. As the understanding of gene expression in sepsis grows, however, so does the potential to move sepsis care into the era of precision medicine. Immunomodulatory therapies have failed when applied broadly but better biomarkers that quantitatively stratify patients will allow for clinical trials based on predictive and prognostic enrichment, which will save costs and increase positive trial outcomes. Furthermore, this better understanding of the underlying immune dysregulation will allow different classes of septic patients to be treated differently, ultimately reducing morbidity and mortality. Much has been learned and validated already. However, more research is needed in targeted validation of proposed gene sets and data-driven microarray studies of sepsis severity and organ-specific outcomes.

## REFERENCES

1. Lagu T, Rothberg MB, Shieh MS, et al. Hospitalizations, costs, and outcomes of severe sepsis in the United States 2003 to 2007. Crit Care Med 2012; 40:754–61.
2. Dellinger RP, Levy MM, Rhodes A, et al. Surviving sepsis campaign: international guidelines for management of severe sepsis and septic shock, 2012. Intensive Care Med 2013;39:165–228.
3. Cohen J, Vincent JL, Adhikari NK, et al. Sepsis: a roadmap for future research. Lancet Infect Dis 2015;15:581–614.
4. Temple R. Enrichment of clinical study populations. Clin Pharmacol Ther 2010;88:774–8.
5. Scicluna BP, Klein Klouwenberg PM, van Vught LA, et al. A molecular biomarker to diagnose community-acquired pneumonia on intensive care unit admission. Am J Respir Crit Care Med 2015;192(7):826–35.
6. Seok J, Warren HS, Cuenca AG, et al. Genomic responses in mouse models poorly mimic human inflammatory diseases. Proc Natl Acad Sci U S A 2013;110:3507–12.
7. Prucha M, Ruryk A, Boriss H, et al. Expression profiling: toward an application in sepsis diagnostics. Shock 2004;22:29–33.
8. Johnson SB, Lissauer M, Bochicchio GV, et al. Gene expression profiles differentiate between sterile SIRS and early sepsis. Ann Surg 2007;245:611–21.
9. Sweeney TE, Shidham A, Wong HR, et al. A comprehensive time-course-based multicohort analysis of sepsis and sterile inflammation reveals a robust diagnostic gene set. Sci Transl Med 2015; 7:287ra271.
10. Pachot A, Lepape A, Vey S, et al. Systemic transcriptional analysis in survivor and non-survivor septic shock patients: a preliminary study. Immunol Lett 2006;106:63–71.
11. Tsalik EL, Langley RJ, Dinwiddie DL, et al. An integrated transcriptome and expressed variant analysis of sepsis survival and death. Genome Med 2014;6:111.
12. Almansa R, Heredia-Rodríguez M, Gomez-Sanchez E, et al. Transcriptomic correlates of organ failure extent in sepsis. J Infect 2015;70:445–56.
13. Parnell GP, Tang BM, Nalos M, et al. Identifying key regulatory genes in the whole blood of septic patients to monitor underlying immune dysfunctions. Shock 2013;40:166–74.
14. Wong HR, Shanley TP, Sakthivel B, et al. Genome-level expression profiles in pediatric septic shock indicate a role for altered zinc homeostasis in poor outcome. Physiol Genomics 2007;30:146–55.
15. Parnell G, McLean A, Booth D, et al. Aberrant cell cycle and apoptotic changes characterise severe influenza A infection–a meta-analysis of genomic signatures in circulating leukocytes. PLoS One 2011;6:e17186.
16. Dolinay T, Kim YS, Howrylak J, et al. Inflammasome-regulated cytokines are critical mediators of acute lung injury. Am J Respir Crit Care Med 2012;185: 1225–34.
17. Severino P, Silva E, Baggio-Zappia GL, et al. Patterns of gene expression in peripheral blood mononuclear cells and outcomes from patients with sepsis secondary to community acquired pneumonia. PLoS One 2014;9:e91886.
18. Pankla R, Buddhisa S, Berry M, et al. Genomic transcriptional profiling identifies a candidate blood biomarker signature for the diagnosis of septicemic melioidosis. Genome Biol 2009;10:R127.
19. Cazalis MA, Lepape A, Venet F, et al. Early and dynamic changes in gene expression in septic shock patients: a genome-wide approach. Intensive Care Med Exp 2014;2(1):20.
20. Desai KH, Tan CS, Leek JT, et al. Dissecting inflammatory complications in critically injured patients by within-patient gene expression changes: a longitudinal clinical genomics study. PLoS Med 2011;8: e1001093.
21. Wong HR, Weiss SL, Giuliano JS Jr, et al. Testing the prognostic accuracy of the updated pediatric sepsis biomarker risk model. PLoS One 2014;9:e86242.

22. Wong HR, Weiss SL, Giuliano JS Jr, et al. The temporal version of the pediatric sepsis biomarker risk model. PLoS One 2014;9:e92121.

23. Wong HR, Lindsell CJ, Pettilä V, et al. A multibiomarker-based outcome risk stratification model for adult septic shock*. Crit Care Med 2014; 42:781–9.

24. Kwan A, Hubank M, Rashid A, et al. Transcriptional instability during evolving sepsis may limit biomarker based risk stratification. PLoS One 2013;8:e60501.

25. Cobb JP, Moore EE, Hayden DL, et al. Validation of the riboleukogram to detect ventilator-associated pneumonia after severe injury. Ann Surg 2009;250: 531–9.

26. McDunn JE, Husain KD, Polpitiya AD, et al. Plasticity of the systemic inflammatory response to acute infection during critical illness: development of the riboleukogram. PLoS One 2008;3:e1564.

27. Yan S, Tsurumi A, Que YA, et al. Prediction of multiple infections after severe burn trauma: a prospective cohort study. Ann Surg 2015;261:781–92.

28. Xiao W, Mindrinos MN, Seok J, et al. A genomic storm in critically injured humans. J Exp Med 2011; 208:2581–90.

29. Gentile LF, Cuenca AG, Efron PA, et al. Persistent inflammation and immunosuppression: a common syndrome and new horizon for surgical intensive care. J Trauma Acute Care Surg 2012;72:1491–501.

30. Vanzant EL, Lopez CM, Ozrazgat-Baslanti T, et al. Persistent inflammation, immunosuppression, and catabolism syndrome after severe blunt trauma. J Trauma Acute Care Surg 2014;76:21–9 [discussion: 29–30].

31. Pena OM, Pistolic J, Raj D, et al. Endotoxin tolerance represents a distinctive state of alternative polarization (M2) in human mononuclear cells. J Immunol 2011;186:7243–54.

32. Pena OM, Hancock DG, Lyle NH, et al. An endotoxin tolerance signature predicts sepsis and organ dysfunction at initial clinical presentation. EBioMedicine 2014;1:64–71.

33. Chen Y, Shi JX, Pan XF, et al. DNA microarray-based screening of differentially expressed genes related to acute lung injury and functional analysis. Eur Rev Med Pharmacol Sci 2013;17:1044–50.

34. Howrylak JA, Dolinay T, Lucht L, et al. Discovery of the gene signature for acute lung injury in patients with sepsis. Physiol Genomics 2009;37:133–9.

35. Kangelaris KN, Prakash A, Liu KD, et al. Increased expression of neutrophil-related genes in patients with early sepsis-induced ARDS. Am J Physiol Lung Cell Mol Physiol 2015;308:L1102–13.

36. Basu RK, Standage SW, Cvijanovich NZ, et al. Identification of candidate serum biomarkers for severe septic shock-associated kidney injury via microarray. Crit Care 2011;15:R273.

37. Maslove DM, Tang BM, McLean AS. Identification of sepsis subtypes in critically ill adults using gene expression profiling. Crit Care 2012;16:R183.

38. Wynn JL, Guthrie SO, Wong HR, et al. Post-natal age is a critical determinant of the neonatal host response to sepsis. Mol Med 2015;21:496–504.

39. Wong HR, Cvijanovich NZ, Allen GL, et al. Validation of a gene expression-based subclassification strategy for pediatric septic shock. Crit Care Med 2011;39:2511–7.

40. Shen-Orr SS, Tibshirani R, Khatri P, et al. Cell type-specific gene expression differences in complex tissues. Nat Methods 2010;7:287–9.

41. Boyd JH, McConechy M, Walley KR. Acute organ injury is associated with alterations in the cell-free plasma transcriptome. Intensive Care Med Exp 2014;2:5.

# Development and Implementation of Sepsis Alert Systems

Andrew M. Harrison, PhD[a], Ognjen Gajic, MD, MSc[b],
Brian W. Pickering, MB, BCh, MSc, FFARCSI[c],
Vitaly Herasevich, MD, PhD, MSc[c],*

## KEYWORDS

- Sepsis • Automated alert systems • Critical care • Intensive care unit • Hospital

## KEY POINTS

- Barriers to implementation of sepsis alert systems include evolving clinical definitions of sepsis, delayed availability of data through the electronic medical record, information overload, and alert fatigue.
- To be clinically useful, alert systems of the future will need to be more reliable with lower rates of false-positive alerts and be much better integrated into clinical workflow.
- Emerging concepts and strategies that may increase the clinical utility of alerts include wearable physiologic monitoring devices; cognitive ergonomics; human-centered interface design; use of more sophisticated mathematical modeling and machine learning techniques; and integrated prevention, patient education, and public awareness.

## INTRODUCTION

Development and implementation of sepsis alert systems has occurred primarily in acute care settings, such as the intensive care unit (ICU) and emergency department (ED).[1] The development and implementation of these systems outside the acute care setting (ICU and ED) is limited for a variety of reasons. As a critical care syndrome,[2,3] the pathogenesis of sepsis has been studied. Thus, the basic pathophysiology of sepsis is best understood primarily in this context.[4,5] Sophisticated technologies and large quantities of data present in the acute care setting, combined with relatively short lengths of stay and clear outcomes (eg, mortality), provide a natural environment for clinical informatics research in general.[6] However, sepsis is not limited to the ICU setting. As a result of advances in the technology and data granularity underlying clinical informatics systems, it is now possible to consider the development and implementation of sepsis alert systems within and outside the ICU.

Funding Sources: AHRQ, R36 HS022799 (A.M. Harrison); NHLBI, U01 HL125119 (O. Gajic and V. Herasevich).
Conflict of Interest: None (A.M. Harrison); AWARE is patent pending (US 2010/0198622, 12/697861, PCT/US2010/022750). Sepsis sniffer is patent number 20110137852. The Mayo Clinic have a financial interest relating to licensed technology described in this article. This research has been reviewed by the Mayo Clinic Conflict of Interest Review Board and is being conducted in compliance with Mayo Clinic Conflict of Interest Policies (O. Gajic, V. Herasevich, and B.W. Pickering).
[a] Medical Scientist Training Program, Mayo Clinic, 200 First Street Southwest, Rochester, MN 55905, USA; [b] Division of Pulmonology and Critical Care Medicine, Mayo Clinic, 200 First Street Southwest, Rochester, MN 55905, USA; [c] Department of Anesthesiology, Mayo Clinic, 200 First Street Southwest, Rochester, MN 55905, USA
* Corresponding author.
E-mail address: Herasevich.Vitaly@mayo.edu

Clin Chest Med 37 (2016) 219–229
http://dx.doi.org/10.1016/j.ccm.2016.01.004
0272-5231/16/$ – see front matter

The reason for considering electronic sepsis surveillance is ultimately to facilitate timely and error-free treatment through early recognition and decision support. However, multiple barriers prevent the development and implementation of hospital-wide sepsis alert systems. These barriers and potential solutions to these barriers are explored. A vision of alert systems of the future is presented.

## DEVELOPMENT AND IMPLEMENTATION OF SEPSIS ALERT SYSTEMS

Early sepsis alert systems were developed primarily for clinical trial enrollment purposes. In 2003, Thompson and colleagues[7] published a sepsis alert and diagnostic system for integrating clinical systems to enhance study coordinator efficiency. In 2005, Embi and colleagues[8] published the effects of a clinical trial alert system on physician participation in clinical trial recruitment. In 2008, Herasevich and colleagues[9] published a computer-based screening engine for severe sepsis and septic shock, which was subsequently used to enroll patients in the critical care setting into a time sensitive clinical study.[10] The development of these early alert systems generated considerable interest in how to best use electronic data to find and treat critically ill patients,[11] as well as lay the foundation for the implementation of sepsis alert systems in the ICU setting (**Table 1**).[12–15]

The first methodologically rigorous clinical trials have failed to demonstrate improvements in clinically significant endpoints. In the first study, Hooper and colleagues[15] deployed a modified systemic inflammatory response syndrome (SIRS) detection algorithm within an ICU setting. They randomized subjects to groups monitored with the algorithm and those who were not. When modified SIRS criteria were met, clinicians were notified via text message. The hypothesis being tested was that automated notification would facilitate a diagnosis of sepsis and shorten the time to initiation of antibiotics, fluid administration, and other sepsis-related cares. The study demonstrated the feasibility and safety of the approach but failed to demonstrate a difference in the time to administration of appropriate cares. In 2015, the same Vanderbilt group, Semler and colleagues,[16] performed another randomized trial of an electronic tool for the evaluation and treatment of sepsis in the ICU. This system combined their existing automated, electronic monitoring system with a clinical decision support system. As with their previous study, this system did not improve clinically significant outcomes in the ICU setting, including length

of stay in the hospital or ICU, and timely completion of appropriate interventions.

At Mayo Clinic, an ICU-specific patient viewer has been clinically validated and implemented in the medical ICU setting.[17–19] In this context, Harrison and colleagues[20] developed a surveillance system for the detection of failure to recognize and treat severe sepsis. The rationale for this system was to not only detect sepsis but also to prevent clinically important deterioration and complications due to failure to treat this underlying illness in a timely manner (failure to rescue).[21,22] However, the validity of this or any other implementation approach has yet to be tested in a clinical trial.

## BARRIERS TO DEVELOPMENT AND IMPLEMENTATION OF CLINICALLY USEFUL SEPSIS ALERT SYSTEMS

In addition to real-time availability of accurate electronic data, the ability of a sepsis detection algorithm to reliably identify sepsis is influenced by many external factors. Critically, algorithms are developed using current knowledge of the condition of sepsis and on data derived from a particular health care setting or patient population. The performance is optimized for those conditions and will be unpredictably altered if used in any other context. In the face of evolving definitions of sepsis and treatment guidelines, changing patient populations or clinical settings, the performance of sepsis algorithms must be continuously monitored and tweaked. Even small changes in the sensitivity or specificity of these algorithms can lead to high rates of false-positive or negative alerts. These changes can undermine confidence in the alert and render it ineffective in clinical practice (**Fig. 1**).

### Clinical Diagnostic Cues Not Available in the Electronic Medical Record

Often, the critical rate-limiting step for efficacy of sepsis alert systems is the availability of real-time data in the electronic medical record (EMR). The data have to be in the record before the algorithm can register it and make a prediction about whether the patient is at risk of sepsis. Delayed data entry or validation, lack of interconnectivity of EMR department systems, and infrequent sampling times all contribute to patchy, absent, or much delayed data availability in the EMR. Furthermore, the clinical diagnosis of sepsis often relies on judgments and measurements not easily captured in the EMR. These measurements can range from physical findings (eg, patient not looking good, rigors, increased capillary refill time, bounding pulse, or increased work of breathing) to physiologic markers (eg, low blood pressure and shock index) or molecular biomarkers (eg, lactate, C-reactive protein, and procalcitonin).[23] Currently, clinical algorithms to detect sepsis are blinded to many of the cues a bedside clinician takes for granted. The result is that, from the perspective of the clinician, sepsis detection alerts will often fire late. Late alerts are nuisance alerts and, understandably, are very poorly tolerated by clinicians.

## Algorithm Alert Performance

Changing definitions of sepsis and its treatment, in addition to patient and health setting characteristics, have a significant impact on the performance of algorithms developed to detect sepsis. Evolving clinical definitions of sepsis are particularly difficult to deal with using the current model of algorithm development, which is largely based on these definitions.[24,25] Alerts developed carefully on the best available evidence, often during an extended period, become obsolete when the definitions on which they are based change. The guidelines for the management of severe sepsis and septic shock by the international Surviving Sepsis Campaign have evolved[26–28] and have been challenged by independent, international, multicenter, randomized controlled trials (**Table 2**).[29–31]

Typically, alerting algorithms are developed on a fixed dataset. The performance of the clinical algorithm is tweaked to perform best on that data set. Depending on the characteristics of the patient population and health care setting, the derived clinical algorithm may not perform as expected in different environments. The health care delivery systems differ significantly between different clinical settings.[32] As an example, in nonemergency settings, nursing ratios are lower, vital sign capture is less frequent, and clinicians are less tuned to rapid intervention with limited information on the floor compared with the ICU. In addition, there are important differences in the clinical characteristics and demographics of the patients in each of these settings.[33–35] These factors combine to make the pretest probability a patient in the ICU has sepsis much higher than that of a floor patient. This alone may be sufficient to skew the performance of an alert developed on an ICU cohort of patients but deployed on the hospital floor. Finally, even if the alert is optimized to perform well in a specific population and environment, if the patient mix and health care delivery system change over time, performance may drift from the original optimum.

Sepsis alert systems must, therefore, possess the flexibility to adapt to changes in definitions that affect the clinical management and treatment of sepsis, changing patient population characteristics, and evolving health settings. Evolution in medicine is not new but the incorporation of new knowledge into practice is potentially greatly accelerated by electronic alerts and clinical decision support systems. Such systems require constant updating if they are not to have an unexpected negative impact on clinicians and patients.

## Information Overload and Alert Fatigue

Sophisticated technology and increasingly large quantities of data are currently flowing into existing, imperfect EMR systems in the acute care setting. This inevitable application of big data to health care cannot and should not be avoided.[36] However, the development and implementation of sepsis alert systems without consideration of the rise of big data in clinical practice has the potential to result in alert fatigue,[37] interruption,[38] human error,[39] and information overload.[40,41] The recognition of the importance of alert fatigue in the hospital setting has increased significantly in recent years.[42] Thus, implementation of any automated alert system must be performed in the context of information overload and complex task interruption.[43,44] It is known that information overload can alter alert perception in the medical setting.[45] This can cause clinicians to perceive alert systems negatively and deter future use.[46,47]

The task of generating clinically meaningful alerts while concurrently minimizing information overload and task interruption is challenging.[48] Successful sepsis alert systems must be designed to minimize alert fatigue, interruption, human error, and information overload.

## Variability in the Systems of Health Care Delivery

The primary purpose of any alert system should be to elicit a response from the clinical team that would otherwise not occur or would be delayed. As might be expected, what a team does with an alert has a tremendous impact on the efficacy of an automated alerting system. Variability in resource availability, leadership engagement, and clinical stakeholder buy-in has a fundamental impact on whether an alert will deliver its intended impact on outcomes. A poorly planned implementation can have a devastating effect on performance.[49] Perhaps the best illustration of this comes from an examination of a computer provider order entry implementation in a pediatric hospital that resulted in an unanticipated doubling in ICU standardized mortality ratio.[50] Subsequent

**Table 1**
Sepsis alert system studies in the acute care setting

| Reference | Stage | Subjects | Number | Design | Setting | Illness | Primary Outcome | Result |
|---|---|---|---|---|---|---|---|---|
| Thompson et al,[7] 2003 | Early development | Patients | 203 | Retrospective & prospective | Medical & surgical ICU | Sepsis | Time (study coordinator screening) | Study coordinator screening time was reduced |
| Embi et al,[8] 2005 | Early development | Physicians | 114 | Prospective | Ambulatory & outpatient | Diabetes (not sepsis) | Rate (trial participation) & time (recruitment) | Physician participation and trial recruitment rates increased |
| Herasevich et al,[9] 2008 | Early development | Patients | 320 | Prospective | Medical ICU | Severe sepsis & septic shock | Feasibility (computerized screening) | Feasibility of automatic screening was demonstrated |
| Herasevich et al,[10] 2011 | Recent development | Patients | 8609 | Before–after | Medical, surgical, & mixed ICU | Severe sepsis & septic shock | Rate (time sensitive study enrollment) | Automated screening improved enrollment efficiency |
| Sawyer,[12] 2011 | Recent development | Patients | 300 | Observational & interventional | Nonintensive medical wards | Sepsis | Rate (early therapeutic & diagnostic intervention) | Early therapeutic and diagnostic interventions increased |

| | | | | | | | |
|---|---|---|---|---|---|---|---|
| Nelson,[13] 2011 | Recent development | Patients 33,460 | Before–after & prospective | ED | Severe sepsis | Rate & Time (interventions) | Frequency and timeliness of some ED interventions increased |
| LaRosa,[14] 2012 | Recent development | Patients 58 | Interventional | Mixed ICU | Severe sepsis & septic shock | Rate (treatment compliance) & outcomes (mortality) | Potential to improve treatment compliance and mortality was demonstrated |
| Hooper,[15] 2012 | Recent development | Patients 442 | Interventional (randomized & controlled) | Medical ICU | Early sepsis (SIRS criteria) | Rate (treatment compliance) & outcomes (mortality) | Measurements of interest were not influenced |
| Selmer et al,[16] 2015 | Current implementation | Patients 407 | Interventional (randomized & controlled) | Medical & surgical ICU | Sepsis (admission diagnosis) | Feasibility (electronic evaluation & management tool) | Measurements of interest were not influenced |
| Harrison,[20] 2015 | Current implementation | Patients 587 | Diagnostic performance (observational) | Medical ICU | Severe sepsis & septic shock | Time & accuracy (failed to recognize & treat) | Feasibility of failure to recognize and treat was demonstrated |

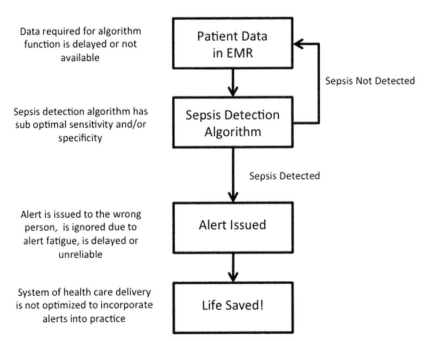

**Fig. 1.** Sepsis alert: The expected outcome is that a sepsis detection algorithm will reduce time to recognition of sepsis prompt clinicians to intervene earlier than they might otherwise. Some potential points of failure are noted.

root cause analysis implicated a highly flawed implementation process as the main contributor to these unanticipated outcomes.

## POTENTIAL SOLUTIONS TO DEVELOPMENT AND IMPLEMENTATION OF CLINICALLY USEFUL SEPSIS ALERT SYSTEMS

The difference between success and failure is often due to very small modifications in approach. Slightly better algorithm performance, more frequent data, ergonomic user interfaces, and well-defined responses all contribute to the overall efficacy of an alert (**Fig. 2**).

### Improved Alert Performance: Mathematical Modeling and Machine Learning

In addition to more ergonomic design, sepsis alert systems of the future must be more accurate. Advanced mathematical modeling and complex machine learning techniques have already been applied to sepsis detection. Machine learning algorithms are already in use for the classification of human physical activity from on-body accelerometers.[51] Thus, the use of these methodologies in sepsis alert systems to improve the clinical management and treatment of sepsis is forthcoming.

The syndromic nature of critical illness,[3] such as sepsis, can result in disruption of homeostasis with inflammation and shock (inadequate oxygen supply and/or demand). In the context of evolving definitions and gold standards of sepsis, it is frequently important to recognize and treat with or without confirmation of infection. Given the current inability to diagnose invasive infection, as exemplified in the gut microbiome hypothesis of sepsis syndrome,[52] measures for infection control must be introduced empirically and deescalated if no infection is identified. Although these factors may seem to initially reduce to potential accuracy of any sepsis alert system, global awareness of homeostasis in sepsis alert systems of the future will increase the accuracy of these systems. This approach is the basis for the ICU-specific patient viewer that has already been clinically validated and implemented in the medical ICU setting at Mayo Clinic.[19]

### Alert Delivery and Integration into Workflow

In parallel with advances in proxy measurements for the diagnosis, prognosis, management, and treatment of sepsis, there is a need to optimize delivery of alerts for these proxy measurements and suspicion of sepsis to clinicians. Studies of methods of alert delivery for clinical information and clinical trial enrollment have been performed outside the ICU setting.[53,54] Increasingly sophisticated electronic decision support systems are

**Table 2**
Overview of studies of the evolving clinical definitions of sepsis and recommended treatment

| Reference | Institutions | Number | Design | Setting | Illness | Primary Outcome | Result |
|---|---|---|---|---|---|---|---|
| Bone,[24] 1992 | US | NA | Consensus conference | NA | Sepsis | Formal definition of sepsis | Consensus definition established |
| Rivers,[25] 2001 | 1 US | 263 | Interventional (randomized) | ED | Severe sepsis & septic shock | EGDT | EGDT demonstrated to significantly reduce mortality |
| Dellinger,[26] 2004 | International | NA | Consensus guidelines | NA | Severe sepsis & septic shock | Surviving Sepsis Campaign, 2004 | Consensus definition established |
| Dellinger,[27] 2008 | International | NA | Consensus guidelines | NA | Severe sepsis & septic shock | Surviving Sepsis Campaign, 2008 | Consensus definitions updated |
| Dellinger,[28] 2013 | International | NA | Consensus guidelines | NA | Severe sepsis & septic shock | Surviving Sepsis Campaign, 2012 | Consensus definitions updated |
| Yealy,[29] 2014 | 31 US | 1341 | Interventional (randomized & controlled) | ED | Early septic shock | Reevaluation of EGDT | E, demonstrated to reduce mortality but not GD |
| Peake,[30] 2014 | 51 Australia & New Zealand | 1600 | Interventional (randomized & controlled) | ED | Early septic shock | Reevaluation of EGDT | E, demonstrated to reduce mortality but not GD |
| Mouncey,[31] 2015 | 56 England | 1260 | Interventional (randomized & controlled) | Any (post-ED admission) | Early septic shock | Reevaluation of EGDT | E, demonstrated to reduce mortality but not GD |
| Kaukonen,[61] 2015 | 172 Australia & New Zealand | 109,663 | Retrospective | ICU | Severe sepsis | Diagnostic value of SIRS criteria | A significant portion of severe sepsis patients are SIRS negative |

*Abbreviations:* E, early; EGDT, early goal-directed therapy; GD, goal-directed; NA, not applicable; US, United States.

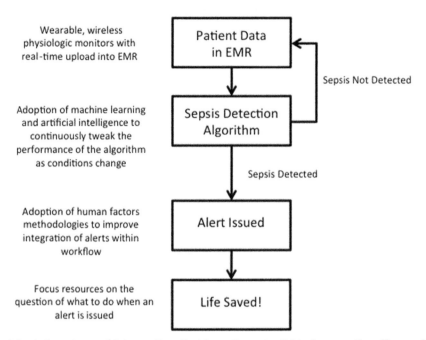

**Fig. 2.** Potential solutions: types of interventions that have the potential to improve the efficacy of sepsis alert systems.

developed with specific consideration of human factors.[55]

The best methods of alert delivery (text paging, EMR systems, email, phone calls, and/or text messaging) for urgent and nonurgent alerts in the hospital setting are poorly understood.[56] Likewise, investigation into the most appropriate clinician recipient (attending physicians, fellows, residents, and/or nurse practitioners or physician assistants) for alert delivery is limited.[57,58] As multidisciplinary response teams have been demonstrated to improve the process of care and mortality in septic shock,[59] an appropriate trigger for multidisciplinary team activation needs to be determined for each individual setting. In the medical ICU of the Mayo Clinic, the electronic sepsis alert is currently sent to a single team member who, if appropriate, activates a multidisciplinary response team (physicians, nurses, respiratory therapists, pharmacists, and laboratory technicians) in charge of rapid execution of time-sensitive interventions.

### Reengineering the Hospital Environment

Another potential strategy to remove the barriers of sepsis alert system implementation is the use of new models of care delivery. Models that recognize the limitations of the current generation of alert systems but that also exploit their potential to provide a safety net for the busy bedside clinician are needed. As more experience is gained in the use of telemedicine, this may prove to be a useful way to incorporate a wide range of alerts into health systems. In this model, a dedicated clinician with the appropriate information tools would e-monitor the entire hospital, validate or silence alerts, and trigger appropriate responses for true positive alerts. A similar approach has already been used by Kahn and colleagues[60] in which remotely located nurse screening and prompting for appropriate evidence-based interventions improved processes and outcomes of ICU patients.

### SUMMARY

Development and implementation of sepsis alert systems began in the acute care setting. Evolving clinical definitions of sepsis, insufficient accuracy and timeliness of current alerts, information overload, alert fatigue, and inadequate consideration of clinician workflow present important barriers for clinical implementation of sepsis alert systems. Outside the ICU, additional barriers include differences in care delivery models, information density, and charting behaviors. Wearable physiologic monitoring devices and the use of advanced mathematical modeling and complex machine learning techniques are likely to improve the accuracy and precision of electronic screening. Advanced informatics tools based on clear understanding of clinician workflow, integrated decision support, and onsideration of alternative care models are being evaluated in clinical studies. Although current evidence does not support the routine use of sepsis alert systems, continuous improvement in accuracy combined with decision support, quality improvement surveillance, and smoother integration into clinical workflow will help translate theoretic advantages into measurable patient benefit.

## REFERENCES

1. Harrison AM, Park JG, Herasevich V. Septic shock electronic surveillance. septic shock - risk factors, management and prognosis. New York: Nova Science Publishers; 2015. p. 1–26.
2. Vincent JL, Korkut HA. Defining sepsis. Clin Chest Med 2008;29:585–90, vii.
3. Adhikari NK, Fowler RA, Bhagwanjee S, et al. Critical care and the global burden of critical illness in adults. Lancet 2010;376:1339–46.
4. Annane D, Bellissant E, Cavaillon JM. Septic shock. Lancet 2005;365:63–78.
5. Schultz S. Homeostasis, humpty dumpty, and integrative biology. Physiology 1996;11:238–46.
6. Pinsky MR, Dubrawski A. Gleaning knowledge from data in the ICU. Am J Respir Crit Care Med 2014; 190(6):606–10.
7. Thompson DS, Oberteuffer R, Dorman T. Sepsis alert and diagnostic system: integrating clinical systems to enhance study coordinator efficiency. Comput Inform Nurs 2003;21:22–6 [quiz: 27–8].
8. Embi PJ, Jain A, Clark J, et al. Effect of a clinical trial alert system on physician participation in trial recruitment. Arch Intern Med 2005;165:2272–7.
9. Herasevich V, Afessa B, Chute CG, et al. Designing and testing computer based screening engine for severe sepsis/septic shock. AMIA Annu Symp Proc 2008;966.
10. Herasevich V, Pieper MS, Pulido J, et al. Enrollment into a time sensitive clinical study in the critical care setting: results from computerized septic shock sniffer implementation. J Am Med Inform Assoc 2011;18:639–44.
11. Singal G, Currier P. How can we best use electronic data to find and treat the critically ill?*. Crit Care Med 2012;40:2242–3.
12. Sawyer AM, Deal EN, Labelle AJ, et al. Implementation of a real-time computerized sepsis alert in non-intensive care unit patients. Crit Care Med 2011;39: 469–73.
13. Nelson JL, Smith BL, Jared JD, et al. Prospective trial of real-time electronic surveillance to expedite early care of severe sepsis. Ann Emerg Med 2011; 57:500–4.
14. Larosa JA, Ahmad N, Feinberg M, et al. The use of an early alert system to improve compliance with sepsis bundles and to assess impact on mortality. Crit Care Res Pract 2012;2012:980369.
15. Hooper MH, Weavind L, Wheeler AP, et al. Randomized trial of automated, electronic monitoring to facilitate early detection of sepsis in the intensive care unit*. Crit Care Med 2012;40:2096–101.
16. Semler MW, Weavind L, Hooper MH, et al. An electronic tool for the evaluation and treatment of sepsis in the ICU: a randomized controlled trial. Crit Care Med 2015;43(8):1595–602.
17. Pickering BW, Herasevich V, Ahmed A, et al. Novel representation of clinical information in the ICU: Developing user interfaces which reduce information overload. Appl Clin Inform 2010;1(2):116–31.
18. Ahmed A, Chandra S, Herasevich V, et al. The effect of two different electronic health record user interfaces on intensive care provider task load, errors of cognition, and performance. Crit Care Med 2011;39:1626–34.
19. Pickering BW, Dong Y, Ahmed A, et al. The implementation of clinician designed, human-centered electronic medical record viewer in the intensive care unit: a pilot step-wedge cluster randomized trial. Int J Med Inform 2015;84(5):299–307.
20. Harrison AM, Thongprayoon C, Kashyap R, et al. Developing the surveillance algorithm for detection of failure to recognize and treat severe sepsis. Mayo Clin Proc 2015;90:166–75.
21. Silber JH, Williams SV, Krakauer H, et al. Hospital and patient characteristics associated with death after surgery. A study of adverse occurrence and failure to rescue. Med Care 1992;30:615–29.
22. Silber JH, Rosenbaum PR, Schwartz JS, et al. Evaluation of the complication rate as a measure of quality of care in coronary artery bypass graft surgery. JAMA 1995;274:317–23.
23. Pierrakos C, Vincent JL. Sepsis biomarkers: a review. Crit Care 2010;14:R15.
24. Bone RC, Balk RA, Cerra FB, et al. Definitions for sepsis and organ failure and guidelines for the use of innovative therapies in sepsis. The ACCP/SCCM Consensus Conference Committee. American College of Chest Physicians/Society of Critical Care Medicine. Chest 1992;101:1644–55.
25. Rivers E, Nguyen B, Havstad S, et al. Early goal-directed therapy in the treatment of severe sepsis and septic shock. Gajic review. N Engl J Med 2001;345:1368–77.
26. Dellinger RP, Carlet JM, Masur H, et al. Surviving Sepsis Campaign guidelines for management of severe sepsis and septic shock. Crit Care Med 2004; 32:858–73.
27. Dellinger RP, Levy MM, Carlet JM, et al. Surviving Sepsis Campaign: international guidelines for management of severe sepsis and septic shock: 2008. Crit Care Med 2008;36:296–327.

28. Dellinger RP, Levy MM, Rhodes A, et al. Surviving sepsis campaign: international guidelines for management of severe sepsis and septic shock. Crit Care Med 2012;2013(41):580–637.

29. Yealy DM, Kellum JA, Huang DT, et al. A randomized trial of protocol-based care for early septic shock. N Engl J Med 2014;370:1683–93.

30. Peake SL, Delaney A, Bailey M, et al. Goal-directed resuscitation for patients with early septic shock. N Engl J Med 2014;371:1496–506.

31. Mouncey PR, Osborn TM, Power GS, et al. Trial of early, goal-directed resuscitation for septic shock. N Engl J Med 2015;372(14):1301–11.

32. Afessa B, Keegan MT, Hubmayr RD, et al. Evaluating the performance of an institution using an intensive care unit benchmark. Mayo Clin Proc 2005;80:174–80.

33. Seferian EG, Afessa B. Demographic and clinical variation of adult intensive care unit utilization from a geographically defined population. Crit Care Med 2006;34:2113–9.

34. Iwashyna TJ, Netzer G, Langa KM, et al. Spurious inferences about long-term outcomes: the case of severe sepsis and geriatric conditions. Am J Respir Crit Care Med 2012;185:835–41.

35. Rubenfeld GD. Does the hospital make you older faster? Am J Respir Crit Care Med 2012;185:796–8.

36. Murdoch TB, Detsky AS. The inevitable application of big data to health care. JAMA 2013;309:1351–2.

37. Singh H, Spitzmueller C, Petersen NJ, et al. Information overload and missed test results in electronic health record-based settings. JAMA Intern Med 2013;173(8):702–4.

38. Hodgetts HM, DMarc J. Reminders, alerts and pop-ups: The cost of computer-initiated interruptions. In: Jacko JA, editor. Human-Computer Interaction: Interaction Design & Usability. Beijing: Springer; 2007. p. 818–26.

39. Bates DW, Leape LL, Cullen DJ, et al. Effect of computerized physician order entry and a team intervention on prevention of serious medication errors. JAMA 1998;280:1311–6.

40. Stokstad E. Information overload hampers biology reforms. Science 2001;293:1609.

41. Dennis C. Information overload. Nature 2002; 417:14.

42. Herasevich V, Kor DJ, Subramanian A, et al. Connecting the dots: rule-based decision support systems in the modern EMR era. J Clin Monit Comput 2013;27(4):443–8.

43. Losee RM Jr. Minimizing information overload: the ranking of electronic messages. J Inform Sci 1989; 15:179–89.

44. Eppler MJ, Mengis J. The concept of information overload: a review of literature from organization science, accounting, marketing, MIS, and related disciplines. Inform Soc 2004;20:325–44.

45. Glassman PA, Belperio P, Simon B, et al. Exposure to automated drug alerts over time: effects on clinicians' knowledge and perceptions. Med Care 2006;44:250–6.

46. van der Sijs H, Aarts J, Vulto A, et al. Overriding of drug safety alerts in computerized physician order entry. J Am Med Inform Assoc 2006;13:138–47.

47. Chopra V, McMahon LF Jr. Redesigning hospital alarms for patient safety: alarmed and potentially dangerous. JAMA 2014;311(12):1199–200.

48. Shojania KG, Jennings A, Mayhew A, et al. The effects of on-screen, point of care computer reminders on processes and outcomes of care. Cochrane Database Syst Rev 2009;(3):CD001096.

49. Harrison AM, Herasevich V, Gajic O. Automated sepsis detection, alert, and clinical decision support: act on it or silence the alarm? Crit Care Med 2015;43:1776–7.

50. Han YY, Carcillo JA, Venkataraman ST, et al. Unexpected increased mortality after implementation of a commercially sold computerized physician order entry system. Pediatrics 2005;116:1506–12.

51. Mannini A, Sabatini AM. Machine learning methods for classifying human physical activity from on-body accelerometers. Sensors (Basel) 2010;10: 1154–75.

52. Alverdy JC, Chang EB. The re-emerging role of the intestinal microflora in critical illness and inflammation: why the gut hypothesis of sepsis syndrome will not go away. J Leukoc Biol 2008; 83:461–6.

53. Wagner MM, Eisenstadt SA, Hogan WR, et al. Preferences of interns and residents for E-mail, paging, or traditional methods for the delivery of different types of clinical information. Proc AMIA Symp 1998;140–4.

54. Embi PJ, Jain A, Harris CM. Physicians' perceptions of an electronic health record-based clinical trial alert approach to subject recruitment: a survey. BMC Med Inform Decis Mak 2008;8:13.

55. Zachariah M, Phansalkar S, Seidling HM, et al. Development and preliminary evidence for the validity of an instrument assessing implementation of human-factors principles in medication-related decision-support systems–I-MeDeSA. J Am Med Inform Assoc 2011;18(Suppl 1):i62–72.

56. Gill PS, Kamath A, Gill TS. Distraction: an assessment of smartphone usage in health care work settings. Risk Manag Healthc Policy 2012;5:105–14.

57. Donchin Y, Gopher D, Olin M, et al. A look into the nature and causes of human errors in the intensive care unit. Crit Care Med 1995;23:294–300.

58. Zhang J, Johnson TR, Patel VL, et al. Using usability heuristics to evaluate patient safety of medical devices. J Biomed Inform 2003;36:23–30.

59. Schramm GE, Kashyap R, Mullon JJ, et al. Septic shock: a multidisciplinary response team and

weekly feedback to clinicians improve the process of care and mortality. Crit Care Med 2011; 39:252–8.

60. Kahn JM, Gunn SR, Lorenz HL, et al. Impact of nurse-led remote screening and prompting for evidence-based practices in the ICU*. Crit Care Med 2014;42:896–904.

61. Kaukonen KM, Bailey M, Pilcher D, et al. Systemic inflammatory response syndrome criteria in defining severe sepsis. N Engl J Med 2015;372(17):1629–38.

# Goal-Directed Resuscitation in Septic Shock: A Critical Analysis

Daniel J. Henning, MD, MPH[a],*, Nathan I. Shapiro, MD, MPH[b]

## KEYWORDS

• Severe sepsis • Septic shock • Goal-directed therapy • Resuscitation

## KEY POINTS

• The Early Goal-Directed Therapy versus Standard Care in 2001 suggested mortality could be reduced by using physiologic goals to guide patient care in septic shock.
• In 2014 and 2015, 3 multicenter, randomized trials did not demonstrate the superiority of goal-directed therapy over unstructured standard care.
• Sepsis mortality seems to be decreasing with early and meticulous care, including early identification, fluid resuscitation, antibiotics, and restoration of blood pressure.

## A BRIEF HISTORY OF GOAL-DIRECTED RESUSCITATION

The term goal-directed resuscitation or goal-directed therapy is used to describe care that targets a physiologic or hemodynamic goals or endpoints. Although the approach is more recently associated with a treatment algorithm based on the 2001 study by Dr Rivers and colleagues[1] for the care of patients with severe sepsis, the concept of goal-directed resuscitation perhaps began in high-risk surgical patients in the form of supranormal oxygen delivery.[2] A 1988 single-center, 88 patient study by Shoemaker and colleagues[2] found that patients treated with a pulmonary artery catheter protocol, aimed to facilitate supranormal oxygen delivery, had a 4% mortality compared with 23% for those receiving nonprotocolized pulmonary catheter care and 33% in a no pulmonary catheter group. These findings were replicated in a study by Boyd and colleagues[3] of 107 high-risk surgery patients where a pulmonary catheter was used to target physiologic goals of supranormal oxygen delivery, demonstrating a significant mortality decrease compared with non-protocolized care (5.7% vs 22.2%). Together these 2 studies ushered in an era of supranormal oxygen delivery titrated to targeted physiologic goals.[3]

This treatment approach continued until 1995 when Gattinoni and colleagues[4] published the results of a multinational 56 center study in 762 patients that failed to find mortality benefit when supranormal oxygen delivery was targeted. In fact, in a subsequent 1994 study by Hayes and associates[5] that included 100 patients at 2 centers, the treatment arm actually had a higher mortality compared with the control arm (54% vs 34%; $P = .04$). Thus, the practice of targeting supranormal oxygen delivery fell out of favor.

A subsequent metaanalysis was performed to assess the hemodynamic optimization studies.[6] Interestingly, when stratified by interventions

Disclosure Statement: Dr N.I. Shapiro has received research funding from Thermo-Fischer and Cheetah Medical, and has been a consultant on an advisory board for Cheetah-Medical.
[a] Division of Emergency Medicine, Harborview Medical Center, University of Washington School of Medicine, 325 9th Avenue, Box 359702, Seattle, WA 98104, USA; [b] Department of Emergency Medicine, Beth Israel Deaconess Medical Center, Harvard Medical School, One Deaconess Road, W-CC2, Boston, MA 02215, USA
* Corresponding author.
E-mail address: henning2@uw.edu

Clin Chest Med 37 (2016) 231–239
http://dx.doi.org/10.1016/j.ccm.2016.01.016
0272-5231/16/$ – see front matter © 2016 Elsevier Inc. All rights reserved.

chestmed.theclinics.com

occurring "before" or "at" the onset of organ dysfunction, as opposed to "after" organs began to fail, studies with treatment initiated early showed mortality benefit, whereas those initiated after onset of organ failure did not. A similar meta-analysis by Jones and colleagues[7] conducted later had similar findings.

This is perhaps the point in history for the Rivers trial of early goal-directed therapy (EGDT), which operationalized the early implementation of goal-directed resuscitation in emergency department patients with sepsis. Published in 2001, the Rivers study found a 16% absolute mortality reduction in patients with severe sepsis and septic shock resuscitated using goal-directed therapy,[1] and it established a new expectation that the mortality of this patient population could be improved with early, focused interventions. A number of subsequent pre–post trials supported these findings[8–13] and quality assurance initiatives such as the Surviving Sepsis Campaign's guidelines[14] endorsed widespread implementation of EGDT.

Although the Rivers trial was a single-center trial, a prospective, multicenter, randomized validation trial was not immediately pursued. In 2014, 13 years after the Rivers trial, the first of 3 large randomized controlled clinical trials comparing EGDT with standard care was published.[15–17] These trials all used similar inclusion and exclusion criteria as the Rivers trial. The Protocol-Based Care for Early Septic Shock (ProCESS) trial, performed in the United States (1351 patients, 31 sites), showed no difference in 60-day in-hospital mortality among patients randomized to EGDT (21.0% mortality), a noninvasive protocol targeted to physiologic goals (18.2% mortality), or usual care (18.9% mortality; $P = .52$).[16] Later in 2014, results from the ARISE trial (1600 patients, 51 sites), conducted in Australia and New Zealand, were published, which did not demonstrate a difference in 90-day all-cause mortality between EGDT and standard care groups (18.6% vs 18.8% mortality; $P = .90$).[15] Last, in early 2015, the Protocolised Management in Sepsis (ProMISe) trial (1260 patients, 56 sites), conducted in England, likewise failed to show a significant difference in all-cause 90-day mortality rates between treatment and usual care (29.5% vs 29.2%; $P = .90$).[15,17] A final metaanalysis evaluating the randomized, controlled studies of EGDT versus standard care seems to be the last argument that EGDT does not confer a mortality benefit over usual care.[18]

The ProCESS, Australasian Resuscitation in Sepsis Evaluation (ARISE), and ProMISe triad of studies do not establish the superiority of standard care over EGDT. However, although these trials sought primarily to assess the mortality benefit of EGDT compared with standard care, they also provide a window to understand the care currently being provided by acute care providers across 3 continents. Likewise, in establishing the equivalence between EGDT and standard care groups, these trials provide new data to update the clinical care of patients with septic shock. By examining the processes of care used across these studies, we can identify the practice patterns, in both treatment and usual care groups, now associated with mortality rates recognized as lower than previously realized.[19,20]

## Early Identification, Intravenous Fluid Resuscitation, and Empiric Antibiotics

An important note about the conduct of the trials is that the inclusion criteria mandated early enrollment (and thus, early identification, namely, within 2.5 hours), an initial fluid bolus of roughly 1 L or 20 to 30 mL/kg of intravenous fluids before randomization, and the majority of patients received early antibiotics as well. Thus, the usual care arms in the 3 validation studies should be interpreted in the backdrop of early identification, early fluid loading, and early antibiotics.

### Early identification

Identifying patients with severe sepsis and septic shock in the early stages of their disease has become increasingly emphasized,[21,22] because septic shock is categorized as a time-critical disease.[23] Even the protocol name—early goal-directed therapy—emphasizes the expected timing of interventions. However, identifying patients with septic shock is often difficult because different disease processes can cause an inflammatory response, resulting in overlapping clinical presentations. For instance, fever may occur in patients without infection, and many patients with septic shock will not exhibit hyperthermia or hypothermia.[24–26] Owing to the high frequency of sepsis as the cause for shock,[27] clinicians should have a low threshold for suspecting sepsis as a cause of shock and initiating appropriate care so that critical interventions are not delayed.

### Intravenous fluid resuscitation

A trial of intravenous fluids to correct hypoperfusion (hypotension or increased lactate) has become the standard of care for septic shock. An early resuscitation with intravenous fluids, which may be regarded as "vigorous," is supported by the practice patterns seen in the ProCESS, ARISE, and ProMISe trials, where the average intravenous fluid given to each patient from before randomization fluids out to 6 hours after randomization was slightly more than 4 L

(Fig. 1). In fact, in these studies and the Rivers trial, patients were not enrolled until they demonstrated persistent hemodynamic or lactate abnormalities after this step had been completed, making each studies' findings contingent on a trial of fluid resuscitation first. Although the volume of intravenous fluids will vary by clinical scenario, the average show in Fig. 1 provides a general appreciation of the intravenous fluid volume a patient received during early resuscitation in the trials.

Although an initial dose of intravenous fluid has become commonplace, and there seems to have been a movement toward a more vigorous resuscitation, there is scarce outcomes-based evidence to support the practice.[28] In fact, there remains an ongoing debate as to whether aggressive or restrictive fluid administration strategies will yield the best outcomes, with data emerging that suggest that overresuscitation may have detrimental effects. For example, using patients from the Vasopressin and Septic Shock Trial (VASST) trial, all of whom had vasopressor-dependent septic shock, Boyd and colleagues[29] found that patients within the upper 2 quartiles of fluid balance at 12 hours after presentation had higher mortality rates. Similarly, in a single-center retrospective review of 325 patients with septic shock, Micek and colleagues[30] found that patients within the highest quartile of fluid balance at 24 hours after presentation had significantly higher 28-day mortality compared with lowest quartile of fluid ($P<.001$). These studies advocate for a more restrictive fluid administration strategy. On the other hand, a retrospective, 24-center study by Waechter and colleagues[31] suggested that lower intravenous fluid volumes, in particular less than 0.5 L in the first hour and less than 1 L in hours 1 to 6 of resuscitation, were associated with higher mortality. Unfortunately, these studies are not the randomized trials, which will be needed to truly test the impact of intravenous fluid quantity or fluid balance on patient outcomes. The initial approach fluid resuscitation will continue to be a refined, yet for now, providing 20 to 30 mL/kg (or the more pragmatic 2 L) of intravenous fluids remains the clinical expectation for septic shock.

## Empiric antibiotics

Empiric antibiotics, similar to intravenous fluids, were a standard aspect of care in the 3 EGDT studies. Although the rates of antibiotics administration were not reported in the ARISE or ProMISe trials, the ProCESS trial reported antibiotics administration rates of 97.5% and 97.2% for the EGDT and standard care groups, respectively. As with intravenous fluids, these trials cannot assess the usefulness of early antibiotics, but the broad use of empiric antibiotics does reflect a pattern of practice seen in the care of most patients with septic shock, and this practice has been reinforced by a number of observational studies showing an association between early, appropriate antibiotics and improved survival[32–34] as well as the Surviving Sepsis Campaign.[21] These data withstanding, a recent metaanalysis by Sterling and colleagues[35] failed to find a mortality benefit based on a specific time threshold for antibiotics; however, this does not mitigate the importance of administering appropriate antibiotics as early as possible.

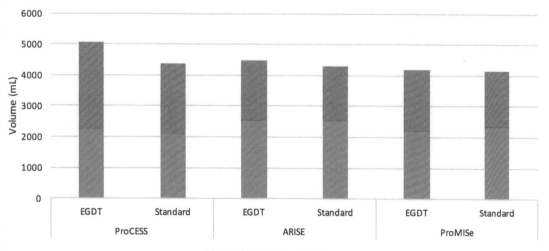

Fig. 1. Intravenous fluid administration before and after randomization up to 6 hours. ARISE, Australasian Resuscitation in Sepsis Evaluation; EGDT, early goal-directed therapy; ProCESS, Protocol-Based Care for Early Septic Shock; ProMISE, Protocolised Management in Sepsis.

## Optimizing Preload

The first goal within EGDT involved achieving a central venous pressure (CVP) of 8 to 12 mm Hg to ensure adequate preload. This was accomplished in the EGDT trial by administering sequential 500-mL boluses of crystalloid every 30 minutes until this target was met. Whether the CVP truly reflects preload, total intravascular fluid, or fluid responsiveness has been contested intensely, and limitations surrounding CVP have been extensively reviewed in the literature.[36–39]

Although rates of CVP measurement were not assessed directly in the ProCESS, ARISE, and ProMISe trials, central venous catheters were placed in 57% of patients in the standard care group, precluding the ability to measure CVP in a large proportion of patients (**Fig. 2**). The lines were placed typically for vasopressor administration as opposed to titrate therapy. Of note, this selective rate of central venous catheter placement also supports the ability of clinicians to select patients for central access, given that mortality remained the same between groups in each of these studies.

There are other alternatives to targeting CVP goals as a method for optimizing preload that have been proposed. These alternatives are sought perhaps owing to the inconsistent relationship between CVP and fluid responsiveness[36,37] and relating a CVP of less than 8 mm Hg to lower mortality.[29] Such alternative strategies for guiding

fluid administration include inferior vena cava ultrasonography[40–45] and dynamic measures of volume responsiveness through passive leg raises or fluid loading.[39,46] Especially in light of the potential harms of overresuscitation with intravenous fluids,[29,30,47] using such measures to determine fluid responsiveness is emphasized increasingly in early resuscitation.[46] Although assessing fluid responsiveness is an intuitive strategy for optimizing preload while mitigating potential harm, none of these modalities have been shown to reduce mortality in large outcomes based clinical trials.

## Vasopressor Support

Hypotension occurs in sepsis as a result of the relative hypovolemia typically caused by a combination of vasoplegia, capillary leak, and myocardial depression.[48] If hypotension persists despite optimizing preload, then vasopressor agents are used to augment vasomotor tone, thereby addressing pathologic vasodilation. Reestablishing a blood pressure adequate for perfusion is critical to maintaining organ function.

The second step of EGDT stipulates that vasopressors are initiated to maintain a mean arterial pressure (MAP) of greater than 65 mm Hg. In the original EGDT trial, vasopressor administration rates in the standard care and EGDT groups were equivalent (30.3% vs 27.4%; $P = .62$) in the first 6 hours after randomization. Interestingly,

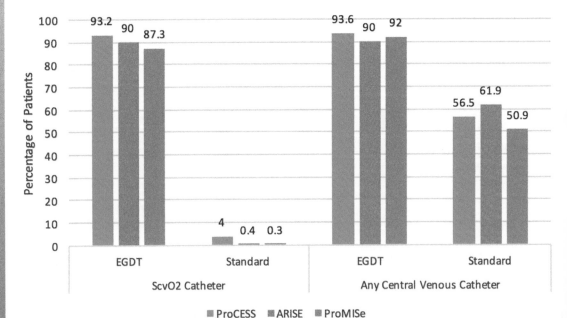

**Fig. 2.** Rates of central venous catheterization in early goal-directed therapy (EGDT) and standard care groups by study. Rates for central venous oxygen saturation ($S_{cv}O_2$) and any central venous catheter placement are shown.

vasopressor administration rates among the both the EGDT standard care groups in ProCESS, ARISE, and ProMISe were much higher than in the Rivers trial (**Fig. 3**), although the total average of vasopressor use across these studies in the EGDT arm (59.4%) was more frequent than in the standard care arm (51.7%). Overall, the increase in vasopressor use compared with the original EGDT study may represent a lower tolerance for hypotension or increased comfort with using vasoactive medications. This comparison also suggests a minimal clinically important difference when vasopressor use was determined by protocol versus clinical discretion.

The therapeutic goal of vasopressor support from the EGDT trial was a MAP of 65 mm Hg, meant to meet the requirements to achieve renal perfusion.[49] However, vasopressors also increase systemic vascular resistance and may impede perfusion in patients with a low cardiac output.[49,50] A recent study did compare MAP goals of 65 to 70 mm Hg versus 80 to 85 mm Hg, and showed no difference in mortality at 28 days.[51] This suggests that increasing the systemic blood pressure with vasopressors does not increase perfusion beyond the limit of autoregulation. This concept was demonstrated in a study showing that sublingual microvascular perfusion remained constant across systolic blood pressures beyond 90 mm

Hg.[52] As in EGDT, the most recent evidence supports the use of a MAP above renal arteriole autoregulation, 65 mm Hg, as a target in vasopressor use. In patients with chronic hypertension, this level may be higher,[51] but otherwise, target levels higher than the autoregulation threshold has not shown benefit.

The use of vasopressors has become a common indication for establishing central venous access, although many patients will be started on peripheral vasopressors before central line placement. However, a recent metaanalysis of case reports of central and peripheral vasopressor adverse events suggests that shorter duration and more proximal peripheral intravenous lines are associated with a low rate of complications and supports the use of a peripheral line for short-term vasopressor administration. Although further confirmatory studies are needed, this approach is potentially practice changing.

## Assessing Oxygen Delivery and the Use of Packed Red Blood Cells and Dobutamine

The final step of EGDT and major component tested within the Rivers Trial involves measuring a central venous (or superior venous) oxygen saturation ($S_{CV}O_2$) to assess whether oxygen delivery was meeting the metabolic needs of the tissues.

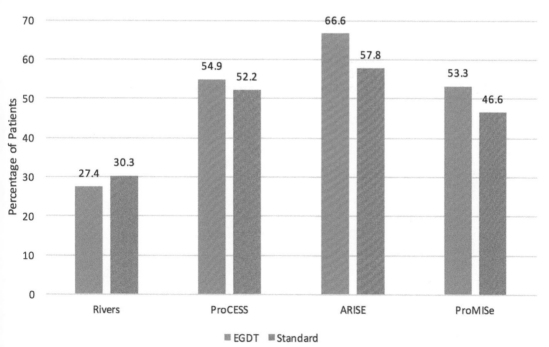

**Fig. 3.** Rates of vasopressor administration. ARISE, Australasian Resuscitation in Sepsis Evaluation; EGDT, early goal-directed therapy; ProCESS, Protocol-Based Care for Early Septic Shock; ProMISE, Protocolised Management in Sepsis.

The physiologic premise assumes that patients with low $S_{CV}O_2$ have increased oxygen extraction compared with delivery, and thus require interventions to increase oxygen delivery. For patients with an $S_{CV}O_2$ of less than 70%, signifying a need to increase oxygen delivery, the first intervention is transfusion of packed red blood cells to achieve a hematocrit of at least 30% to ensure adequate oxygen-carrying capacity. The second intervention, once all other EGDT criteria are fulfilled, is to administer dobutamine to increase cardiac output until $S_{CV}O_2$ is raised above the 70% threshold. In the Rivers trial, $S_{CV}O_2$-guided interventions occurred frequently: EDGT patients received far more blood transfusions (64.1% vs 18.5%; $P<.001$) and dobutamine infusions (13.7% vs 0.8%; $P<.001$) compared with standard care in the first 6 hours after randomization. Although these interventions tended to be used more frequently in the protocol versus control groups of the triad of validation studies, the degree to which they were used in either group tended to be much less compared with the original EGDT trial (**Figs. 4** and **5**).

In 2010, Jones and colleagues[24] assessed the usefulness of $S_{CV}O_2$ versus lactate clearance to trigger red blood cell transfusion and dobutamine in the form of a randomized trial. This trial found no differences for in-hospital mortality between patients randomized to $S_{CV}O_2$ measurements versus those randomized to serial lactate levels. This finding supports the use of lactate clearance as an alternative to using $S_{CV}O_2$ monitoring. Interestingly, despite using the same inclusion and exclusion criteria as Rivers, the number of patients meeting criteria for either packed red blood cells ($S_{CV}O_2$ 3% vs lactate clearance 7%) or dobutamine ($S_{CV}O_2$ 5% vs lactate clearance 3%) were

far below the rates in the original EGDT trial, and the mortality rate in both the lactate clearance and $S_{CV}O_2$ groups (17% vs 23%) was similar to the triad of validation trials, all of which were much lower than the original EGDT trial.

The ProCESS, ARISE, and ProMISe trials showed similar rates of $S_{CV}O_2$-directed interventions in the EGDT groups (see **Figs. 3** and **4**) as the Jones trial, reaffirming that few patients met the $S_{CV}O_2$ criteria that were more common in the Rivers trial. Furthermore, in comparison with patients in the EGDT groups, those treated by standard care used significantly less packed red blood cells and dobutamine, and had very low numbers of $S_{CV}O_2$ catheters placed. These studies demonstrate significantly greater resource use in the EGDT groups, triggered by $S_{CV}O_2$ monitoring. Last, the near absence of $S_{CV}O_2$ catheter placement suggests that very few clinicians are using this measure, without any detriment to patients (see **Fig. 2**).

Although the Jones trial offered lactate clearance as an alternative resuscitation endpoint to $S_{CV}O_2$ monitoring,[24] the true role of lactate measurements as a resuscitation goal remains incompletely defined. In the context of the subsequent triad of trials, it is plausible that the equivalence of $S_{CV}O_2$ monitoring and lactate clearance in the Jones trial is potentially a result of neither intervention having a significant effect on outcomes, as opposed to equivalence between the measurements in guiding therapy. There is reasonable observational evidence that lactate concentrations[53] and clearance patterns[54–56] are useful in prognostication. Persistently abnormal values of lactate should, however, at least trigger a clinical reassessment of the resuscitation.

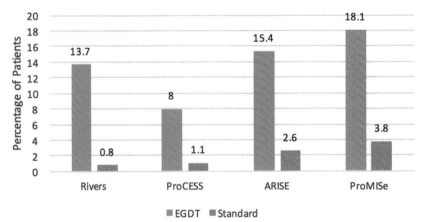

**Fig. 4.** Rates of dobutamine administration between EGDT and standard care groups. ARISE, Australasian Resuscitation in Sepsis Evaluation; EGDT, early goal-directed therapy; ProCESS, Protocol-Based Care for Early Septic Shock; ProMISE, Protocolised Management in Sepsis.

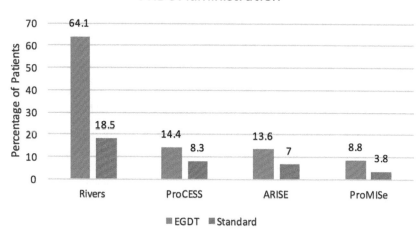

**Fig. 5.** Rates of packed red blood cell (PRBC) transfusion in EGDT and standard care groups. ARISE, Australasian Resuscitation in Sepsis Evaluation; EGDT, early goal-directed therapy; ProCESS, Protocol-Based Care for Early Septic Shock; ProMISE, Protocolised Management in Sepsis.

## Moving Forward

Since the time that Rivers' protocol was published, studies support a declining mortality rate for severe sepsis and septic shock.[19,20] We cannot truly identify why this mortality reduction has occurred; however, it is reasonable to postulate that there has been an increase in early recognition and timely intervention over this time period. This potential emphasis on the early aspects of care, inspired in a large part by the Rivers study, has created a number of quality assurance initiatives such as the Surviving Sepsis Campaign that have reinforced the concept of early, meticulous care in septic shock.[21,22] The EGDT protocol encouraged physicians to be diligent in their surveillance of septic patients, aggressive in the early resuscitation of these patients, and to reassess the effect of their interventions. However, although trials demonstrate that the EGDT protocol did not confer a mortality benefit when compared with standard clinical care, the level of standard clinical care may be considered to be "high quality." It is also important to note that EGDT did not show harm; thus, it is still a reasonable treatment strategy.

It is likely that new approaches to septic shock will be developed. Questions remain regarding multiple aspects of care including methods for early identification, the amount of fluids that should be given, methods to monitor fluid responsiveness, and how to monitor tissue perfusion. The research that is available currently does not provide distinct solutions that can be applied broadly to improve these aspects of care. However, the introduction of novel biomarkers,[57–59] dynamic monitoring of fluid responsiveness,[46,60] and novel techniques for monitoring changes in tissue perfusion during resuscitation[61,62] may provide the next steps forward in sepsis care. Until then, the concepts of early and meticulous care demonstrated in ProCESS, ARISE, and ProMISe trials provide us with the most current standard of clinical care for the treatment of severe sepsis and septic shock.

## REFERENCES

1. Rivers E, Nguyen B, Havstad S, et al. Early goal-directed therapy in the treatment of severe sepsis and septic shock. N Engl J Med 2001;345(19): 1368–77.
2. Shoemaker WC, Appel PL, Kram HB, et al. Prospective trial of supranormal values of survivors as therapeutic goals in high-risk surgical patients. Chest 1988;94(6):1176–86.
3. Boyd O, Grounds RM, Bennett ED. A randomized clinical trial of the effect of deliberate perioperative increase of oxygen delivery on mortality in high-risk surgical patients. JAMA 1993;270(22): 2699–707.
4. Gattinoni L, Brazzi L, Pelosi P, et al. A trial of goal-oriented hemodynamic therapy in critically ill patients. SvO2 Collaborative Group. N Engl J Med 1995;333(16):1025–32.
5. Hayes MA, Timmins AC, Yau EH, et al. Elevation of systemic oxygen delivery in the treatment of critically ill patients. N Engl J Med 1994;330(24): 1717–22.
6. Kern JW, Shoemaker WC. Meta-analysis of hemodynamic optimization in high-risk patients. Crit Care Med 2002;30(8):1686–92.

7. Jones AE, Brown MD, Trzeciak S, et al. The effect of a quantitative resuscitation strategy on mortality in patients with sepsis: a meta-analysis. Crit Care Med 2008;36(10):2734–9.

8. Trzeciak S, Dellinger RP, Abate NL, et al. Translating research to clinical practice: a 1-year experience with implementing early goal-directed therapy for septic shock in the emergency department. Chest 2006;129(2):225–32.

9. Jones AE, Focht A, Horton JM, et al. Prospective external validation of the clinical effectiveness of an emergency department-based early goal-directed therapy protocol for severe sepsis and septic shock. Chest 2007;132(2):425–32.

10. Nguyen HB, Corbett SW, Menes K, et al. Early goal-directed therapy, corticosteroid, and recombinant human activated protein c for the treatment of severe sepsis and septic shock in the emergency department. Acad Emerg Med 2006;13(1):109–13.

11. Nguyen HB, Corbett SW, Steele R, et al. Implementation of a bundle of quality indicators for the early management of severe sepsis and septic shock is associated with decreased mortality. Crit Care Med 2007;35(4):1105–12.

12. Micek ST, Roubinian N, Heuring T, et al. Before-after study of a standardized hospital order set for the management of septic shock. Crit Care Med 2006; 34(11):2707–13.

13. Shapiro NI, Howell MD, Talmor D, et al. Implementation and outcomes of the multiple urgent sepsis therapies (MUST) protocol. Crit Care Med 2006;34(4): 1025–32.

14. Dellinger RP, Levy MM, Carlet JM, et al. Surviving sepsis campaign: international guidelines for management of severe sepsis and septic shock: 2008. Crit Care Med 2008;36(1):296–327.

15. ARISE Investigators, ANZICS Clinical Trials Group, Peake SL, et al. Goal-directed resuscitation for patients with early septic shock. N Engl J Med 2014; 371(16):1496–506.

16. Investigators TP. A randomized trial of protocol-based care for early septic shock. N Engl J Med 2014;370(18):1683–93.

17. Mouncey PR, Osborn TM, Power GS, et al. Trial of early, goal-directed resuscitation for septic shock. N Engl J Med 2015;372(14):1301–11.

18. Angus DC, Barnato AE, Bell D, et al. A systematic review and meta-analysis of early goal-directed therapy for septic shock: the ARISE, ProCESS and ProMISe Investigators. Intensive Care Med 2015;41:1–12.

19. Kaukonen K-M, Bailey M, Suzuki S, et al. Mortality related to severe sepsis and septic shock among critically ill patients in Australia and New Zealand, 2000-2012. JAMA 2014;311(13):1308–16.

20. Stevenson EK, Rubenstein AR, Radin GT, et al. Two decades of mortality trends among patients with severe sepsis. Crit Care Med 2014;42(3):625–31.

21. Dellinger RP, Levy MM, Rhodes A, et al. Surviving sepsis campaign: international guidelines for management of severe sepsis and septic shock. Crit Care Med 2013;41(2):580–637.

22. Levy MM, Rhodes A, Phillips GS, et al. Surviving sepsis campaign: association between performance metrics and outcomes in a 7.5-year study. Intensive Care Med 2014;40(11):1623–33.

23. Perman SM, Goyal M, Gaieski DF. Initial emergency department diagnosis and management of adult patients with severe sepsis and septic shock. Scand J Trauma Resusc Emerg Med 2012;20(1):41.

24. Jones AE, Shapiro NI, Trzeciak S, et al. Lactate clearance vs central venous oxygen saturation as goals of early sepsis therapy: a randomized clinical trial. JAMA 2010;303(8):739–46.

25. Kaukonen K-M, Bailey M, Pilcher D, et al. Systemic inflammatory response syndrome criteria in defining severe sepsis. N Engl J Med 2015;372(17):1629–38.

26. Young PJ, Saxena M, Beasley R, et al. Early peak temperature and mortality in critically ill patients with or without infection. Intensive Care Med 2012; 38(3):437–44.

27. Finfer SR, Vincent J-L, De Backer D. Circulatory shock. N Engl J Med 2013;369(18):1726–34.

28. Hilton AK, Bellomo R. A critique of fluid bolus resuscitation in severe sepsis. Crit Care 2012;16(1):302.

29. Boyd JH, Forbes J, Nakada TA, et al. Fluid resuscitation in septic shock: a positive fluid balance and elevated central venous pressure are associated with increased mortality. Crit Care Med 2011;39(2): 259–65.

30. Micek ST, McEvoy C, McKenzie M, et al. Fluid balance and cardiac function in septic shock as predictors of hospital mortality. Crit Care 2013;17(5):R246.

31. Waechter J, Kumar A, Lapinsky SE, et al. Interaction between fluids and vasoactive agents on mortality in septic shock. Crit Care Med 2014;42(10):2158–68.

32. Ferrer R, Martin-Loeches I, Phillips G, et al. Empiric antibiotic treatment reduces mortality in severe sepsis and septic shock from the first hour. Crit Care Med 2014;42(8):1749–55.

33. Funk DJ, Kumar A. Antimicrobial therapy for life-threatening infections: speed is life. Crit Care Clin 2011;27(1):53–76.

34. Kumar A, Zarychanski R, Light B, et al. Early combination antibiotic therapy yields improved survival compared with monotherapy in septic shock: a propensity-matched analysis. Crit Care Med 2010; 38(9):1773–85.

35. Sterling SA, Miller WR, Pryor J, et al. The impact of timing of antibiotics on outcomes in severe sepsis and septic shock: a systematic review and meta-analysis. Crit Care Med 2015;43(9):1907–15.

36. Marik PE, Baram M, Vahid B. Does central venous pressure predict fluid responsiveness? Chest 2008;134(1):172.

37. Marik PE, Cavallazzi R. Does the central venous pressure predict fluid responsiveness? An updated meta-analysis and a plea for some common sense. Crit Care Med 2013;41(7):1774–81.

38. Vellinga NA, Ince C, Boerma EC. Elevated central venous pressure is associated with impairment of microcirculatory blood flow in sepsis: a hypothesis generating post hoc analysis. BMC Anesthesiol 2013;13:17.

39. Westphal GA. How to guide volume expansion in severe sepsis and septic shock patients? possibilities in the real world. Shock 2013;39:38–41.

40. Barbier C, Loubières Y, Schmit C, et al. Respiratory changes in inferior vena cava diameter are helpful in predicting fluid responsiveness in ventilated septic patients. Intensive Care Med 2004;30(9):1740–6.

41. Charbonneau H, Riu B, Faron M, et al. Predicting preload responsiveness using simultaneous recordings of inferior and superior vena cavae diameters. Crit Care 2014;18(5):473.

42. Machare-Delgado E, Decaro M, Marik PE. Inferior vena cava variation compared to pulse contour analysis as predictors of fluid responsiveness: a prospective cohort study. J Intensive Care Med 2011; 26(2):116–24.

43. Moretti R, Pizzi B. Inferior vena cava distensibility as a predictor of fluid responsiveness in patients with subarachnoid hemorrhage. Neurocrit Care 2010; 13(1):3–9.

44. Muller L, Bobbia X, Toumi M, et al. Respiratory variations of inferior vena cava diameter to predict fluid responsiveness in spontaneously breathing patients with acute circulatory failure: need for a cautious use. Crit Care 2012;16(5):R188.

45. Zhang Z, Xu X, Ye S, et al. Ultrasonographic measurement of the respiratory variation in the inferior vena cava diameter is predictive of fluid responsiveness in critically ill patients: systematic review and meta-analysis. Ultrasound Med Biol 2014;40(5): 845–53.

46. Marik PE, Monnet X, Teboul J-L. Hemodynamic parameters to guide fluid therapy. Ann Intensive Care 2011;1(1):1.

47. Smith SH, Perner A. Higher vs. lower fluid volume for septic shock: clinical characteristics and outcome in unselected patients in a prospective, multicenter cohort. Crit Care 2012;16(3):R76.

48. Jones AE, Puskarich MA. Sepsis-induced tissue hypoperfusion. Crit Care Clin 2009;25(4):769–79.

49. Magder SA. The highs and lows of blood pressure: toward meaningful clinical targets in patients with shock. Crit Care Med 2014;42(5):1241–51.

50. Boerma EC, Ince C. The role of vasoactive agents in the resuscitation of microvascular perfusion and tissue oxygenation in critically ill patients. Intensive Care Med 2010;36(12):2004–18.

51. Asfar P, Meziani F, Hamel J-F, et al. High versus low blood-pressure target in patients with septic shock. N Engl J Med 2014;370(17):1583–93.

52. Filbin MR, Hou PC, Massey M, et al. The microcirculation is preserved in emergency department low-acuity sepsis patients without hypotension. Acad Emerg Med 2014;21(2):154–62.

53. Howell MD, Donnino M, Clardy P, et al. Occult hypoperfusion and mortality in patients with suspected infection. Intensive Care Med 2007;33(11):1892–9.

54. Puskarich MA, Trzeciak S, Shapiro NI, et al. Prognostic value and agreement of achieving lactate clearance or central venous oxygen saturation goals during early sepsis resuscitation. Acad Emerg Med 2012;19(3):252–8.

55. Marty P, Roquilly A, Vallée F, et al. Lactate clearance for death prediction in severe sepsis or septic shock patients during the first 24 hours in intensive care unit: an observational study. Ann Intensive Care 2013;3(1):3.

56. Arnold RC, Shapiro NI, Jones AE, et al. Multicenter study of early lactate clearance as a determinant of survival in patients with presumed sepsis. Shock 2009;32(1):35–9.

57. Day DE, Oedorf K, Kogan S, et al. The utility of inflammatory and endothelial markers to identify infection in emergency department patients. Shock 2015; 44(3):215–20.

58. Limper M, de Kruif MD, Duits AJ, et al. The diagnostic role of procalcitonin and other biomarkers in discriminating infectious from non-infectious fever. J Infect 2010;60(6):409–16.

59. Tsalik EL, Jaggers LB, Glickman SW, et al. Discriminative value of inflammatory biomarkers for suspected sepsis. J Emerg Med 2012;43(1):97–106.

60. Saugel B, Kirsche SV, Hapfelmeier A, et al. Prediction of fluid responsiveness in patients admitted to the medical intensive care unit. J Crit Care 2013; 28(4):537.e1–9.

61. Hernandez G, Boerma EC, Dubin A, et al. Severe abnormalities in microvascular perfused vessel density are associated to organ dysfunctions and mortality and can be predicted by hyperlactatemia and norepinephrine requirements in septic shock patients. J Crit Care 2013;28(4):538.e9–14.

62. van Genderen ME, Klijn E, Lima A, et al. Microvascular perfusion as a target for fluid resuscitation in experimental circulatory shock. Crit Care Med 2014;42(2):e96–105.

# Sepsis Resuscitation
## Fluid Choice and Dose

Matthew W. Semler, MD*, Todd W. Rice, MD, MSc

## KEYWORDS

- Fluid resuscitation • Sepsis • Crystalloids • Colloids • Albumin • Early goal-directed therapy

## KEY POINTS

- Fluid resuscitation to correct hypovolemia and support organ perfusion is central to current management of severe sepsis and septic shock.
- Recent randomized trials have not confirmed a benefit for targeting invasive physiologic parameters; the ideal fluid volume and end points in sepsis resuscitation remain unknown.
- Increased fluid balance is associated with increased mortality in early and late sepsis; whether conservative fluid management can improve sepsis outcomes requires further study.
- Hydroxyethyl starch increases risk of acute kidney injury and may increase mortality in patients with sepsis.
- Whether albumin or physiologically balanced crystalloids improve clinical outcomes in sepsis remains the focus of ongoing study.

## INTRODUCTION

Sepsis is an inflammatory response to severe infection characterized by hypovolemia and vasodilation and treated with early antibiotics and fluid resuscitation.[1] In the United States, sepsis with organ dysfunction (severe sepsis) or fluid-resistant hypotension (septic shock) accounts for 2% of hospital admissions and 10% of intensive care unit (ICU) admissions.[1] In-hospital mortality rates have decreased from 80% in the early years of intensive care to 20% to 30% in the modern era[2–4] through improved surveillance, early treatment of underlying infection, and advances in support for failing organs. Despite the central role intravenous (IV) fluid administration has played in sepsis management for the last 15 years,[5,6] fundamental questions regarding "which fluid" and "in what amount" remain unanswered. This article addresses the physiologic principles and scientific evidence available to help clinicians address those questions in practice.

## PHYSIOLOGY OF FLUID RESUSCITATION IN SEPSIS

Patients with early sepsis are frequently hypovolemic from decreased intake and increased insensible losses. In addition, inflammation alters vascular resistance, venous capacitance, and vascular leak generating a "relative hypovolemia." Resultant decreases in stroke volume and cardiac output imbalance oxygen delivery and demand, precipitating tissue hypoxia, anaerobic metabolism, and lactic acidosis.

The classic physiologic rationale for fluid resuscitation in sepsis is to restore intravascular volume, cardiac output, and oxygen delivery. Volume and choice of resuscitation fluids have largely been predicated on this model. Resuscitation end points, such as central venous pressure (CVP), inferior vena cava filling, mixed venous oxygen saturation, and lactate, are used to restore preload independence and match oxygen demand and supply. Selection of colloids over crystalloids is

Funding: When this review was prepared, Dr M.W. Semler was supported by a National Heart, Lung, and Blood Institute T32 award (HL087738 09).
Conflicts of Interest: The authors have no potential conflicts of interest.
Division of Allergy, Pulmonary, and Critical Care Medicine, Vanderbilt University Medical Center, Medical Center North, T-1218, Nashville, TN 37232-2650, USA
* Corresponding author.
E-mail address: matthew.semler@vanderbilt.edu

chestmed.theclinics.com

intended to optimize volume expansion through colloid retention in the intravascular space.

It is increasingly clear, however, that the hemodynamic response to fluid administration is determined by an intricate interaction of mean systemic filling pressure, right atrial pressure, venous resistance, and ventricular compliance, which makes predicting a critically ill patient's response to fluid challenging.[7] Impaired oxygen use and nonhypoxemic causes of lactic acidosis may elevate lactate levels despite adequate perfusion. Perhaps most importantly, the century-old Starling model conceptualizing maintenance of vascular volume as the balance of hydrostatic and oncotic pressure gradients between the vessel lumen and interstitial space has been challenged by the recent recognition of the importance of the endothelial glycocalyx (**Fig. 1**).[8] Because it is a primary determinant of membrane permeability, damage to the glycocalyx during sepsis may alter patients' response

to fluid resuscitation. Although the clinical implications of these findings are not yet fully understood, they argue against an overly simplified approach to fluid dose ("fill the tank") and fluid choice ("colloids stay in the vasculature").

## FLUID DOSE
### Fluid Administration in Sepsis Resuscitation

Fluid resuscitation is currently considered an essential component of early sepsis management.[1] Prompt IV fluid administration for patients with sepsis was advanced by a 2001 study of early goal-directed therapy (EGDT).[5] In that landmark trial, 263 patients with sepsis and hypoperfusion were randomized to either standard therapy or EGDT. Standard therapy involved arterial and central venous catheterization and a protocol targeting CVP of 8 to 12 mm Hg, mean arterial pressure (MAP) at least 65 mm Hg, and urine output at

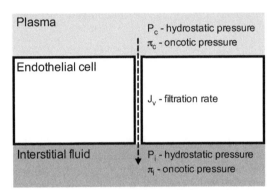

$$J_v = \kappa_f(P_c - P_i) - \sigma(\pi_c - \pi_i)$$

## Original Starling Principle

• Intravascular volume consists of plasma and cells

• Fluid is driven from the arteriolar capillaries to the interstitial space by a hydrostatic pressure gradient

• Fluid is resorbed from the low-protein interstitial space into venous capillaries by an oncotic pressure gradient

• Higher plasma oncotic pressure enhances absorption of fluid from interstitial space to plasma

• Colloids distribute through the plasma volume

• Crystalloids distribute through the extracellular volume

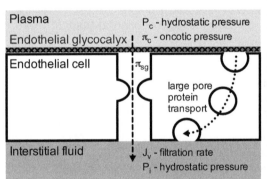

$$J_v = \kappa_f(P_c - P_i) - \sigma(\pi_c - \pi_{sg})$$

## Glycocalyx model

• Endothelial glycocalyx layer is semi-permeable to proteins causing low oncotic pressure in sub-glycocalyx

• Intravascular volume consists of plasma volume, glycocalyx volume, and cells

• Transcapillary flow is driven by a hydrostatic gradient and the difference in oncotic pressure between the plasma and subglycocalyx, not the interstitial space

• Plasma oncotic pressure does not cause absorption, the major route of return to the circulation is lymph

• Colloids initially distribute through plasma volume, crystalloids through intravascular volume

**Fig. 1.** Models of transvascular fluid exchange. In the original Starling model, the gradient of hydrostatic pressure from the capillary ($P_c$) to the interstitium ($P_i$) is opposed by the gradient of oncotic pressure from the capillary ($\pi_c$) to the interstitium ($\pi_i$), with filtration ($K_f$) and reflection ($\sigma$) coefficients. Understanding the web of membrane-bound glycoproteins and proteoglycans on the luminal side of endothelial cells (endothelial glycocalyx layer) suggests the low oncotic pressure under this semipermeable membrane ($\pi_{sg}$) is a more important regulator of transcapillary flow than the interstitial oncotic pressure.

east 0.5 mL/kg/h. EGDT included all elements of standard therapy in addition to a catheter measuring central venous oxygen saturation (SvO$_2$), 6 hours of treatment in the emergency department before admission, and protocolized administration of 500 mL of IV crystalloid every 30 minutes to achieve CVP goals, vasopressors and vasodilators to maintain MAP goals, and blood transfusion or dobutamine to achieve SvO$_2$ at least 70%. During the 6 hours of intervention, EGDT patients received more IV fluid (5.0 vs 3.5 L; $P$<.001), red-cell transfusions (64.1% vs 18.5%; $P$<.001), and dobutamine (13.7% vs 0.8%; $P$<.001). In-hospital mortality was 16% lower with EGDT compared with standard therapy (46.5% vs 30.5%; $P$ = .009).

The remarkable improvement in mortality propelled early, protocolized fluid resuscitation to the forefront of sepsis management. Based on the 2001 EGDT study, an EGDT trial at eight Chinese centers, and dozens of before-after studies of EGDT implementation, the Surviving Sepsis Campaign (SSC) promoted incorporation of goal-directed fluid resuscitation into early sepsis management globally.[6] The most recent version of the SSC guidelines recommends "protocolized, quantitative resuscitation of patients with sepsis-induced tissue hypoperfusion" beginning with an "initial fluid challenge…to achieve a minimum of 30 mL/kg of crystalloids" targeting CVP, blood pressure, urine output, and venous oxygen saturation goals outlined in the 2001 EGDT trial.[6]

More than a decade after the original EGDT study, three large, multicenter trials attempted to confirm the benefit of EGDT. The ProCESS,[2] ARISE,[3] and ProMISe[4] trials all compared EGDT with usual care in which invasive management was optional (eg, central venous access in ProCESS) or forbidden (eg, SvO$_2$ measurement in ARISE). Fluid resuscitation in the first 6 hours of each EGDT trial is shown in **Fig. 2**. There were no differences in any clinical outcome between EGDT and usual care among the 4201 patients in these trials. Understanding the implications of these new EGDT trials for fluid resuscitation presents several challenges. First, the largest separation between arms in fluid administration in the first 6 hours was a 1-L difference between modified protocol-based standard therapy (3.3 L) and usual care (2.2 L), less than the 1.5-L difference in the original trial. Advocates of EGDT would suggest that routine sepsis care has shifted to resemble the intervention arm of the original trial, but patients in both arms of the modern trials actually received less IV fluid than either arm of the original trial (see **Fig. 2**). Although the modern trials enrolled patients later after presentation, the

pre-enrollment fluids were similar to the 20 to 30 mL/kg required before inclusion in the original trial. Patients in the modern trials were less severely ill than patients in the original trial, potentially limiting the impact of early intervention. Ultimately, ancillary aspects of critical care have changed so dramatically in the decade between trials[9] that comparing fluid management across EGDT studies may not yield firm conclusions about the optimal approach to early fluid resuscitation.

Although broad adoption of EGDT in developed countries complicates the study of sepsis resuscitation, provocative data have emerged elsewhere. The Fluid Expansion as Supportive Therapy (FEAST) study[10] randomized 3170 African children with sepsis to weight-based fluid boluses with 0.9% saline, 5% albumin, or no bolus. The median volume of fluid received by 1 and 8 hours was 20.0 and 40.0 mL/kg for the bolus groups compared with 1.2 and 10.1 mL/kg in the no bolus group. By 48 hours, 10.5% of children in the fluid bolus groups had died compared with 7.3% in the no bolus group ($P$ = .003). Receipt of fluid was harmful in all subgroups. Although shock resolved more frequently in the bolus groups, excess mortality was evident regardless of blood pressure response.[11] Similarly, the Simplified Severe Sepsis Protocol (SSSP) trial[12] randomized 112 African adults with sepsis and organ dysfunction to usual care or an algorithm of simplified, goal-directed resuscitation. Patients in the intervention arm received 1.3 L more fluid in the first 6 hours (2.9 vs 1.6 L; $P$<.001) with no differences in vasopressors, transfusions, or antibiotics. In-hospital mortality was 64.2% with fluid resuscitation compared with 60.7% without when the study was stopped early for high mortality among patients with baseline respiratory failure randomized to the intervention.[12] The Simplified Severe Sepsis Protocol-2 (SSSP-2) trial currently enrolling patients with septic shock in Zambia (NCT01663701) may provide more definitive data on the impact of fluid compared with little or no resuscitation for early sepsis in this population.

---

**Recommendation for clinical practice**

For patients with severe sepsis and septic shock, early administration of IV fluids to correct hypovolemia and potentially improve blood pressure and tissue perfusion remains standard of care. The optimal amount, rate, and end point for fluid administration in early sepsis are unknown. Fluid resuscitation beyond euvolemia may be detrimental.

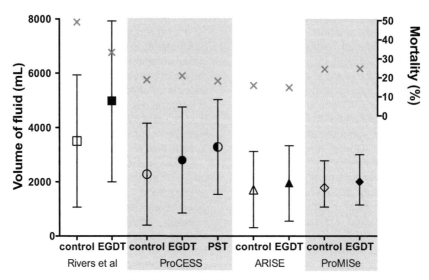

**Fig. 2.** Fluid administration in EGDT trials. Volume of IV fluid during the first 6 hours in each EGDT trial. Volume of fluid (*black*) is mean and standard deviation for all trials except ProMISe, which is median and interquartile range. Mortality (*gray X*) is through 60 days in ProCESS and 28 days in all other trials. PST, protocol-based standard therapy.

## Fluid Management in Sepsis After Resuscitation

In contrast to the intense focus on fluid in the first 6 to 12 hours of sepsis, little attention has been dedicated to optimal fluid management after resuscitation. There is broad agreement that fluid management may differ between different phases of sepsis, but the factors delineating each phase and the optimal fluid strategy for each phase remain largely undefined. The 2012 SSC guidelines recommend a fluid challenge approach for patients requiring hemodynamic support wherein fluid boluses are continued as long as there is hemodynamic improvement.[6] Frequently in clinical practice this has meant administering IV fluids to patients for changes in heart rate, blood pressure, or urine output. Recognizing the limitations of these traditional indices in assessing intravascular volume status and fluid responsiveness, researchers and clinicians have sought dynamic predictors of response to fluid administration.[13,14] Cardiac output monitoring,[15] pulse pressure and stroke volume variation,[16] and interior vena cava diameter and stroke volume assessment by echocardiography[13] have all been advocated to guide fluid administration. However, many dynamic measures cannot be used for patients who are spontaneously breathing or receiving low tidal-volume ventilation. Moreover, no clear evidence yet correlates improvement in short-term physiologic parameters with improvements in longer-term clinical outcomes.

Historically, patients with sepsis have received significant volumes of fluid throughout their ICU stay. Observational studies report positive fluid balances of 5 to 11 L in the week after presentation.[17,18] After resuscitation, potential benefits of fluid are balanced against risks of pulmonary edema, renal parenchymal edema, and effects of the IV fluid constituents themselves. Observational studies have associated fluid receipt and positive fluid balance with mortality. Among 778 patients with septic shock in the Vasopressin in Septic Shock Trial (VASST), odds of mortality doubled for patients with the highest cumulative fluid balance.[17] For 1177 patients with sepsis in the Sepsis Occurrence in Acutely Ill Patients (SOAP) study, each additional liter of fluid balance at 72 hours was associated with a 10% increase in the odds of death.[19] These observational studies are inherently limited by the indication bias that patients with higher severity of illness may be more likely to die and have fluid administered by providers. The Fluid and Catheter Treatment Trial (FACTT) controlled postresuscitation fluid management for 1000 patients with acute respiratory distress syndrome (ARDS), of whom 70% had underlying infection. Fluid management emphasizing diuretics and limiting fluid administration increased ventilator-free days and ICU-free days without precipitating cardiovascular or renal dysfunction.[20] The 2012 SSC recommends conservative fluid management for patients with sepsis and ARDS after the resolution of shock.[6]

Whether a conservative approach to fluid management after resuscitation can improve outcomes for patients with sepsis without ARDS is being evaluated in ongoing randomized trials (NCT02079402, NCT02159079, and NCT01309724).

---

**Recommendation for clinical practice:**

For patients beyond the early phase of sepsis, the risks and benefits of further IV fluid administration should be weighed. Hypervolemia should be avoided and consideration should be given to targeting a net even-to-negative fluid balance.

---

## FLUID CHOICE

Since the advent of IV fluids, there has been debate as to which fluid is best for patients critically ill from infection.[21] The ideal sepsis resuscitation fluid would increase intravascular volume without accumulating in tissues, contain a chemical composition similar to plasma, and improve patient outcomes in a cost-effective manner. No such fluid exists currently. Available IV fluids are categorized as crystalloid or colloid solutions (**Table 1**).

### Crystalloids

Crystalloids are solutions of ions that determine fluid tonicity but are freely permeable through capillary membranes. Isotonic crystalloids are the most commonly administered IV fluid internationally[22] and the recommended first-line fluid for sepsis resuscitation.[6] Crystalloid solutions were first prepared in response to the cholera pandemic in 1832.[21] Early solutions comprised of sodium, chloride, and bicarbonate in water[21] evolved over the following century into two basic categories of isotonic crystalloid: sodium chloride and physiologically balanced solutions. Normal saline (0.9% sodium chloride) is the most common crystalloid globally, with more than 200 million liters administered annually in the United States alone. With 154 mmol/L each of sodium and chloride, normal saline is isotonic to extracellular fluid but contains a chloride concentration significantly higher than plasma. In contrast, so-called balanced crystalloids derived from the original Hartmann and Ringer solutions may be slightly hypotonic to extracellular fluid but provide anions that more closely approximate plasma pH (see **Table 1**).

### Hyperchloremic metabolic acidosis

The difference in chloride content between saline and balanced crystalloids causes hyperchloremia and metabolic acidosis among critically ill patients.[23] In the Stewart physicochemical approach,[24] hydrogen ion concentration is determined by carbon dioxide; weak acids; and the balance of sodium, potassium, magnesium, calcium, chloride, and lactate (strong ion difference). The increased concentration of chloride with saline infusion decreases the strong ion difference, increases dissociation of water into hydrogen ions, and induces a nonanion gap metabolic acidosis.[23] Whether metabolic acidosis associated with saline infusion influences patient outcomes remains unclear.

### Acute kidney injury

Crystalloid chloride content also regulates renal blood flow and may contribute to acute kidney injury (AKI). Delivery of chloride to the macula densa drives mesangial contraction and decreases glomerular filtration. Denervated dog kidneys infused with chloride-rich solutions demonstrate renal vasoconstriction.[25] Human volunteers experience decreased renal blood flow with high-chloride fluids,[26] and surgery patients have decreased urine output after saline administration.[27] A before-after study of 1400 patients in an ICU transitioning from higher to lower chloride solutions found an association between higher chloride fluid and development of AKI.[28] However, subsequent analyses suggested unidentified confounders beyond fluid choice may have contributed to the difference in AKI.[29] A meta-analysis of high- versus low-chloride IV fluid in critically ill patients found increased AKI but not mortality.[30]

### Isotonic crystalloids in sepsis

Animal models of sepsis link saline administration to acidosis, inflammation, and mortality. An observational study of adults with septic shock associated higher chloride and increased mortality,[31] with a dose-response curve for chloride that seems independent of volume of fluid received.[32] A recent meta-analysis linked balanced crystalloids to reduced mortality in sepsis,[33] although another suggested no relationship between chloride content and renal-replacement therapy.[34] Ongoing randomized trials (ACTRN12613001370796, NCT02444988) comparing saline with balanced crystalloids in critically ill populations may definitively establish the impact of crystalloid choice on AKI and mortality among patients with sepsis.

**Table 1**
Composition of common sepsis resuscitation fluids

| | | Crystalloid | | | | Colloid | | | | | | | | | |
| | | | | | | Human | | Hydroxyethyl Starch | | | | | | Gelatin | |
| | Plasma | 0.9% Sodium Chloride | Ringer Lactate | Hartmann Solution | Plasma-Lyte | 4% Albumin | 20% Albumin | 10% (200/0.5) (Hemohes) | 6% (450/0.7) (Hextend) | 6% (130/0.4) (Voluven) | 6% (130/0.4) (Volulyte) | 6% (130/0.42) (Venofundin) | 6% (130/0.42) (Tetraspan) | 4% Succinylated Gelatin (Gelofusine) | 3.5% Urea-Linked Gelatin (Haemaccel) |
|---|---|---|---|---|---|---|---|---|---|---|---|---|---|---|---|
| Sodium | 135–145 | 154 | 130 | 131 | 140 | 130–160 | 48–100 | 154 | 143 | 154 | 137 | 154 | 140 | 154 | 145 |
| Potassium | 4.5–5.0 | — | 4.0 | 5.4 | 5.0 | — | — | — | 3.0 | — | 4.0 | — | 4.0 | — | 5.1 |
| Calcium | 2.2–2.6 | — | 1.5 | 1.8 | — | — | — | — | 5.0 | — | — | — | 2.5 | — | — |
| Magnesium | 0.8–1.0 | — | — | — | 1.5 | — | — | — | 0.9 | — | 1.5 | — | 1.0 | — | — |
| Chloride | 94–111 | 154 | 109 | 112 | 98 | 128 | 19 | 154 | 124 | 154 | 110 | 154 | 118 | 120 | 145 |
| Acetate | — | — | — | — | 27 | — | — | — | — | — | 34 | — | 24 | — | — |
| Lactate | 1–2 | — | 28 | 28 | — | — | — | — | 28 | — | — | — | — | — | — |
| Malate | — | — | — | — | — | — | — | — | — | — | — | — | 5.0 | — | — |
| Gluconate | — | — | — | — | 23 | — | — | — | — | — | — | — | — | — | — |
| Bicarbonate | 23–27 | — | — | — | — | — | — | — | — | — | — | — | — | — | — |
| Octanoate | — | — | — | — | — | 6.4 | 32.0 | — | — | — | — | — | — | — | — |
| Osmolarity | 291 | 308 | 273 | 277 | 294 | 250 | 210–260 | 308 | 304 | 308 | 286 | 308 | 296 | 274 | 301 |

All values are given in mmol/L except osmolarity, which is in mOsm/L. Electrolyte concentrations of intravenous fluid preparations may differ by manufacturer: information is given for Hartmann solution (B. Braun Melsungen AG, Melsungen, Germany). Plasma-Lyte 148 (Baxter, Deerfield, IL, USA), and Albumex 20 (CSL Behring, King of Prussia, PA, USA). HES solutions are described with regard to their concentration (6%–10%), mean molecular weight (70–480 kDa), and degree of molar substitution (range, 0–1; tetrastarch 0.4, pentastarch 0.5, hexastrach 0.6).

---

**Recommendation for clinical practice:**

For patients with sepsis, administration of normal saline contributes to metabolic acidosis and may increase the risk of AKI. Whether use of balanced crystalloids can prevent AKI and decrease mortality remains unknown.

---

## Colloids

Colloids are suspensions of molecules in a carrier fluid with high enough molecular weight to prevent crossing of healthy capillary membranes. Available colloids include derivatives of human plasma (albumin solutions) and semisynthetic colloids (gelatins, dextrans, and hydroxyethyl starches [HES]). The physiologic rationale favoring colloids over crystalloids is that colloids may more effectively expand intravascular volume by remaining in the intravascular space and maintaining colloid oncotic pressure.

### Albumin

Human serum albumin is a small protein synthesized by the liver and maintained in the vasculature through a dynamic equilibrium of leak into the interstitium matched by lymphatic return. Beyond providing 75% of plasma colloid oncotic pressure, albumin binds nitric oxide, protects against lipid peroxidation, and regulates inflammation, leading to the enticing proposition that albumin solutions might expand intravascular volume and directly mediate sepsis pathogenesis.

Administration of human albumin was introduced in World War II for victims of traumatic and thermal injury. Commercial preparations of isotonic 4% to 5% albumin solution for fluid replacement and hyperoncotic 20% to 25% albumin solution to support colloidal pressure led to expanded use in civilian operating rooms, emergency departments, and ICUs. Fifty years after the introduction of albumin into clinical practice, the first systematic evaluation of albumin's effect on clinical outcomes reported an alarming 6% increase in the risk of death with albumin use[35] and calls were made for large, rigorously conducted trials of albumin administration in critical illness.

Three large trials now inform the utility of albumin administration for patients with sepsis.[36–38] The Saline versus Albumin Fluid Evaluation (SAFE) Study randomized nearly 7000 critically ill adults to 4% albumin versus 0.9% sodium chloride for fluid resuscitation throughout the ICU stay.[36] The albumin group received slightly less fluid input but demonstrated similar heart rate and MAP. Overall there was no difference in 28-day mortality between albumin and saline. However, analysis of a prespecified subgroup of patients with severe sepsis (N = 1218) suggested reduced in-hospital mortality with albumin (relative risk, 0.87; 95% confidence interval, 0.74–1.02).[36] In contrast to the SAFE study of 4% albumin for fluid resuscitation, the Albumin Italian Outcome Sepsis (ALBIOS) study examined daily administration of 20% albumin targeting a serum albumin level of 3 g/L.[37] Among 1818 ICU patients with sepsis, albumin administration resulted in higher serum albumin levels, lower net fluid balance, lower heart rate, higher MAP, and more rapid freedom from vasopressors. The 28-day mortality was identical in the two groups but a post hoc subgroup analysis suggested fewer deaths with albumin among patients in shock (relative risk, 0.87; 95% confidence interval, 0.77–0.99; P interaction = .03). The third trial, Early Albumin Resuscitation during Septic Shock (EARSS; available only in abstract form), randomized patients with septic shock within 6 hours of vasopressor initiation to receive 100 mL of 20% albumin or 100 mL of 0.9% saline every 8 hours for 3 days. Among 798 patients, vasopressor-free days were higher with albumin without improvement in 28-day mortality (24.1% vs 26.3%).[38] (Although the Colloids vs Crystalloids for the Resuscitation of the Critically Ill (CRISTAL) trial allowed use of 4% or 20% albumin, albumin administration was too similar between the colloid and crystalloid arms (20.4% vs 16.5%) to allow inferences about the relative effects of albumin[39]).

Despite no overall benefit in each of the individual trials, multiple meta-analyses[33,40–42] have suggested improved mortality with albumin administration in sepsis (**Fig. 3**). The SCC in 2012 continued to recommend crystalloids as the initial sepsis resuscitation fluid, but advised consideration of albumin "when patients require substantial amounts of crystalloids."[6] Given albumin's cost and a more recent meta-analysis showing no impact on sepsis mortality,[43] ongoing trials evaluating earlier albumin administration (NCT01337934, NCT00819416) need to demonstrate clear mortality benefit for albumin to replace crystalloids as the gold standard fluid for sepsis resuscitation.

### Semisynthetic colloids

The expense and limited availability of human albumin has prompted the development of semisynthetic colloid solutions (gelatins, dextrans, and HES) (see **Table 1**). Gelatins are prepared by hydrolysis of bovine collagen, dextrans

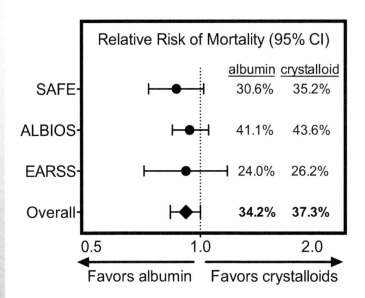

**Fig. 3.** Mortality of patients with sepsis in trials of albumin administration. Relative risks of death by 28 days with albumin (N = 603) versus saline (N = 615) for patients with severe sepsis in the SAFE study, death by 90 days with albumin (N = 888) versus crystalloid (N = 893) in the AL-BIOS study, and death by 28 days with albumin (N = 399) versus saline (N = 393) in the EARSS study are displayed with accompanying 95% confidence intervals (CI). (*Data from* Refs.[36–38,42].)

biosynthesized from sucrose by bacteria, and HES synthesized from the maize-derived D-glucose polymer amylopectin. Each colloid's duration of volume expansion is governed by rate of loss from the circulation (determined by molecular weight) and metabolism (determined by chemical properties, such as molar substitution). Each colloid has been linked to a unique profile of adverse events: increased risk of AKI (HES, gelatin), allergic reactions (gelatins, dextrans), and bleeding (dextrans, HES).

HES is the only semisynthetic colloid for which large trials enrolling patients with sepsis have been conducted. The 2004 Efficacy of Volume Substitution and Insulin Therapy in Severe Sepsis (VISEP) trial comparing Ringer lactate with 10% HES 200/0.5 among 537 patients with severe sepsis was stopped early for increased AKI (34.9% vs 22.8%; $P = .002$) and a trend toward increased 90-day mortality (41.0% vs 33.9%; $P = .09$) with HES.[44] Based on a reportedly improved safety profile for starches with lower molecular weight and molar substitution, 6% HES 130/0.4 was compared with 0.9% sodium chloride among 196 patients with sepsis in the CRYSTMAS study.[45] Differences between HES and 0.9% sodium chloride in mortality (31.0% vs 25.3%) and AKI (24.5% vs 20.0%) failed to reach statistical significance. However, in the larger Scandinavian Starch for Severe Sepsis/Septic Shock (6S) trial in which 804 patients with severe sepsis were resuscitated with 6% HES 130/4.2 or Ringer acetate, renal-replacement therapy (22% vs 16%; $P = .04$) and 90-day mortality (51% vs 43%; $P = .03$) were significantly higher with HES.[46] Among 7000 critically ill adults (1937 with sepsis) in the Crystalloid versus

Hydroxyethyl Starch Trial (CHEST) trial, those randomized to 6% HES 130/0.4 received more renal-replacement therapy (7.0% vs 5.8%; $P = .04$) with similar 90-day mortality (18.0% vs 17.0%). A subsequent meta-analysis confirmed an association between HES and both AKI and mortality.[47] In contrast, the CRISTAL trial found similar short-term mortality and improved ventilator-free days and long-term mortality with colloids compared with crystalloids.[39] The CRISTAL trial randomized 2857 adult ICU patients (55% with sepsis) to resuscitation with colloids or crystalloids. Patients in the colloid arm received less 0.9% saline and Ringer lactate, more gelatins and HES, and a similar amount of albumin to patients in the crystalloid arm. The 28-day mortality was 25.4% with colloids compared with 27.0% with crystalloids ($P = .26$), a difference that increased to favor colloids at 90 days (30.7% vs 34.2%; $P = .03$). Given the preponderance of data linking HES to AKI and the relatively high use of albumin in both arms of the CRISTAL trial, unless the improvement in long-term mortality seen in CRISTAL is replicated, the cost and potential risks prevent colloids from replacing crystalloids as first-line fluid therapy in sepsis.[6]

---

**Recommendation for clinical practice:**

Colloid solutions should not be used as first-line fluid therapy for patients with sepsis. HES seems to increase AKI and potentially mortality; the safety of other semisynthetic colloids is not established. Unless the potential beneficial effects of albumin infusion are confirmed by further trials, cost precludes its routine use.

## SUMMARY

Sepsis remains a common and lethal illness with few effective therapies. Since the 2001 EGDT trial, fluid resuscitation targeting hemodynamic parameters in sepsis has been disseminated globally. Recent trials have not confirmed the benefits of EGDT and question reliance on resuscitation targets, but leave unanswered how fluid should be dosed in sepsis. Trials in the Third World examining outcomes of early fluid therapy compared with limited sepsis resuscitation are ongoing. Conservative fluid management after sepsis resuscitation is being studied in the United States and Europe. Pending further evidence, an initial 20 mL/kg IV fluid bolus for patients with severe sepsis or septic shock will remain common practice; the optimal volume and end points of additional fluid administration are unclear.

Crystalloids remain the first-line sepsis resuscitation fluid because they are widely available, inexpensive, and have not been shown to result in worse outcomes. Whether balanced crystalloids result in better organ function or outcomes is the focus of ongoing trials. Despite extensive study, the effect of albumin solutions on sepsis outcomes remains unclear. HES is the only semisynthetic colloid robustly studied in sepsis and increases the incidence of AKI and potentially mortality. Ongoing research on the endothelial glycocalyx, balanced crystalloids, and early albumin administration hold the potential to further improve sepsis survival.

## REFERENCES

1. Angus DC, van der Poll T. Severe sepsis and septic shock. N Engl J Med 2013;369:840–51.
2. Investigators ProCESS, Yealy DM, Kellum JA, et al. A randomized trial of protocol-based care for early septic shock. N Engl J Med 2014;370:1683–93.
3. ARISE Investigators, ANZICS Clinical Trials Group, Peake SL, et al. Goal-directed resuscitation for patients with early septic shock. N Engl J Med 2014; 371:1496–506.
4. Mouncey PR, Osborn TM, Power GS, et al. Trial of early, goal-directed resuscitation for septic shock. N Engl J Med 2015;372:1301–11.
5. Rivers E, Nguyen B, Havstad S, et al. Early goal-directed therapy in the treatment of severe sepsis and septic shock. N Engl J Med 2001;345:1368–77.
6. Dellinger RP, Levy MM, Rhodes A, et al. Surviving sepsis campaign: international guidelines for management of severe sepsis and septic shock: 2012. Crit Care Med 2013;41:580–637.
7. Marik PE, Cavallazzi R. Does the central venous pressure predict fluid responsiveness? an updated meta-analysis and a plea for some common sense. Crit Care Med 2013;41:1774–81.
8. Woodcock TE, Woodcock TM. Revised Starling equation and the glycocalyx model of transvascular fluid exchange: an improved paradigm for prescribing intravenous fluid therapy. Br J Anaesth 2012; 108:384–94.
9. Kaukonen K-M, Bailey M, Suzuki S, et al. Mortality related to severe sepsis and septic shock among critically ill patients in Australia and New Zealand, 2000-2012. JAMA 2014;311:1308–16.
10. Maitland K, Kiguli S, Opoka RO, et al. Mortality after fluid bolus in African children with severe infection. N Engl J Med 2011;364:2483–95.
11. Maitland K, George EC, Evans JA, et al. Exploring mechanisms of excess mortality with early fluid resuscitation: insights from the FEAST trial. BMC Med 2013;11:68.
12. Andrews B, Muchemwa L, Kelly P, et al. Simplified severe sepsis protocol: a randomized controlled trial of modified early goal-directed therapy in Zambia. Crit Care Med 2014;42:2315–24.
13. Feissel M, Michard F, Faller JP, et al. The respiratory variation in inferior vena cava diameter as a guide to fluid therapy. Intensive Care Med 2004;30:1834–7.
14. Marik PE, Monnet X, Teboul JL. Hemodynamic parameters to guide fluid therapy. Ann Intensive Care 2011;1:1.
15. Alhashemi JA, Cecconi M, Hofer CK. Cardiac output monitoring: an integrative perspective. Crit Care 2011;15:214.
16. Yang X, Du B. Does pulse pressure variation predict fluid responsiveness in critically ill patients? a systematic review and meta-analysis. Crit Care 2014; 18:650.
17. Boyd JH, Forbes J, Nakada T, et al. Fluid resuscitation in septic shock: a positive fluid balance and elevated central venous pressure are associated with increased mortality. Crit Care Med 2011;39: 259–65.
18. Micek ST, McEvoy C, McKenzie M, et al. Fluid balance and cardiac function in septic shock as predictors of hospital mortality. Crit Care 2013;17:R246.
19. Vincent J-L, Sakr Y, Sprung CL, et al. Sepsis in European intensive care units: results of the SOAP study. Crit Care Med 2006;34:344–53.
20. National Heart, Lung, and Blood Institute, Acute Respiratory Distress Syndrome (ARDS) Clinical Trials Network, Wiedemann HP, Wheeler AP, et al. Comparison of two fluid-management strategies in acute lung injury. N Engl J Med 2006;354:2564–75.
21. Awad S, Allison SP, Lobo DN. The history of 0.9% saline. Clin Nutr 2008;27(2):179–88.
22. Finfer S, Liu B, Taylor C, et al. Resuscitation fluid use in critically ill adults: an international cross-sectional study in 391 intensive care units. Crit Care 2010;14:R185.

23. Yunos NM, Kim IB, Bellomo R, et al. The biochemical effects of restricting chloride-rich fluids in intensive care. Crit Care Med 2011;39:2419–24.

24. Stewart PA. Modern quantitative acid-base chemistry. Can J Physiol Pharmacol 1983;61:1444–61.

25. Wilcox CS. Regulation of renal blood flow by plasma chloride. J Clin Invest 1983;71:726–35.

26. Chowdhury AH, Cox EF, Francis ST, et al. A randomized, controlled, double-blind crossover study on the effects of 2-L infusions of 0.9% saline and Plasma-Lyte® 148 on renal blood flow velocity and renal cortical tissue perfusion in healthy volunteers. Ann Surg 2012;256:18–24.

27. Wilkes NJ, Woolf R, Mutch M, et al. The effects of balanced versus saline-based hetastarch and crystalloid solutions on acid-base and electrolyte status and gastric mucosal perfusion in elderly surgical patients. Anesth Analg 2001;93:811–6.

28. Yunos NM, Bellomo R, Hegarty C, et al. Association between a chloride-liberal vs chloride-restrictive intravenous fluid administration strategy and kidney injury in critically ill adults. JAMA J Am Med Assoc 2012;308:1566–72.

29. Yunos NM, Bellomo R, Glassford N, et al. Chloride-liberal vs. chloride-restrictive intravenous fluid administration and acute kidney injury: an extended analysis. Intensive Care Med 2015;41:257–64.

30. Krajewski ML, Raghunathan K, Paluszkiewicz SM, et al. Meta-analysis of high- versus low-chloride content in perioperative and critical care fluid resuscitation. Br J Surg 2015;102:24–36.

31. Raghunathan K, Shaw A, Nathanson B, et al. Association between the choice of IV crystalloid and in-hospital mortality among critically ill adults with sepsis*. Crit Care Med 2014;42:1585–91.

32. Shaw AD, Raghunathan K, Peyerl FW, et al. Association between intravenous chloride load during resuscitation and in-hospital mortality among patients with SIRS. Intensive Care Med 2014;40:1897–905.

33. Rochwerg B, Alhazzani W, Sindi A, et al. Fluid resuscitation in sepsis: a systematic review and network meta-analysis. Ann Intern Med 2014;161:347–55.

34. Rochwerg B, Alhazzani W, Gibson A, et al. Fluid type and the use of renal replacement therapy in sepsis: a systematic review and network meta-analysis. Intensive Care Med 2015;41(9):1561–71.

35. Cochrane Injuries Group Albumin Reviewers. Human albumin administration in critically ill patients: systematic review of randomised controlled trials. BMJ 1998;317:235–40.

36. Finfer S, Bellomo R, Boyce N, et al. A comparison of albumin and saline for fluid resuscitation in the intensive care unit. N Engl J Med 2004;350:2247–56.

37. Caironi P, Tognoni G, Masson S, et al. Albumin replacement in patients with severe sepsis or septic shock. N Engl J Med 2014;370:1412–21.

38. Charpentier, J & Mira, JP. Efficacy and tolerance of hyperoncotic albumin administration in septic shock patients: the EARSS study [abstract] Intensive Care Med 2011,37(Suppl 2):S115–S438.

39. Annane D, Siami S, Jaber S, et al. Effects of fluid resuscitation with colloids vs crystalloids on mortality in critically ill patients presenting with hypovolemic shock: the CRISTAL randomized trial. JAMA 2013; 310:1809–17.

40. Delaney AP, Dan A, McCaffrey J, et al. The role of albumin as a resuscitation fluid for patients with sepsis: a systematic review and meta-analysis. Crit Care Med 2011;39:386–91.

41. Bansal M, Farrugia A, Balboni S, et al. Relative survival benefit and morbidity with fluids in severe sepsis: a network meta-analysis of alternative therapies. Curr Drug Saf 2013;8:236–45.

42. Wiedermann CJ, Joannidis M. Albumin replacement in severe sepsis or septic shock. N Engl J Med 2014;371:83.

43. Patel A, Laffan MA, Waheed U, et al. Randomised trials of human albumin for adults with sepsis: systematic review and meta-analysis with trial sequential analysis of all-cause mortality. BMJ 2014;349:g4561.

44. Brunkhorst FM, Engel C, Bloos F, et al. Intensive insulin therapy and pentastarch resuscitation in severe sepsis. N Engl J Med 2008;358:125–39.

45. Guidet B, Martinet O, Boulain T, et al. Assessment of hemodynamic efficacy and safety of 6% hydroxyethyl starch 130/0.4 vs. 0.9% NaCl fluid replacement in patients with severe sepsis: the CRYSTMAS study. Crit Care 2012;16:R94.

46. Perner A, Haase N, Guttormsen AB, et al. Hydroxyethyl starch 130/0.42 versus Ringer's acetate in severe sepsis. N Engl J Med 2012;367:124–34.

47. Zarychanski R, Abou-Setta AM, Turgeon AF, et al. Association of hydroxyethyl starch administration with mortality and acute kidney injury in critically ill patients requiring volume resuscitation: a systematic review and meta-analysis. JAMA 2013;309:678–88.

# Vasopressors During Sepsis: Selection and Targets

Jean P. Gelinas, MD[a], James A. Russell, MD[a,b],*

## KEYWORDS

- Vasopressors • Norepinephrine • Epinephrine • Vasopressin • Dobutamine • Milrinone
- Septic shock • Sepsis

## KEY POINTS

- Urgent resuscitation using intravenous fluids and vasopressors is a universally accepted early intervention in septic shock.
- Randomized controlled trials (RCTs) have compared different types of vasopressors, use of vasopressors with inotropic agents, and mean arterial pressure targets.
- RCTs of early goal-directed therapy (EGDT) to optimize oxygen delivery by use of fluids, vasopressors, inotropic agents, and red blood cell transfusion(s) have been studied extensively.
- Recent negative EGDT RCTs have put into question fundamental treatment paradigms of severe sepsis and septic shock such as $SvO_2$ monitoring to titrate resuscitation.
- Better biomarkers of sepsis diagnosis, biomarkers of improved response to vasoactive agents, and biomarkers of prognosis are needed to stratify patients in trials and in clinical care.

## INTRODUCTION

Septic shock is the most serious complication of sepsis and requires emergent recognition and treatment. Considerable efforts have been made to evaluate different therapies for septic shock, but consensus is far from established. Coinciding with improvements in optimal management of septic shock, there is a trend toward improved survival of septic patients.[1–3] Many different strategies of fluid replacement,[4] monitoring[5,6] vasopressor use, and combinations of therapies or goal-directed therapies have now been assessed in large pivotal randomized controlled trials (RCTs). The complexity of the literature prompted various groups to create the Surviving Sepsis Campaign Guidelines in 2004.[7] The most recent version of The Surviving Sepsis Campaign guidelines attempt to organize available information up to 2012 into practical guidelines and bundles.[1] More recent updates can be found at www.survivingsepsis.org. Herein, we review questions, answers, and clinical application for selection of vasopressor support in septic shock. We focus on high-level evidence RCTs despite concerns that such evidence does not routinely lead to changes in practice.[8,9] We then proceed to discuss exciting new targets under investigation.

## HYPOTENSION, SHOCK, AND MEASUREMENT OF ARTERIAL PRESSURE

Sepsis-mediated hypotension is the clinical manifestation of the interactions of venous and arterial vasoplegia, hypovolemia and myocardial depression.

Financial Disclosures: Canadian Institutes of Health Research, Grant number: MCT 44152, Registration: ISRCTN94845869.
[a] Centre for Heart Lung Innovation, St. Paul's Hospital, Department of Medicine, University of British Columbia, 1081 Burrard Street, Vancouver, British Columbia V6Z 1Y6, Canada; [b] Division of Critical Care Medicine, St. Paul's Hospital, University of British Columbia, 1081 Burrard Street, Vancouver, British Columbia V6Z 1Y6, Canada
* Corresponding author. Centre for Heart Lung Innovation, St. Paul's Hospital, 1081 Burrard Street, Vancouver, British Columbia V6Z 1Y6, Canada.
E-mail address: Jim.Russell@hli.ubc.ca

Clin Chest Med 37 (2016) 251–262
http://dx.doi.org/10.1016/j.ccm.2016.01.008
0272-5231/16/$ – see front matter © 2016 Elsevier Inc. All rights reserved.

chestmed.theclinics.com

The 2001 Society of Critical Care Medicine/European Society of Intensive Care Medicine/American College of Chest Physicians/American Trauma Society/Surgical Infection Society International Sepsis Definitions Conference defined severe sepsis as sepsis complicated by organ dysfunction. Septic shock refers to a state of acute circulatory failure characterized by persistent arterial hypotension unexplained by other causes. In this 2001 consensus hypotension is defined by a systolic arterial pressure of less than 90 mm Hg, a mean arterial pressure (MAP) of less than 60, or a decrease in systolic blood pressure of 40 mm Hg from baseline, despite adequate volume resuscitation, in the absence of other causes for hypotension.[10]

How should arterial pressure be measured and monitored?[1,11,12] The 2013 Surviving Sepsis Guidelines recommend that patients who are receiving vasopressors have an arterial catheter[1] yet 2 very recent large RCT of early goal-directed therapy (EGDT) did not mandate this in their study protocol.[13,14] Arterial catheters are often suggested because pressure measured invasively can differ from noninvasive blood pressure measurement and this can, therefore, alter clinical decisions. These differences between invasive versus noninvasive arterial pressure are somewhat minimized by using MAP.[15,16] Dorman and colleagues[17] showed that patients receiving high doses of norepinephrine could have clinically meaningful differences in MAP and systolic arterial pressure when comparing invasive radial and femoral blood pressures. Using femoral instead of radial arterial pressure resulted in frequent and meaningful reductions in vasopressor support.[17] Furthermore, nurses and physicians in the intensive care unit (ICU) sometimes chose to disregard radial arterial pressure readings in favor of noninvasive blood pressure when radial artery catheters gave 'positional readings' or were otherwise deemed unreliable. Few if any of the studies mentioned in this review seem to have mentioned or taken into consideration faulty radial artery blood pressure measurements in their interpretation of the data. This seems a little surprising, considering that so much emphasis is put on that one hemodynamic measurement.

### Recommendation for Clinical Practice

Noninvasive blood pressure monitoring is indicated for most patients requiring vasopressors.

## WHAT IS THE TARGET MEAN ARTERIAL PRESSURE FOR SEPTIC SHOCK?

Recent reviews and guidelines have recommended 65 mm Hg as the threshold MAP below which

therapies to increase MAP should be started[1,11,12] based on knowledge of physiology and expert opinion. A scenario-based questionnaire reported in 2011 of Canadian Intensivists seemed to demonstrate that intensivists are using vasopressors in a relatively homogenous way. MAP was the most commonly used and initiation of vasopressors was usually begun when the MAP was less than 60 mm Hg and target MAP was about 65 mm Hg. Intensivists almost uniformly raised targeted MAP for patients with severe chronic hypertension and past cerebrovascular injury with known vascular stenosis. MAP target modifications for other comorbidities were less frequent or less consistent. Digital cyanosis or livido reticularis prompted almost one-half of clinicians to lower vasopressors, whereas low urine output and the doubling of the creatinine motivated about one-third of respondents to increase vasopressors.[18]

Because blood pressure target recommendations were historically based on low quality evidence Asfar and colleagues[19] designed and completed an important large multicenter RCT of 776 patients with septic shock randomized to a high target MAP (80–85 mm Hg) or to a low target MAP group (60–65 mm Hg) for 5 days. Fluid administration was equivalent in both groups and significantly higher doses of vasopressors were used in the high MAP target group. Both the low and high MAP groups exceeded their target MAP. Survival at 28 days (primary end point) and 90 days was not different. Atrial fibrillation was more frequent in the high MAP group, but strokes were not evaluated as an endpoint. In the prospectively defined group of patients with hypertension (about 40% of enrolled patients had baseline hypertension), those that were assigned to the high MAP group had significantly less renal dysfunction and renal replacement therapy.[19] This RCT leads us to suggest that routinely targeting a high MAP in septic shock is not warranted because high MAP target did not lower mortality but increased de novo atrial fibrillation.[20] Second, a high MAP target may decrease incidence of acute kidney injury and need for renal replacement therapy (number needed to treat of 9.5 to prevent 1 patient from needing renal replacement therapy) in patients with hypertension. Interestingly, fluid resuscitation varies widely between RCTs of septic shock. Asfar and colleagues[19] used less fluid and higher doses of norepinephrine than was used in some other trials,[21,22] but used less norepinephrine and similar fluids when compared with 1 other trial.[23] This variability in fluid use suggests that, as with vasopressors and many things in septic shock management, optimal fluid use is far from an exact science.

## Recommendation for Clinical Practice

The target MAP for septic shock is 60 to 65 mm Hg, except in patients with preexisting hypertension in whom a target MAP of 80 to 85 mm Hg is recommended because of less need of renal replacement therapy, but with some increased risk of atrial fibrillation.

## COMPARISONS OF VASOPRESSORS FOR SEPTIC SHOCK

An extensive 2011 Cochrane review of vasopressors for hypotensive shock analyzed data from 23 RCTs in 3212 patients (overall mortality rate of 50%; **Fig. 1, Table 1**). Six different vasopressors, alone or in combination with dobutamine or dopexamine, were studied in different comparisons. Norepinephrine versus dopamine, the largest comparison in 1400 patients from 6 RCTs, yielded similar mortality. Dopamine increased the risk of arrhythmias. Vasopressors used as add-on therapy in comparison with placebo were not effective either. The authors concluded that there was not sufficient evidence to prove that any of the vasopressors were superior to others and that the choice of a specific vasopressor may, therefore, be individualized and left to the discretion of the treating physicians. When discussing the implications for future research the Cochrane authors suggested that, "Maybe a more suitable approach to the treatment of shock is not the choice of a specific vasopressor but a goal directed approach (Rivers 2001). To the best of our knowledge this has not yet been assessed in a systematic way."[24] (A very recent systematic review and meta-analysis of EGDT as well as an invited accompanying editorial were reported [ICM 2105 in press] see below Early Goal-Directed Therapy for more detail.)

The 2013 Surviving Sepsis Guidelines are more prescriptive than the Cochrane Review. Norepinephrine is recommended as first choice vasopressor based on high-quality evidence. Epinephrine may be added to or substituted for norepinephrine when an additional agent is needed to maintain adequate blood pressure based on less clear evidence.[1] A Canadian intensivists' survey found that norepinephrine was the most commonly used first-line vasopressor (95% of respondents). About 80% of the respondents who selected norepinephrine as a first-line agent chose vasopressin as an alternate first-line agent.[18]

In addition to well-known adverse effects of beta-adrenergic agents on arrhythmias, tachycardia, and peripheral ischemia at high doses, there is a growing body of literature linking powerful beta-adrenergic agonists (including epinephrine) to type 2 lactic acidosis.[25–27] The recent intriguing placebo-controlled RCT showing that the beta-blocker esmolol seemed to decrease mortality of septic shock highlights the potential adverse effects of beta-adrenergic agents and the potential efficacy of esmolol.[28,29] Further multicenter RCTs of esmolol are needed before recommending it for routine clinical care.

There is a profound deficiency of vasopressin early in septic shock because of decreased output of vasopressin from the posterior pituitary gland.

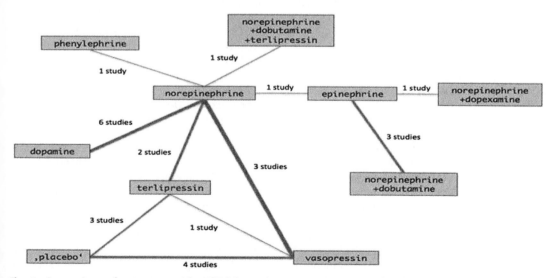

**Fig. 1.** Comparison of vasopressor identified from the systematic review. The 26 comparisons come from 23 studies. Line thickness is proportional to the number of included patients. (*From* Havel C, Arrich J, Losert H, et al. Vasopressors for hypotensive shock. Cochrane Database Syst Rev 2011;(5):CD003709; with permission.)

**Table 1**
**Pivotal RCTs of vasopressors in septic shock**

| Author, Year | Treatment (n) | Control Intervention (n) | Treatment Mortality Rate (%) | Control Mortality Rate (%) | P |
|---|---|---|---|---|---|
| De Backer et al,[23] 2010 | Dopamine | Norepinephrine | 52.5 | 48.5 | .10 |
| Russell et al,[22] 2008 | Vasopressin + norepinephrine | Norepinephrine | 35.4 | 39.3 | .26 |
| Annane et al,[51] 2007 | Norepinephrine + dobutamine | Epinephrine | 34 | 40 | .31 |
| Myburgh et al,[21] 2008 | Epinephrine | Norepinephrine | 30.4 | 34.3 | .49 |

Vasopressin has potential advantages to augment vasopressors in septic shock because small studies showed that vasopressin decreased need for vasopressors in septic shock through its direct V1a-mediated vasopressor action and indirectly because vasopressin increases responsiveness to adrenergic agents (such as norepinephrine). In the Vasopressin versus Norepinephrine Infusion in Patients with Septic Shock (VASST) study, vasopressin plus norepinephrine had similar mortality to norepinephrine-treated patients.[22] Vasopressin is recommended as a second agent in patients who are not responsive to norepinephrine.[1] In VASST and subsequent substudies, vasopressin plus norepinephrine[22] seemed to decrease mortality in patients who had less severe septic shock and decrease risk of acute kidney injury and need for renal replacement therapy in patients at risk of acute kidney injury.[30] Furthermore, there is an interaction of vasopressin and corticosteroids (the combination was beneficial) in VASST[31] that is being validated in an ongoing RCT.[32] The Surviving Sepsis Guidelines state that vasopressin is not recommended as the single initial vasopressor and vasopressin doses higher than 0.03 to 0.04 U/min should be reserved for use when MAP targets are not attained with other vasopressor agents. We suggest that higher doses of vasopressin (>0.04 U/min) should be used only in research studies to better define the safety of these doses. No level of conviction as to the strength of the Surviving Sepsis Guidelines recommendation evidence was given despite publication of VASST, a large pivotal blinded multicenter RCT of vasopressin plus norepinephrine versus norepinephrine. Vasopressin should be titrated and weaned after a period of some hours off other vasopressors such as norepinephrine, in decrements of 0.01/U.min over 30 to 90 minutes.

A large RCT of dopamine versus norepinephrine in shock found no difference in mortality, but dopamine use was associated with increased risk of arrhythmias and increased heart rate.[23] Accordingly, dopamine should be reserved for use as an alternative vasopressor agent to norepinephrine only in highly selected patients, such patients with bradycardia and at low risk of developing arrhythmia. Phenylephrine is not recommended except in uncommon specific circumstances like norepinephrine-induced arrhythmias. Finally, low-dose dopamine should not be used for renal protection[1] because of a lack of efficacy.[33,34]

### Recommendation for Clinical Practice

We recommend norepinephrine as the first-line vasopressor with epinephrine or vasopressin as a reasonable second-line vasopressor(s).

## GOAL-DIRECTED THERAPIES

Clinicians and investigators have used therapies with defined goals for resuscitation, so-called EGDT of septic shock (**Table 2**). This is relevant herein because vasopressor use is embedded in EGDT so we narrow the focus of this discussion to what we have learned about vasopressors in RCTs of EGDT. In the 1990s, RCTs of supraphysiologic oxygen delivery proved unrewarding; all were negative or showed harm[35] of supraphysiologic oxygen delivery. That supernormal oxygen delivery showed no value and possibly harmful[35–37] forced reevaluation of resuscitation of septic shock. Perhaps interventions were neither early nor aggressive enough.[38–40]

Rivers and colleagues' single-center RCT compared 6 hour emergency department-initiated EGDT versus standard care (MAP >65 mm Hg, CVP 8–12 mm Hg, and urine output > 0.5 mL/kg/h). In the EGDT group, a target continuous superior vena cava oxygen saturation (SvO$_2$ $\geq$70%) was added. Interventions to achieve central venous oxygen saturation (ScvO$_2$) target included RBC

**Table 2**
Goal-directed therapy in randomized controlled trials

| Study | Trial and Characteristics | Hypothesis Tested | Therapeutic Intervention | Pressure Target(s) | Hb/Hct Target(s) | Trial Results |
|---|---|---|---|---|---|---|
| Supernormal oxygen delivery ($DO_2$) Hayes et al,[35] 1994 | 2 center RCT n = 109 critically ill patients | Supernormal $DO_2$ | Volume Dobutamine Dopamine | MAP >80 | Hb 10 | Increased mortality in intervention group |
| Goal-oriented hemodynamic therapy Gattinoni et al,[36] 1995 | Multicentre n = 762 critically ill patients | Supernormal $DO_2$ (PAC CO) vs $SvO_2$ >70 vs normal cardiac index | Volume Dobutamine Dopamine) Nitroprusside Nitrates) Epinephrine Norepinephrine | MAP >60 Wedge <18 CVP 8–12 | Hct 30 | No difference in mortality |
| EGDT Rivers et al,[38] 2001 | Single center n = 263 severe sepsis | 6-h ER EGDT (continuous $SvO_2$) vs usual care | $SvO_2$ ≥70% dobutamine CVP 8–12 MAP ≥65 norepinephrine Epinephrine, dopamine, or phenylephrine | MAP >65 CVP 8–12 | If $SvO_2$ <70% 1. RBC to Htc >30 2. Dobutamine | Mortality lower in EGDT group |
| Lactate clearance vs $SvO_2$ in early sepsis Jones et al,[85] 2010 | 3-center RCT n = 300 septic | $ScvO_2$ goals vs Serial lactate clearance | Crystalloids, dopamine, or norepinephrine Dobutamine depending on $SvO_2$ vs lactate clearance | MAP ≥65 CVP ≥8 | If $SvO_2$ <70% RBC if Hct <30 Lactate clearance group: if lactate not decreasing RBC if Hct <30 | No difference in mortality |
| Protocol-Based Care for Early Septic Shock The ProCESS Investigators,[13] 2014 | 31 centers n = 1351 severe septic patients | EGTD $SvO_2$ vs clinical protocol vs usual care (no protocol) | $SvO_2$ threshold 70% dobutamine vs ProCESS protocol: clinical protocol vs usual care | EGDT MAP ≥65 CVP 8–12 ProCESS protocol: SAP ≥100 Shock index ≥0.8 Usual care | EGDT Hct ≥30 ProCESS protocol: Hb ≥7.5 Usual care | No difference in mortality |

(continued on next page)

**Table 2**
*(continued)*

| Study | Trial and Characteristics | Hypothesis Tested | Therapeutic Intervention | Pressure Target(s) | Hb/Hct Target(s) | Trial Results |
|---|---|---|---|---|---|---|
| Goal-Directed Resuscitation in Early Septic Shock Mouncey[14], 2015 | 51 centers n = 1600 severe sepsis patients | EGDT SvO2-guided protocol vs usual care | EGDT: SvO2 >70% dobutamine vs usual care | EGDT: MAP >65 CVP ≥8 (spontaneous ventilation) CVP ≥12 (mechanical ventilation) Usual care | EGDT: SvO2 <70% RBC if: Hb <100 or Htc <30 Usual care | No difference in mortality |
| Early, Goal-Directed Resuscitation for Septic Shock ProMISe Trial Investigators,[14] 2015 | 56 centers n = 1243 severe sepsis patients | EGDT SvO2 vs usual care | EGDT SvO2 >70% dobutamine vs usual care | EGDT MAP >65 SBP >90 CVP ≥8 Usual care | EGDT: SvO2<70% RBC if Hb <100 or dobutamine if Hb ≥100 Usual care | No difference in mortality |
| Levosimendan Morellia et al,[80] 2010 | 1 center 50 septic shock patients | Levisimendan (n = 20) vs comparator (dobutamine 5 µg·kg⁻¹ min⁻¹; control (n = 20) | Levisimendan (n = 20) vs comparator (dobutamine 5 µg·kg⁻¹ min⁻¹; control (n = 20) | NA | NA | Microcirculatory flow higher in levosimendan |
| Milrinone Wang et al,[84] 2015 | 1 center 90 severe sepsis patients control (n = 30), milrinone (n = 30), and milrinone-esmolol (n = 30) | control (n = 30) vs milrinone (n = 30) vs milrinone-esmolol (n = 30) | control (n = 30) vs milrinone (n = 30) vs milrinone-esmolol (N = 30) | NA | NA | ME lower 28-day mortality |

*Abbreviations:* CO, cardiac output; CVP, central venous pressure; EGDT, early goal-directed therapy; ER, emergency room; Hb, hemoglobin; Hct, hematocrit; MAP, mean arterial pressure; NA, not applicable; PAC, pulmonary artery catheter; RBC, red blood cells; RCT, randomized controlled trial; SAP, systolic arterial pressure; ScvO2, central venous oxygen saturation; SvO2, mixed venous oxygen saturation; Wedge, pulmonary capillary wedge pressure.

transfusions (target Hct >30) and dobutamine. The EGDT group had significantly decreased hospital mortality (30.5 vs 46.5%; $P = .009$).

How did the intervention differ from standard care group regarding vasopressors? Vasopressors were equivalent in both groups (EGDT patients received more crystalloids, blood, and inotropic agents) during the first 6 hours. Specific vasopressor selection was not controlled or evaluated.[38] The 2008 Surviving Sepsis Guidelines incorporated EGDT and before/after case control nonrandomized trials suggested that EGDT decreased mortality.[41–43]

Rivers' EGDT was controversial because it was single center, the control mortality rate was high, and the baseline $ScvO_2$ was about 50%. Three subsequent multicenter RCTs of EGDT compared with usual care found no differences in mortality. ProCESS[13] (US-based) compared EGDT with 2 control groups (protocol-based resuscitation and usual care). The 'ProCESS protocol-based group' had a central venous catheter inserted if peripheral access was inadequate. Administration of fluids and vasopressors was guided by blood pressure targets and shock index (heart rate/systolic blood pressure). Regarding vasopressors, vasopressor choice was not prespecified. Mortality rates were similar in all groups. More vasopressors were given to the ProCESS and EGDT protocol groups than the usual care group and dobutamine was administered more in the EGDT group (8%) then in the ProCESS (1.1%) or the usual care groups (0.9%). Regarding later times, vasopressor and dobutamine use was similar from 6 to 72 hours.[13]

ARISE[44,45] (Australia/New Zealand [ANZICS]-based) RCT used Rivers' EGDT algorithm until 6 hours after randomization. Vasopressors (not guided by protocol) could include norepinephrine, epinephrine, dopamine, vasopressin, metaraminol, or phenylephrine. Prerandomization vasopressors in the EGDT and usual care groups were similar. Regarding later vasopressors, the EGDT group received more vasopressors (66.6% vs 57.8%; duration did not differ significantly) and more dobutamine (15.4% vs 2.6%) during the first 6 hours. From 6 to 72 hours, the EGDT group received more vasopressors (58.8% vs 51.5%) and dobutamine (9.5% vs 5.0%). Mortality at 28 and 90 days was similar in the EGDT and the usual-care groups (18.6% and 18.8%, respectively).

The ProMISe[14] (UK-based) RCT of $ScvO_2$ monitoring versus usual care[14] harmonized with ProCESS and ARISE for metaanalysis.[13,44] The EGDT group received more 'advanced cardiovascular support' (presumably vasopressors) and had longer ICU stay, but there was no difference in mortality (29.5% EGDT vs 29.2% usual care).

## Recommendation for Clinical Practice

Recent negative EGDT RCTs have put into question the fundamental treatment paradigms of severe sepsis and septic shock, such as $SvO_2$ monitoring to titrate resuscitation.

## IMPROVED OUTCOMES OF SEPSIS AND SEPTIC SHOCK

There is growing evidence of improved outcomes of severe sepsis and septic shock. A very large observational cohort study showed that patients in Australia and New Zealand suffering from severe sepsis and septic shock have had a remarkable improvement in outcome (from 35% to 18.4% mortality rates) over the last 12 years.[2] In the United States, Stevenson and colleagues[3] analyzed the outcomes of patients in the 'usual care' control arms of 36 severe sepsis RCTs dating back to 1991. Patients in the control arms have had progressively better outcomes over time (from 46.9% to 29%). The authors also evaluated 1993 to 2009 discharge data from Nationwide Inpatient Sample and that validated that severe sepsis mortality was decreasing.[3]

The reasons for this generalized trend toward improved survival of severe sepsis and septic shock are unclear. Levy and colleagues[46] demonstrated that patients from hospitals that had higher success rates of adoption of the Surviving Sepsis Guidelines and Bundles have improved survival compared with patients from hospitals that were less successful in the implementation of the Sepsis Guidelines and Bundles.

Some authors have questioned whether the recent decreases in mortality rates of severe sepsis and septic shock are real and only reflect changes in coding of severe sepsis in administrative databases.[47–49] Changes in hospital accreditation after publication of Rivers RCT included much greater emphasis on quality of early sepsis care in the emergency room and that could have led to much more inclusion of less severe cases of sepsis that would have been missed in prior reviews. Another possibility could be that patients with terminal diseases are now more readily given access to palliative care and are therefore no longer considered candidates for ICU admission. This would make it more likely that their deaths are classified or coded as caused by their primary terminal conditions and not sepsis. This systemic exclusion of patients with a certain upcoming mortality would significantly improve survival rates for those patients who do get admitted to an ICU.[50] Needless to say, it remains controversial whether, by how much, and why sepsis outcomes have improved.

## Recommendation for Clinical Practice

Mortality of septic shock has decreased. It remains controversial whether, by how much, and why sepsis outcomes have improved.

## INOTROPIC AGENT USE WHILE ON VASOPRESSORS

The Surviving Sepsis Guidelines recommend that inotropic agents should not be used to increase cardiac index to supranormal levels but that "a trial of dobutamine infusion up to 20 μg/kg/min be administered or added to vasopressors (if in use) in the presence of (a) myocardial dysfunction as suggested by elevated cardiac filling pressures and low cardiac output, or (b) ongoing signs of hypoperfusion, despite achieving adequate intravascular volume and adequate MAP." This recommendation is graded 1C (strongly believed recommendation but based on low-quality evidence).[1]

The few RCTs done to evaluate the possible specific benefits of dobutamine in septic shock were structured in way that make interpretation of the role of dobutamine difficult. The biggest dobutamine RCT randomized septic patients to either receive epinephrine (n = 161) or norepinephrine plus dobutamine (n = 169). Comparison of norepinephrine and dobutamine versus epinephrine and a placebo infusion was done using a predetermined titration algorithm. Drug titration was done to maintain: mean blood pressure at 70 mm Hg or more and normal cardiac performance as assessed by various locally selected diagnostic methods (right heart catheterization, Doppler echocardiography, pulse contour cardiac output, or esophageal Doppler ultrasonography). The trial results showed mortality up to 90 days to be nearly identical (50% vs 52%) and that other outcome measures were also nearly identical in both groups. The group of patients receiving epinephrine did have persistently lower pH levels and higher initial lactic acid levels then the norepinephrine and dobutamine group.[51] Other studies comparing epinephrine administration versus a combination of norepinephrine and dobutamine (or dopexamine) were very small and provide limited clinically outcome measures that could meaningfully help to determine the usefulness of dobutamine (or dopexamine) in septic shock management.[52–54]

## Recommendation for Clinical Practice

Dobutamine (or another inotropic agents such as milrinone) are needed in a minority of patients who have ventricular dysfunction during septic shock.

## MONITORING PATIENTS WHO REQUIRE VASOPRESSORS

Determining which patients could potentially benefit from increased fluid administration and/or inotropic support is often difficult to decide when based only on clinical information. Because of these limitations, methods to assist in the evaluation of blood pressure and cardiac output responses to various therapeutic interventions are important and have become integral components in the treatment of septic patients. These measuring and monitoring techniques range from the very simple and easy to perform to the complex and highly specialized. A detailed analysis of these different methodologies is beyond the scope of this review, but the authors feel that this topic is so intimately associated with the use of inotropic agents that we need to at least touch on it. At the 'easy, cheap and simple' end of the diagnostic methodology spectrum the passive leg raising test, a noninvasive test, is reasonably accurate and reliable to evaluate fluid challenge responsiveness.[55] At the other end of the technology spectrum, echocardiography can be a valuable tool for the titration of fluid, vasopressor, and inotropic agents. The precise role of echocardiography in septic shock management is still not clearly established, however, because of a lack of large, rigorous, multicenter RCTs powered for mortality. Optimal selection of septic patients who should or could potentially benefit from echocardiographic assessment is limited in part by delays in availability of the equipment and variable 'around the clock' technical expertise to interpreting the images. These and other barriers have limited more widespread use of this potentially powerful technology.[56–60]

Echocardiography and other noninvasive cardiac output measurement systems are inherently safer than pulmonary artery catheter monitoring. In addition to the specific technical limitations of these systems, it remains to be seen whether 'inotropic hemodynamic optimization' using echocardiographic (or any other technology) will prove to be of significantly greater efficacy and effectiveness than usual care or whether we see a repeat of negative results of inotropic/pulmonary artery catheter–guided RCTs. The vasopressor and inotropic therapies currently recommended and used clinically to optimize hemodynamic status are similar, if not identical, to what were used in the many negative prior RCTs.[35,61,62] Ironically, the Italian esmolol RCT showed that patients given esmolol had improved survival yet cardiac outputs decreased, norepinephrine needs decreased, stroke volume increased, and glomerular filtration rates increased. It is worth noting that patients with cardiac failure (cardiac index $\leq 2.2$ and pulmonary occlusion pressures >18) were excluded from the RCT and that the average baseline cardiac index in the esmolol treated group was 4.0 versus about 3.6 in the control group.[28] Generally, these would not be patients who would be considered candidates for inotropic administration.[1] It is nevertheless difficult to accept that both beta-blockers and beta-agonists could both prove effective in the same septic patient population. Perhaps specific subgroups of patients benefit from these opposing interventions. For example, the evolutionary complexities of the stress response call for different approaches to adrenergic modulation at different stages of sepsis process?[29] More rigorous studies to discover, validate, and precisely define the responsive subgroups for inotropic versus beta-blocker treatment (eg, by clinical or biomarker selection), followed by large, well-powered RCTs are needed to better understand how and when we should use inotropic agents versus beta-blockers in septic shock.

It is also unclear as to how we should monitor inotropic response to treatment in low output states. To the best of our knowledge no RCT has convincingly and reproducibly shown vasoactive therapy guided by a 'cardiac output monitoring system(s)' to be clinically superior in terms of efficacy to decrease mortality in septic patients. Despite this lack of evidence, some now consider echocardiography to be a routine modality for cardiovascular assessment of all ICU patients[63–65] because echocardiography can discover unsuspected clinically relevant diagnostic information[66] in shock[65] and in other serious life-threatening situations.[67–70] That routine echocardiography findings improve outcome is far from certain.[71] A very detailed and comprehensive review of echocardiography in critically ill patients was recently done by The World Interactive Network Focused on Critical UltraSound.[72]

### Recommendation for Clinical Practice

The passive leg raising test, a noninvasive test, is reasonably accurate and reliable to evaluate fluid challenge responsiveness. Echocardiography and other noninvasive cardiac output measurement systems are inherently safer than pulmonary artery catheter monitoring, and echocardiography can discover unsuspected clinically relevant diagnostic information in shock. More studies are required validate and define the responsive subgroups for inotropic versus beta-blocker treatment.

## MILRINONE AND LEVOSIMENDAN TO SUPPLEMENT VASOPRESSORS

Milrinone[73–76] and levosimendan[77,78] are both inotropic agents that have been used, similar to dobutamine, as inotropic agents to supplement vasopressors in patients who have impaired ventricular function. Both are also vasodilators so are sometimes limited by worsening of hypotension. Neither is a beta-adrenergic agent and so do not suffer from beta-adrenergic receptor downregulation and tolerance to beat-adrenergic stimulation.

Levosimendan could have antiinflammatory and antioxidative properties, and can potentially decrease the deleterious effects of reactive oxygen species on the tissues.[79] A small RCT showed that, compared with low-dose dobutamine (5 $\mu g\,kg^{-1}min^{-1}$), levosimendan improved markers of microcirculatory blood flow.[80] Levosimendan has also been shown to control the decrease in cardiac output that can occur after vasopressin in a bovine model of septic shock.[81]

Levosimendan is now undergoing evaluation in a large in the UK.[82] This innovative RCT will assess efficacy of levosimendan to reduce acute organ dysfunction and evaluate its biological mechanisms of action in adult septic shock.

The use of inotropic agents remains controversial also because of observational propensity-scored controlled cohort studies showing that even after adjusting for baseline risks of death, use of inotropic agents is associated with increased mortality rates.[83]

### Recommendation for Clinical Practice

Dobutamine (or another inotropic agents such as milrinone) are needed in a minority of patients who have ventricular dysfunction in sepsis. Levosimendan is now undergoing evaluation in a large in the UK.

## SUMMARY

Regardless of the almost consistently negative RCTs, patients with septic shock may have lower mortality, but the degree and cause(s) of this change remain unknown. Perhaps priorities such as early, appropriate broad-spectrum antibiotics matters more than precise titration of specific vasopressors. We suggest that the clinician still lacks the optimal tools to assess adequacy of resuscitation and, accordingly, the need for, type, and dose(s) of vasopressors. We are aligned with international guidelines in recommending norepinephrine as first vasopressor if fluid resuscitation does not achieve resuscitation goals. Vasopressin or epinephrine may be added as second vasopressors.

Dobutamine (or another inotropic agents, such as milrinone) are needed in a minority of patients who have ventricular dysfunction in sepsis. Regarding EGDT, we recommend that routine use of EGDT including $ScvO_2$ in adult severe sepsis not be used in the developed world. Further studies of EGDT in children, in emerging countries, and/or different endpoints and algorithms would be helpful to clinicians everywhere.

Basic, translational and clinical research should have several complementary aims. First, we need to better define biomarkers of sepsis diagnosis (diagnostic biomarkers), biomarkers of improved response to vasoactive agents (predictive biomarkers), and biomarkers of prognosis (prognostic biomarkers) to better stratify patients in trials and in clinical care. Second, novel interventions such as esmolol require a better understanding of the mechanism of action in septic shock and who to treat (based on new RCTs). Third, we need a better understanding of the molecular and clinical interactions of the combinations of therapies so commonly used in septic shock (ie, vasopressors, inotropic agents, corticosteroids). Finally, we need a further understanding of novel targets to further improve outcomes of septic shock.

## REFERENCES

1. Dellinger RP, Levy MM, Rhodes A, et al. Surviving sepsis campaign: international guidelines for management of severe sepsis and septic shock: 2012. Crit Care Med 2013;41:580–637.
2. Kaukonen K-M, Bailey M, Suzuki S, et al. Mortality related to severe sepsis and septic shock among critically ill patients in Australia and New Zealand, 2000-2012. JAMA 2014;311(13):1308–9.
3. Stevenson EK, Rubenstein AR, Radin GT, et al. Two decades of mortality trends among patients with severe sepsis: a comparative meta-analysis*. Crit Care Med 2014;42(3):625–31.
4. Seymour CW, Angus DC. Making a pragmatic choice for fluid resuscitation in critically ill patients. JAMA 2013;310(17):1803–4.
5. Connors AF, Speroff T, Dawson NV, et al. The effectiveness of right heart catheterization in the initial care of critically ill patients. SUPPORT Investigators. JAMA 1996;276(11):889–97.
6. Rajaram SS, Desai NK, Kalra A. Pulmonary artery catheters for adult patients in intensive care. Cochrane Database Syst Rev 2013;(2):CD003408.
7. Dellinger RP, Carlet JM, Masur H, et al. Surviving Sepsis Campaign guidelines for management of severe sepsis and septic shock. Crit Care Med 2004;32:858–73.
8. Hussey MA, Hughes JP. Design and analysis of stepped wedge cluster randomized trials. Contemp Clin Trials 2007;28(2):182–91.
9. Kalil AC, Sun J. Why are clinicians not embracing the results from pivotal clinical trials in severe sepsis? A bayesian analysis. PLoS One 2008;3(5):e2291.
10. Levy MM, Fink MP, Marshall JC, et al. 2001 SCCM/ESICM/ACCP/ATS/SIS international sepsis definitions conference. Crit Care Med 2003;31:1250–6.
11. Finfer SR, Vincent J-L, De Backer D. Circulatory shock. N Engl J Med 2013;369(18):1726–34.
12. Angus DC, van der Poll T. Severe sepsis and septic shock. N Engl J Med 2013;369(9):840–51.
13. The ProCESS Investigators. A randomized trial of protocol-based care for early septic shock. N Engl J Med 2014;370(18):1683–93.
14. Mouncey PR, Osborn TM, Power GS, et al. Trial of early, goal-directed resuscitation for septic shock. N Engl J Med 2015;372(14):1301–11.
15. Lehman L-WH, Saeed M, Talmor D, et al. Methods of blood pressure measurement in the ICU. Crit Care Med 2013;41(1):34–40.
16. Wax DB, Lin H-M, Leibowitz AB. Invasive and concomitant noninvasive intraoperative blood pressure monitoring: observed differences in measurements and associated therapeutic interventions. Anesthesiology 2011;115(5):973–8.
17. Dorman T, Breslow MJ, Lipsett PA, et al. Radial artery pressure monitoring underestimates central arterial pressure during vasopressor therapy in critically ill surgical patients. Crit Care Med 1998;26(10):1646–9.
18. Lamontagne F, Cook DJ, Adhikari NKJ, et al. Vasopressor administration and sepsis: a survey of Canadian intensivists. J Crit Care 2011;26(5):532.e1–7.
19. Asfar P, Meziani F, Hamel J-F, et al. High versus low blood-pressure target in patients with septic shock. N Engl J Med 2014;370(17):1583–93.
20. Russell JA. Is there a good MAP for septic shock? N Engl J Med 2014;370(17):1649–51.
21. Myburgh JA, Higgins A, Jovanovska A, et al. A comparison of epinephrine and norepinephrine in critically ill patients. Intensive Care Med 2008;34(12):2226–34.
22. Russell JA, Walley KR, Singer J, et al. Vasopressin versus norepinephrine infusion in patients with septic shock. N Engl J Med 2008;358(9):877–87.
23. De Backer D, Biston P, Devriendt J, et al. Comparison of dopamine and norepinephrine in the treatment of shock. N Engl J Med 2010;362(9):779–89.
24. Havel C, Arrich J, Losert H, et al. Vasopressors for hypotensive shock. Cochrane Database Syst Rev 2011;(5):CD003709.
25. Kraut JA, Madias NE. Lactic acidosis. N Engl J Med 2014;371(24):2309–19.
26. Levy B, Desebbe O, Montemont C, et al. Increased aerobic glycolysis through beta2 stimulation is a common mechanism involved in lactate formation during shock states. Shock 2008;30(4):417–21.

27. Dodda V, Spiro P. Albuterol, an uncommonly recognized culprit in lactic acidosis. Chest 2011;140(4_MeetingAbstracts):183A.

28. Morelli A, Ertmer C, Westphal M, et al. Effect of heart rate control with esmolol on hemodynamic and clinical outcomes in patients with septic shock: a randomized clinical trial. JAMA 2013;310(16):1683–91.

29. Pinsky MR. Is there a role for β-blockade in septic shock? JAMA 2013;310(16):1677–8.

30. Gordon AC, Russell JA, Walley KR, et al. The effects of vasopressin on acute kidney injury in septic shock. Intensive Care Med 2010;36(1):83–91.

31. Russell JA, Walley KR, Gordon AC, et al. Interaction of vasopressin infusion, corticosteroid treatment, and mortality of septic shock. Crit Care Med 2009; 37(3):811–8.

32. Gordon AC, Mason AJ, Perkins GD, et al. The interaction of vasopressin and corticosteroids in septic shock: a pilot randomized controlled trial. Crit Care Med 2014;42(6):1325–33.

33. Bellomo R, Chapman M, Finfer S, et al. Low-dose dopamine in patients with early renal dysfunction: a placebo-controlled randomised trial. Australian and New Zealand Intensive Care Society (ANZICS) Clinical Trials Group. Lancet 2000;356(9248):2139–43.

34. Bellomo R, Kellum JA, Ronco C. Acute kidney injury. Lancet 2012;380(9843):756–66.

35. Hayes MA, Timmins AC, Yau EH, et al. Elevation of systemic oxygen delivery in the treatment of critically ill patients. N Engl J Med 1994;330(24):1717–22.

36. Gattinoni L, Brazzi L, Pelosi P, et al. A trial of goal-oriented hemodynamic therapy in critically ill patients. SvO2 Collaborative Group. N Engl J Med 1995;333(16):1025–32.

37. The SvO2 study: general design and results of the feasibility phase of a multicenter, randomized trial of three different hemodynamic approaches and two monitoring techniques in the treatment of critically ill patients. The SvO2 Collaborative Group. Control Clin Trials 1995;16(1):74–87.

38. Rivers E, Nguyen B, Havstad S, et al. Early goal-directed therapy in the treatment of severe sepsis and septic shock. N Engl J Med 2001;345(19):1368–77.

39. Hinds C, Watson D. Manipulating hemodynamics and oxygen transport in critically ill patients. N Engl J Med 1995;333(16):1074–5.

40. Shoemaker WC. Goal-oriented hemodynamic therapy. N Engl J Med 1996;334(12):799–800 [author reply: 800].

41. Ferrer R, Artigas A, Levy MM, et al. Improvement in process of care and outcome after a multicenter severe sepsis educational program in Spain. JAMA 2008;299(19):2294–303.

42. Ferrer R, Artigas A, Suarez D, et al. Effectiveness of treatments for severe sepsis: a prospective, multicenter, observational study. Am J Respir Crit Care Med 2009;180(9):861–6.

43. Gao F, Melody T, Daniels DF, et al. The impact of compliance with 6-hour and 24-hour sepsis bundles on hospital mortality in patients with severe sepsis: a prospective observational study. Crit Care 2005; 9(6):R764–70.

44. The ARISE Investigators, ANZICS Clinical Trials Group. Goal-directed resuscitation for patients with early septic shock. N Engl J Med 2014;371(16):1496–506.

45. ProCESS/ARISE/ProMISe Methodology Writing Committee, Huang DT, Angus DC, et al. Harmonizing international trials of early goal-directed resuscitation for severe sepsis and septic shock: methodology of ProCESS, ARISE, and ProMISe. Intensive Care Med 2013;39(10):1760–75.

46. Levy MM, Rhodes A, Phillips GS, et al. Surviving sepsis campaign. Crit Care Med 2015;43(1):3–12.

47. Lindenauer PK, Lagu T, Shieh M-S, et al. Association of diagnostic coding with trends in hospitalizations and mortality of patients with pneumonia, 2003-2009. JAMA 2012;307(13):1405–13.

48. Hall WB, Willis LE, Medvedev S, et al. The implications of long-term acute care hospital transfer practices for measures of in-hospital mortality and length of stay. Am J Respir Crit Care Med 2012;185(1):53–7.

49. Lagu T, Rothberg MB, Shieh M-S, et al. Hospitalizations, costs, and outcomes of severe sepsis in the United States 2003 to 2007. Crit Care Med 2012; 40(3):754–61.

50. Khandelwal N, Kross EK, Engelberg RA, et al. Estimating the effect of palliative care interventions and advance care planning on ICU utilization: a systematic review. Crit Care Med 2015;43:1102–11.

51. Annane D, Vignon P, Renault A, et al. Norepinephrine plus dobutamine versus epinephrine alone for management of septic shock: a randomised trial. Lancet 2007;370(9588):676–84.

52. Seguin P, Bellissant E, Le Tulzo Y, et al. Effects of epinephrine compared with the combination of dobutamine and norepinephrine on gastric perfusion in septic shock. Clin Pharmacol Ther 2002;71(5):381–8.

53. Levy B, Bollaert PE, Charpentier C, et al. Comparison of norepinephrine and dobutamine to epinephrine for hemodynamics, lactate metabolism, and gastric tonometric variables in septic shock: a prospective, randomized study. Intensive Care Med 1997;23(3):282–7.

54. Seguin P, Laviolle B, Guinet P, et al. Dopexamine and norepinephrine versus epinephrine on gastric perfusion in patients with septic shock: a randomized study [NCT00134212]. Crit Care 2006;10(1):R32.

55. Cavallaro F, Sandroni C, Marano C, et al. Diagnostic accuracy of passive leg raising for prediction of fluid responsiveness in adults: systematic review and meta-analysis of clinical studies. Intensive Care Med 2010;36(9):1475–83.

56. Jozwiak M, Persichini R, Monnet X, et al. Management of myocardial dysfunction in severe sepsis. Semin Respir Crit Care Med 2011;32(2):206–14.

57. Marik PE. Surviving sepsis: going beyond the guidelines. Ann Intensive Care 2011;1(1):17.

58. Landesberg G, Jaffe AS, Gilon D, et al. Troponin elevation in severe sepsis and septic shock: the role of left ventricular diastolic dysfunction and right ventricular dilatation*. Crit Care Med 2014;42(4):790–800.

59. Reynolds TE, Pearse RM. Cardiac troponins in sepsis: an indication for echocardiography?*. Crit Care Med 2014;42(4):975–6.

60. Antonucci E, Fiaccadori E, Donadello K, et al. Myocardial depression in sepsis: from pathogenesis to clinical manifestations and treatment. J Crit Care 2014;29(4):500–11.

61. Heyland DK, Cook DJ, King D, et al. Maximizing oxygen delivery in critically ill patients: a methodologic appraisal of the evidence. Crit Care Med 1996;24(3):517–24.

62. Rhodes A, Cusack RJ, Newman PJ, et al. A randomised, controlled trial of the pulmonary artery catheter in critically ill patients. Intensive Care Med 2002;28(3):256–64.

63. Vieillard-Baron A, Prin S, Chergui K, et al. Hemodynamic instability in sepsis: bedside assessment by Doppler echocardiography. Am J Respir Crit Care Med 2003;168(11):1270–6.

64. Arntfield RT, Millington SJ. Point of care cardiac ultrasound applications in the emergency department and intensive care unit–a review. Curr Cardiol Rev 2012;8(2):98–108.

65. Jones AE, Tayal VS, Sullivan DM, et al. Randomized, controlled trial of immediate versus delayed goal-directed ultrasound to identify the cause of nontraumatic hypotension in emergency department patients. Crit Care Med 2004;32(8):1703–8.

66. Marcelino PA, Marum SM, Fernandes APM, et al. Routine transthoracic echocardiography in a general Intensive Care Unit: an 18 month survey in 704 patients. Eur J Intern Med 2009;20(3):e37–42.

67. Breitkreutz R, Price S, Steiger HV, et al. Focused echocardiographic evaluation in life support and peri-resuscitation of emergency patients: a prospective trial. Resuscitation 2010;81(11):1527–33.

68. Conti RAS, Oppenheim IM. Low-pressure cardiac tamponade masquerading as severe sepsis diagnosed with a bedside ultrasound and as the initial presentation of malignancy. J Community Hosp Intern Med Perspect 2014;4.

69. Durand M, Lamarche Y, Denault A. Pericardial tamponade. Can J Anaesth 2009;56(6):443–8.

70. Denault A, Deschamps A. Abnormal aortic-to-radial arterial pressure gradients resulting in misdiagnosis of hemodynamic instability. Can J Anaesth 2009;56(7):534–6.

71. Via G, Price S, Storti E. Echocardiography in the sepsis syndromes. Crit Ultrasound J 2011;3(2):71–85.

72. Via G, Hussain A, Wells M, et al. International evidence-based recommendations for focused cardiac ultrasound. J Am Soc Echocardiogr 2014;27(7):683.e1–33.

73. Colucci WS. Cardiovascular effects of milrinone. Am Heart J 1991;121(6):1945–7.

74. Barton P, Garcia J, Kouatli A, et al. Hemodynamic effects of IV milrinone lactate in pediatric patients with septic shock: a prospective, double-blinded, randomized, placebo-controlled, interventional study. Chest 1996;109(5):1302–12.

75. Borow KM, Come PC, Neumann A, et al. Physiologic assessment of the inotropic, vasodilator and afterload reducing effects of milrinone in subjects without cardiac disease. Am J Cardiol 1985;55(9):1204–9.

76. Baim DS, McDowell AV, Cherniles J, et al. Evaluation of a new bipyridine inotropic agent — milrinone — in patients with severe congestive heart failure. N Engl J Med 1983;309(13):748–56.

77. Morelli A, De Castro S, Teboul J-L, et al. Effects of levosimendan on systemic and regional hemodynamics in septic myocardial depression. Intensive Care Med 2005;31(5):638–44.

78. Chew MS, Hawthorne WJ, Bendall J, et al. No beneficial effects of levosimendan in acute porcine endotoxaemia. Acta Anaesthesiol Scand 2011;55(7):851–61.

79. Hasslacher J, Bijuklic K, Bertocchi C, et al. Levosimendan inhibits release of reactive oxygen species in polymorphonuclear leukocytes in vitro and in patients with acute heart failure and septic shock: a prospective observational study. Crit Care 2011;15(4):R166.

80. Morelli A, Donati A, Ertmer C, et al. Levosimendan for resuscitating the microcirculation in patients with septic shock: a randomized controlled study. Crit Care 2010;14(6):R232.

81. Rehberg S, Ertmer C, Vincent J-L, et al. Effects of combined arginine vasopressin and levosimendan on organ function in ovine septic shock. Crit Care Med 2010;38(10):2016–23.

82. Orme RML, Perkins GD, McAuley DF, et al. An efficacy and mechanism evaluation study of Levosimendan for the Prevention of Acute oRgan Dysfunction in Sepsis (LeoPARDS): protocol for a randomized controlled trial. Trials 2014;15(1):199.

83. Wilkman E, Kaukonen K-M, Pettilä V, et al. Association between inotrope treatment and 90-day mortality in patients with septic shock. Acta Anaesthesiol Scand 2013;57(4):431–42.

84. Wang Z, Wu Q, Nie X, et al. Combination therapy with milrinone and esmolol for heart protection in patients with severe sepsis: a prospective, randomized trial. Clin Drug Investig 2015;35(11):707–16.

85. Jones AE, Shapiro NI, Trzeciak S, et al. Lactate clearance vs central venous oxygen saturation as goals of early sepsis therapy: a randomized clinical trial. JAMA 2010;303:739–46.

# Endothelial and Microcirculatory Function and Dysfunction in Sepsis

James F. Colbert, MD[a], Eric P. Schmidt, MD[b],*

## KEYWORDS

- Sepsis • Microcirculation • Glycocalyx • Intravital microscopy • Glycosaminoglycans
- Heparan sulfate

## KEY POINTS

- Microcirculatory functions critical for the homeostatic control of infection can become dysregulated and harmful during sepsis.
- Microcirculation dysfunction may arise in part from septic degradation of the endothelial glycocalyx, a substantial, glycosaminoglycan (GAG)-rich layer lining the vascular lumen.
- The microcirculation can be measured at the bedside, either directly via intravital microscopy or indirectly via circulating measures of vascular damage. Such evidence of microcirculatory dysfunction is predictive of sepsis outcomes.
- Additional human studies are needed to determine if sepsis treatments, when titrated to improvement of microvascular function, improve patient outcomes.

## ANATOMY AND FUNCTION OF THE MICROVASCULATURE

The microcirculation, comprised of less than 100 μm–diameter arterioles, capillary beds, and draining venules, performs essential homeostatic functions, including oxygen delivery and solute exchange.[1] Although this simple construct holds true across all human tissues, there is substantial organ specificity of microcirculation structure, reflecting unique functions assigned to different vascular beds. The kidney glomerulus, tasked with plasma ultrafiltration, features afferent and efferent arterioles flanking a capillary network lined with fenestrated endothelium. In contrast, the cerebral and pulmonary vasculature are characterized by tight endothelial barriers (and supporting pericytes), reflecting organ functions that are threatened by interstitial edema. These organ-specific differences in microvascular function are paralleled by tissue-specific endothelial phenotypes, yielding varied mechanisms of endothelial-leukocyte adhesion (eg, pulmonary vs systemic circulations[2]) and organ-specific endothelial glycocalyces.[3]

## THE NORMAL MICROVASCULAR RESPONSE TO INFECTION

To understand dysfunction of the microcirculation during sepsis, it is necessary to appreciate the appropriate microvascular response to infection. The inflammatory response to infection, as described in the first century AD, consists of calor (heat), rubor (redness), dolor (pain), and tumor (swelling).[4] From a microcirculation standpoint, these responses reflect altered regional blood flow, vascular hyperpermeability, leukocyte

Disclosure Statement: The authors have nothing to disclose.
[a] Division of Infectious Diseases, Department of Medicine, University of Colorado School of Medicine, 12700 E. 19th Avenue, Aurora, CO 80045, USA; [b] Division of Pulmonary Sciences and Critical Care Medicine, Department of Medicine, Denver Health Medical Center, University of Colorado School of Medicine, 12700 E. 19th Avenue, Aurora, CO 80045, USA
* Corresponding author. 12700 East 19th Avenue, Research Complex 2, Mail Stop C272, Aurora, CO 80045.
E-mail address: eric.schmidt@ucdenver.edu

Clin Chest Med 37 (2016) 263–275
http://dx.doi.org/10.1016/j.ccm.2016.01.009

recruitment, and coagulation.[1] It is critical to recognize that these physiologic changes are appropriate and effective in the setting of acute infection. A vast majority of viral and bacterial infections are controlled quickly by the host and do not lead to disseminated infection, organ failure, and death. By allowing for the beneficial actions of calor, rubor, dolor, and tumor, the microcirculation facilitates local quarantine of pathogens, targeted delivery of soluble anti-infectious agents (eg, complement and immuno-globulins), and chemotaxis of activated host immune cells.

### Leukocyte Adhesion

The recruitment of leukocytes to areas of infection is a highly regulated process, consisting (in systemic venules) of active leukocyte rolling, adhesion, activation, aggregation, and transmigration, demonstrating the importance of these processes to tissue homeostasis.[5] In the absence of infection, leukocyte-endothelial interactions are limited, occurring primarily in specialized vascular beds (eg, lymph node high endothelial venules). There is great heterogeneity across different vascular beds regarding processes of leukocyte extravasation, with rolling essential for diapedesis from systemic venules but dispensable for extravasation from the pulmonary capillaries.[2,6]

### Tissue Edema

The intense, multiprocess regulation of vascular permeability reflects its critical importance in microvascular function.[7] The targeted extravasation of antibacterial peptides, antibodies, and complement is beneficial to the host response to infection. Barrier dysfunction, however, can become pathologic if transvascular fluid flux overwhelms lymphatic drainage or other tissue-specific safeguards against interstitial edema.[8]

### Coagulation

Microvascular coagulation is important to the host response to infection. Endothelial damage and inflammatory cytokines lead to a procoagulant state in the microvasculature, allowing for the development of microthrombi.[9,10] This response functions to isolate infection and prevent dissemination. Murine studies have shown that anticoagulants facilitate bacterial spread after peritonitis, leading to worsened sepsis outcomes.[11] The failures of activated protein C, antithrombin III, and tissue factor antagonists to improve sepsis outcomes perhaps reflect homoeostatic effects of microvascular coagulation.[12–14]

These and other microcirculatory responses are adaptive and often successful in localizing and eliminating infectious insults.[15–18] In extreme cases of overwhelming infection, however, these processes may contribute to the overall morbidity and mortality of sepsis (**Fig. 1**).

## EVIDENCE OF MICROVASCULAR DYSFUNCTION DURING SEPSIS

Oxygen delivery is a function of both cardiac output and blood oxygen content. Because early sepsis is characterized by a low systemic vascular resistance/high cardiac output state, oxygen delivery is typically elevated in sepsis. The kidney, brain, and heart all experience augmented blood flow during sepsis.[19] Despite this increased bulk delivery of oxygen, tissue hypoxia persists in sepsis and contributes to septic organ injury.[1] This suggests that the defect of sepsis is not a loss of macrovascular blood supply but rather a loss of microvascular function. Therapeutic attempts to augment macrocirculatory oxygen delivery by increasing cardiac output or hemoglobin have failed to improve outcomes in sepsis.[20–24]

This suspected microvascular defect in sepsis has been extensively investigated using animal models,[25] identifying critical pathogenic roles of endothelial barrier dysfunction,[26,27] inappropriate leukocyte adhesion,[28] platelet activation,[29] activation of microvascular coagulation,[9] and aberrant control of vascular tone.[30] These changes broadly mediate injury across numerous organ systems of relevance to sepsis outcomes, including the lung,[31] kidney,[32] and brain.[33]

There is no discrete, readily apparent inflection point at which beneficial microvascular responses to infection change to pathologic contributors to sepsis. Sepsis may arise from numerous microcirculatory changes, including activation of anti-infection responses in vascular beds where no pathogens exist, or a magnitude of anti-infection response that outstrips what is necessary for microbial clearance. This complexity warrants a deeper understanding of the precise changes occurring within an individual during sepsis, potentially allowing for personalization of sepsis therapeutics.

## MEASURING SEPTIC MICROVASCULAR DYSFUNCTION IN HUMANS

Detecting and characterizing microvascular dysfunction in humans is technically challenging, given difficulties in the direct measurement of clinically relevant vascular beds. Systemic, circulating biomarkers of tissue ischemia (eg, central venous oxygenation and lactate) are not sensitive to

## Normal microvascular responses to infection

## Pathologic microvascular responses in sepsis

### Lung

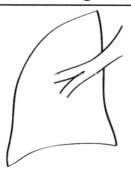

- Focal endothelial activation and adhesion molecule exposure, allowing for targeted neutrophil diapedesis[16]
- Focal leakage of antibacterial plasma proteins[16]
- Hypoxic vasoconstriction shunts blood to aerated alveoli

- Diffuse endothelial adhesion molecule exposure/activation enables untargeted neutrophilia[28]
- Nonfocal/diffuse endothelial hyperpermeability, edema[31]
- Nonhomeostatic, diffuse pulmonary vasoconstriction and consequent pulmonary hypertension[18]

### Kidney

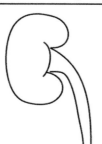

- Focal loss of peritubular microvascular flow induces ischemia and epithelial sloughing, detaching adherent bacteria[15]
- Local extravasation of antimicrobial peptides, leukocytes[17]

- Early vasorelaxation of efferent glomerular arterioles increases total renal blood flow at expense of decreased glomerular filtration[32]
- Tubular microvascular inflammation and interstitial edema trigger tubuloglomerular feedback, decreasing total renal blood flow in established kidney injury[32]

**Fig. 1.** Homeostatic versus pathologic (septic) pulmonary and renal microvascular responses to infection.

microcirculatory defects, given the potential for functional shunting, in which venular $P_{O_2}$ exceeds capillary $P_{O_2}$.[1] Furthermore, the value of therapeutically targeting these markers is uncertain, given recent negative studies of early goal-directed therapy.[22–24] As recently reviewed elsewhere,[27,34] numerous promising biomarkers for capillary endothelial dysfunction (eg, angiopoietins and glycocalyx fragments) have been identified in septic shock. These biomarkers, however, often are not easily measured point of care and have yet to be validated as clinically relevant treatment endpoints.

An alternative approach to rapidly measuring microcirculatory function is direct imaging of microvessels using intravital microscopy.[35] Although nail fold or episcleral vessels can be visualized at the bedside,[35] these vascular beds yield few quantitative data regarding microvascular function without the use of large microscopy systems. The development of microscopy techniques, however, such as orthogonal phase spectrometry (OPS) or sidestream dark field imaging

(SDF), has led to increasing enthusiasm for the bedside imaging of the sublingual microvasculature. OPS and SDF imaging can clearly identify red blood cells (RBCs), due to the absorptive effects of hemoglobin. As such, these techniques can identify RBC-perfused vessels (**Fig. 2**); a lack of visualized sublingual vessels serves as evidence of absent or impaired RBC flow.[36]

This visualized loss of sublingual microvascular RBC perfusion can be quantified via several techniques, either at point of care[37] or during later review of recorded images. Loss of RBC flow yields a heterogeneous loss of vascular density apparent on OPS and SDF imaging, particularly involving small (<20-µm) microvessels. This microvascular dropout can be quantified by using several different validated approaches, including the De Backer score (which uses a stereological-like approach in which vessel density is calculated from intersections with overlying gridlines) or the microvascular flow index (a semiquantitative score determined from the average of qualitative assessments across 4 visual field quadrants; see **Fig. 2**).[36,38]

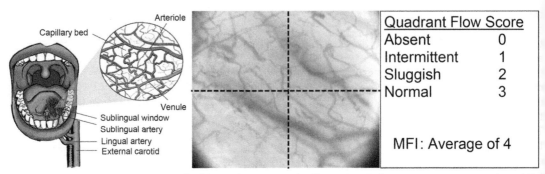

**Fig. 2.** Semiquantitative assessment of sublingual microvascular flow. Intravital microscopy can access the sublingual miscrovasculature (OPS image [*center panel*]). Semiquanitative measurements of flow in each quadrant of image yields an average microvascular flow index (MFI); at least 5 images should be measured. (*Adapted from* Klijn E, Den Uil CA, Bakker J, et al. The heterogeneity of the microcirculation in critical illness. Clin Chest Med 2008;29(4):646; with permission.)

Although consensus statements have detailed standardized approaches to the quantification of intravital measures of microvascular function,[36] there remain several practical challenges to the widespread implementation of these approaches. A major concern is the risk of visual artifacts (eg, capillary dropout) produced from undue pressure of the microscope objective on the sublingual microvessels.[36,39] Even when excluding video clips that have such artifacts, only 30.8% of SDF recordings were found of excellent technical quality.[39] Despite these concerns, a recently published international study (Microcirculatory Shock Occurrence in Acutely Ill Patients [microSOAP]) performed across 36 ICUs performed SDF sublingual microvascular measurements in 501 patients, with low variation in microvascular flow index (MFI) (2%) and De Backer scoring (7%).[40]

An additional concern regarding the sublingual microcirculation is the relevance of this vascular bed during sepsis, particularly given divergent responses of the sublingual microvasculature from vascular beds more proximal to the site of a sepsis-inducing infection (eg, the submucosa of an intestinal ostomy during abdominal sepsis).[41] Convergent findings from multiple groups, however, have linked sublingual microvascular alterations with clinical outcomes in sepsis, providing reassurance for the relevance of these measurements. Using OPS imaging of the sublingual microvasculature, De Backer and colleagues[42] compared 10 healthy volunteers, 16 patients prior to cardiac surgery, 5 nonseptic ICU patients, and 50 patients with sepsis/septic shock. Patients with sepsis had significant loss (or intermittent interruption) of RBC perfusion in small (<20-μm) sublingual microvessels. Perfusion was highly variable in patients with sepsis, and vessel perfusion was lower in nonsurvivors. These changes were independent of measures of macrovascular function, including mean arterial

pressure and need for vasopressor medications. Further studies demonstrated that septic shock survivors tended to have rapid (albeit incomplete) correction of early microvascular dysfunction, as opposed to persistent abnormalities in patients who ultimately died.[43] An increase in small vessel perfusion of greater than 7.8% in the first 24 hours of sepsis was 82% specific for survival.[43] In the microSOAP study, 17% of mixed ICU patients (septic and nonseptic) demonstrated abnormal sublingual microvascular function; in the subgroup of patients with tachycardia, this dysfunction predicted hospital mortality.[40] These studies and others[44–46] support the feasibility (and reproducibility) of bedside measures of sublingual microvascular function and their relevance to sepsis outcomes.

As with any observational human approach, it is difficult to prove that observed changes in microvascular dysfunction during sepsis are causal to, as opposed to a consequence of, organ dysfunction. For example, it is possible that loss of microvascular flow is an appropriate response to decreased tissue metabolic demand. Sepsis-induced suppression of mitochondrial oxidative phosphorylation is expected to decrease cellular oxygen demand, triggering a reactive decrease in microvascular flow and vascular density. This phenomenon, however, is not supported by available experimental data. During sepsis, extravascular tissue $CO_2$ partial pressures (a measure of cellular respiration quantifiable by sublingual capnometery) increase as microvascular flow decreases, suggesting that tissue metabolic activity outstrips microvascular blood supply.[47]

## PATHOGENESIS OF MICROVASCULAR DYSFUNCTION DURING SEPSIS

Given the potential causal importance of microvascular dysfunction during sepsis, the pathogenic mechanisms underlying these changes are attractive therapeutic targets. Likely contributors to these changes include pathophysiologic events typically implicated in septic organ injury, including aberrant vascular tone, inappropriate barrier dysfunction (and consequent tissue edema), inappropriate leukocyte adhesion (and inflammation), and activation of microvascular coagulation.[1] These pathophysiologic events can yield a signature appearance on intravital microscopy, with extraluminal (tissue edema and vasoconstriction) and intraluminal (coagulation and leukocyte adhesion) events conspiring to produce a loss of visualized RBC flow. Loss of RBC flow has physiologic consequence, leading to tissue hypoxia in the setting of tissue injury-amplified metabolic demands. Although loss of microvascular flow can be compensated by increased flow through other vessels, this compensation can produce a functional shunt, in which the high velocity of flow through patent collateral microvessels decreases the capillary dwell time of RBCs, diminishing oxygen diffusion and potentially leading to additional hypoxia surrounding perfused microvessels.[19]

Because many pathophysiologic events contribute to microvascular dysfunction during sepsis, it is unlikely that targeting a discrete contributor to vascular injury would have broad beneficial effects on patient outcomes in sepsis. As such, there has been great effort invested in identifying, and subsequently targeting, unifying mechanisms upstream of endothelial barrier dysfunction, inflammation, and microthrombosis. Particularly intense attention has been dedicated to the immunopathogenesis of sepsis, a broad topic ranging from the initial infection-associated release of pathogen-associated molecular patterns, consequent induction of pattern receptor (eg, toll-like) signaling, downstream induction of inflammatory cytokine production (cytokine storm), leukocyte recruitment, and tissue damage with release of immune-amplifying damage-associated molecular patterns.[48] These events coincide with induction/augmentation of coagulation pathway signaling.[48] These proinflammatory pathways, however, have largely failed to identify clinically effective immunotherapies for sepsis.[49–51] Although these failures may be largely the consequence of practical challenges in therapeutically interrupting hyperacute events driving sepsis onset, it may also reflect an incomplete understanding of the complex immunologic events surrounding sepsis. Recent efforts have highlighted the pathologic significance of anti-inflammatory signaling in severe sepsis and septic shock.[52]

These limitations of the classic cytokine storm theory as a unifying mechanism of microcirculatory dysfunction have raised the need to identify novel pathophysiologic pathways of organ dysfunction (and microcirculatory failure) in sepsis. De Backer and colleagues[42,53] demonstrated that septic sublingual microcirculatory heterogeneity can be completely corrected by the topical administration of vasodilators (eg, acetylcholine). This rapid reversibility suggests that septic microvascular failure may arise largely from pathologic involvement of processes associated with the dynamic regulation of vascular tone. Accordingly, nitric oxide (NO) has been the intense focus of research as a mediator of sepsis and septic organ injury. Unfortunately, NO signaling is highly complex, with context-specific functions that can be both homeostatic and pathologic.[54–56] Human studies of NO-targeted microvascular therapeutics have accordingly been disappointing,[57,58] potentially reflecting broad, nonspecific effects of NO manipulation.[59] These challenges (and opportunities) of NO-based therapies are reviewed in detail elsewhere.[60]

The limitations of systemic, NO-targeted therapeutic approaches in sepsis have raised interest in other, more specific, manipulations of vascular tone. Although many pathways are currently the focus of intense investigation, this review focuses on 1 particularly promising therapeutic target—the endothelial glycocalyx.

## ENDOTHELIAL GLYCOCALYX AND THE SEPTIC MICROCIRCULATION

The endothelial glycocalyx is a layer of GAGs and associated proteoglycans lining the vascular lumen (**Fig. 3**).[61] First described as a 20 nm–thick "endocapillary layer" in 1966, the glycocalyx was long thought to be a structure of trifling significance.[62] This underappreciation of glycocalyx structure/significance likely reflected glycocalyx aberrance in vitro[63] as well as its frequent degradation during tissue fixation.[64] With the advent and optimization of intravital microscopy, it is now apparent that in vivo, negatively charged glycocalyx GAGs sequester water, forming a massive (0.5 $\mu$m–11 $\mu$m) endothelial surface layer (ESL) with measurable rigidity.[61,65,66] The ESL has several homeostatic functions, including maintenance of the endothelial barrier to fluid and protein[67] as well as regulation of leukocyte-endothelial adhesion.[5] The ESL also serves as a mechanotransducer of shear stress: in the presence of sufficient shear, the ESL-replete endothelium activates endothelial NO synthase, leading to vasodilation and accommodation of increased flow.[68] Experimental ESL degradation induces edema,[67] inappropriate leukocyte adhesion,[69]

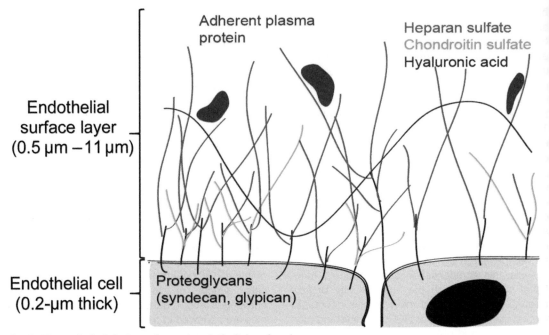

**Fig. 3.** The endothelial glycocalyx and endothelial surface layer.

and loss of microvascular autoregulation.[68] Accordingly, degradation of the ESL in animal models increased microvascular heterogeneity, with some vessels becoming occluded to RBC flow and others becoming hyperemic.[70,71]

Endothelial glycocalyx/ESL integrity is, therefore, highly relevant to septic organ injury and microvascular dysfunction. In experimental models of polymicrobial sepsis, GAG degradation occurred within the pulmonary and renal vascular beds, contributing to both lung edema/inflammation[8,28] as well as loss of glomerular filtration.[72] In a rat model of endotoxemia, loss of intestinal capillary density occurred in association with mesenteric ESL degradation.[73] In humans, several techniques exist for the detection and quantification of glycocalyx degradation in critically ill patients (**Table 1**). Loss of glycocalyx/ESL integrity was apparent within the sublingual microcirculation after endotoxin administration to healthy volunteers, coincident with loss of capillary density.[74] Patients with sepsis demonstrate elevated circulating ESL degradation products, including proteoglycans[75–77] as well as GAGs heparan sulfate, hyaluronic acid, and chondroitin sulfate.[75,78–83] Accordingly, glycocalyx/ESL degradation is predictive of clinical outcomes in critical illness.[78,79] The development of rapid, point-of-care assays for glycocalyx breakdown products (see **Table 1**) may allow for microvascular personalization of sepsis treatment, identifying patients who may benefit the most from vascular-protective therapies.

## THERAPEUTIC TARGETING OF THE MICROCIRCULATION IN SEPSIS

The ability to directly visualize the sublingual microvasculature in human subjects has allowed for hypothesis-generating human studies identifying treatments that, by virtue of rescuing the dysfunctional microvasculature, could serve as clinically effective treatments for sepsis.[89] Such microcirculation-protective therapies, however, have largely failed to improve patient outcomes when broadly applied across large, multicenter trials (**Table 2**).

The failure of activated protein C as a treatment of sepsis is particularly disappointing, due to not only the promising microcirculation-protective effects observed in animal models and preliminary human studies[90] but also the initial success of drotrecogin alfa as reported in the seminal Recombinant Human Activated Protein C Worldwide Evaluation in Severe Sepsis (PROWESS)[91] study. Ultimately, the futility of drotrecogin alfa was demonstrated in the Administration of Drotecogin Alpha [Activated] in Early Stage Severe Sepsis (ADDRESS)[92] and PROWESS-Shock[12] studies, paralleling negative studies of other anticoagulants such as antithrombin III[14] and tissue factor antagonists.[13] A recent meta-analysis suggested, however, a mortality decrease with heparin treatment during sepsis (odds ratio 0.88),[111] although this analysis is derived largely from a single study of low-dose heparin for venous thromboembolism prophylaxis (a dosing regimen of uncertain relevance to the septic microcirculation)

**Table 1**
**Measurement of endothelial glycocalyx/endothelial surface layer degradation in humans**

| Assay | Human Studies | Advantages | Disadvantages |
|---|---|---|---|
| Detection of circulating glycocalyx fragments | | | |
| Dimethylmethylene blue/alcian blue | • Plasma GAGs (via alcian blue binding) increased in septic shock, correlated with mortality[75]<br>• Urinary, plasma GAGs increased in pediatric meningococcemia[83]<br>• Modified dimethylmethylene blue assay feasible in trauma patients[84] | Rapid, inexpensive colorimetric assay | Only detects sulfated GAGs (cannot detect hyaluronic acid) |
| ELISA/latex agglutination assay | • Plasma hyaluronan increased in endotoxin-treated volunteers,[74] patients with septic shock[79,82]<br>• Plasma heparan sulfate increased in septic shock[79]<br>• Plasma syndecan-1 shedding increased in sepsis patients[75,81] | Quantitative measure of proteoglycans, GAGs | Insufficient rapidity to date for bedside use; uncertain specificity of antibody binding to GAGs |
| Mass spectrometry | • Elevated heparan sulfate in patients with severe sepsis[78]<br>• Chondroitin sulfate unchanged in severe sepsis[78,79] | High sensitivity; allows detection of sulfation signatures, potentially identifying tissue source | Expensive, impractical for rapid bedside use |
| Thromboelastography | Trauma patients with thromboelastography evidence of circulating sulfated heparan sulfate fragments had higher plasma syndecan-1, injury severity[85] | Rapid, inexpensive measurement of circulating heparan sulfate fragments with anticoagulant ability | Detection limited to highly sulfated heparan pentasaccharides (or larger) |
| Measurement of whole-body glycocalyx volume | | | |
| Tracer dilution technique[86] | In healthy volunteers, total body glycocalyx volume correlated with sublingual intravital imaging[86] | Can measure whole-body ESL volume based on differences in tracer volumes of distribution | Technical assumptions controversial[87] |
| Intravital microscopy | | | |
| Sublingual SDF imaging | Loss of sublingual glycocalyx thickness in endotoxin-treated volunteers,[74] ICU patients[88] | Rapid, point-of-care assay; allows for simultaneous measurements of microvascular function | Concerns regarding relevance of imaged vascular bed and interobserver variability; need for specialized training |

**Table 2**
**Microcirculation-protective therapies and outcomes in clinical trials of sepsis**

| Intervention | Microcirculation Benefit | Benefit as Sepsis Therapeutic |
|---|---|---|
| **Anticoagulants** | | |
| Activated protein C | 4-h improvement in capillary perfusion; improvement did not persist after drug cessation.[90] | Initial benefit[91] unable to be reproduced in confirmatory studies[12,92] |
| **Vasoactive medications** | | |
| Vasopressors | Mixed benefit of norepinephrine, with studies showing either microvascular benefit of increasing MAP from 65 mm Hg–85 mm Hg[93] or no change[94] | Targeting MAP of 80 mm Hg–85 mm Hg equivalent to MAP of 65 mm Hg–70 mm Hg in septic shock[95] |
| Inotropic agents | Dobutamine (added to patients receiving dopamine ± norepinephrine) improves perfused capillary density.[53] | No benefit from early goal-directed therapy studies, which included dobutamine therapy.[22–24] No benefit and potential harm from supranormal oxygen delivery in established sepsis.[96] |
| **Anti-inflammatory therapy** | | |
| Corticosteroids | Stress dose (50 mg) hydrocortisone improved sublingual microvascular function within 4 h; perfused capillary density remained improved at 24 h.[97] | High-dose steroids without benefit[98,99] and potential harm.[100] Stress dose steroids without benefit.[101] |
| Hemofiltration (endotoxin removal) | • Improved De Backer score during hemofiltration sessions; benefit lost after filtration[102] • MFI improvement during 12 h hemofiltration, persistent for 6 h after session[103] | Potential early mortality benefit of 2 hemofiltration sessions after surgery for intra-abdominal infection; benefit lost at 30 d[104] |
| **Fluid therapy** | | |
| Early goal-directed therapy | Fluid bolus administration early (<24 h) in sepsis improves microvascular function; no such benefit later (72 h) in sepsis.[105] | No benefit from early goal-directed therapy in sepsis.[22–24] This may reflect efficacy/implementation of very early fluid resuscitation (ie, prior to study enrollment). |
| Colloids | Hydroxyethyl starch more effective than saline at improving sublingual MFI in septic patients[106]; albumin equivalent to crystalloid[105] | Although albumin may be beneficial in septic shock (based on post hoc subgroup analyses[107]), hydroxyethyl starch is associated with harm.[108–110] |

in patients receiving activated protein C.[112] Low-dose heparin administration had been previously implicated as detrimental in sepsis studies of antithrombin III[14] and tissue factor antagonists.[13] This complexity may reflect the varied biologic effects of heparin, including the ability of this highly sulfated GAG to inhibit selectins,[113] influence growth factor signaling,[114] and inhibit enzymes implicated in endothelial glycocalyx degradation (ie, heparanase).[28] Many anticoagulants (including activated protein C and antithrombin) have multiple biologic effects; the failure of these agents to improve sepsis outcomes, therefore, cannot be viewed as a direct repudiation of the pathophysiological importance of tissue thrombosis to organ injury.

## NOVEL MICROCIRCULATION-PROTECTIVE THERAPIES

The general failures of microcirculation-targeted therapies to improve patient outcomes highlights a need to identify new therapeutic targets in sepsis. Given the known benefit of early antibiotics n sepsis, studies of the impact of antibiotic administration on microcirculatory function would be instructive as to potential new therapeutic targets.[115] Sheddases implicated in septic glycocalyx degradation may be targeted,[116] including the use of doxycycline[69] or sphingosine-1-phosphate[117] to inhibit matrix metalloproteinases responsible for proteoglycan shedding. Alternatively, coagulant or nonanticoagulant variants of heparin can be used to block heparanase, a heparan sulfate-degrading endoglucuronidase responsible for septic endothelial glycocalyx degradation and lung and kidney injury.[28,72] Furthermore, interventions aimed at promoting glycocalyx reconstitution may hasten a return of microvascular homeostasis. Rosuvastatin improved glycocalyx reconstitution in patients with familial hyperlipidemia[118]; however, a randomized trial of statins failed to show benefit as a sepsis therapeutic.[119]

Although the general failure of microcirculation-protective interventions to improve clinical outcomes may reflect a lack of novel therapeutic targets, a more compelling explanation might lie in the indiscriminant administration of microcirculation-protective therapies in multicenter trials. Microvascular-protective treatments might only benefit patients who demonstrate baseline abnormalities of microvascular function.[89] Ideally, future studies will pursue such microvasculature-targeted, personalized approaches to sepsis resuscitation. This assessment of baseline microvascular status could be based on bedside intravital microscopy (with its accompanying technical limitations) or systemic markers of endothelial damage (with their accompanying logistic concerns as point-of-care tests). The promise of such personalized approaches to infection treatment has been demonstrated in recent studies of pneumonia, in which a benefit of adjunctive corticosteroids existed largely in patients with baseline evidence of systemic inflammation.[120,121]

## SUMMARY

The microcirculation is a promising therapeutic target in sepsis. Although several techniques allow for the detection of microcirculation dysfunction in humans (including intravital imaging and measures of glycocalyx degradation), these approaches have yet to guide sepsis therapeutics in a manner that demonstrably (in phase III studies) improves patient outcomes. Validating, multicenter, patient outcome–focused studies of interventions titrated to improving microcirculation function are needed to create new treatment paradigms in sepsis.

## REFERENCES

1. Ince C. The microcirculation is the motor of sepsis. Crit Care 2005;9(Suppl 4):S13–9.
2. Kuebler WM. Inflammatory pathways and microvascular responses in the lung. Pharmacol Rep 2005;57(Suppl):196–205.
3. Marki A, Esko JD, Pries AR, et al. Role of the endothelial surface layer in neutrophil recruitment. J Leukoc Biol 2015;98(4):503–15.
4. Donaldson IM. Celsus: de medicina, florence 1478. Part 1. J R Coll Physicians Edinb 2014; 44(3):252–4.
5. Schmidt EP, Lee WL, Zemans RL, et al. On, around, and through: neutrophil-endothelial interactions in innate immunity. Physiology (Bethesda) 2011;26(5):334–47.
6. Rossaint J, Zarbock A. Tissue-specific neutrophil recruitment into the lung, liver, and kidney. J Innate Immun 2013;5(4):348–57.
7. Mehta D, Malik AB. Signaling mechanisms regulating endothelial permeability. Physiol Rev 2006; 86(1):279–367.
8. Negrini D, Passi A, Moriondo A. The role of proteoglycans in pulmonary edema development. Intensive Care Med 2008;34(4):610–8.
9. Levi M, van der Poll T, Schultz M. Systemic versus localized coagulation activation contributing to organ failure in critically ill patients. Semin Immunopathol 2012;34(1):167–79.
10. Dixon B. The role of microvascular thrombosis in sepsis. Anaesth Intensive Care 2004;32(5):619–29.
11. Echtenacher B, Weigl K, Lehn N, et al. Tumor necrosis factor-dependent adhesions as a major protective mechanism early in septic peritonitis in mice. Infect Immun 2001;69(6):3550–5.
12. Ranieri VM, Thompson BT, Barie PS, et al. Drotrecogin alfa (activated) in adults with septic shock. N Engl J Med 2012;366(22):2055–64.
13. Abraham E, Reinhart K, Opal S, et al. Efficacy and safety of tifacogin (recombinant tissue factor pathway inhibitor) in severe sepsis: a randomized controlled trial. JAMA 2003;290(2):238–47.
14. Warren BL, Eid A, Singer P, et al. Caring for the critically ill patient. High-dose antithrombin III in severe sepsis: a randomized controlled trial. JAMA 2001;286(15):1869–78.
15. Melican K, Boekel J, Mansson LE, et al. Bacterial infection-mediated mucosal signalling induces local renal ischaemia as a defence against sepsis. Cell Microbiol 2008;10(10):1987–98.
16. Mizgerd JP. Acute lower respiratory tract infection. N Engl J Med 2008;358(7):716–27.
17. Nielubowicz GR, Mobley HL. Host-pathogen interactions in urinary tract infection. Nat Rev Urol 2010;7(8):430–41.
18. Bull TM, Clark B, McFann K, et al. Pulmonary vascular dysfunction is associated with poor

outcomes in patients with acute lung injury. Am J Respir Crit Care Med 2010;182(9):1123–8.

19. Ostergaard L, Granfeldt A, Secher N, et al. Microcirculatory dysfunction and tissue oxygenation in critical illness. Acta Anaesthesiol Scand 2015; 59(10):1246–59.

20. Hayes MA, Timmins AC, Yau EH, et al. Elevation of systemic oxygen delivery in the treatment of critically ill patients. N Engl J Med 1994;330(24): 1717–22.

21. Hebert PC, Wells G, Blajchman MA, et al. A multicenter, randomized, controlled clinical trial of transfusion requirements in critical care. Transfusion Requirements in Critical Care Investigators, Canadian Critical Care Trials Group. N Engl J Med 1999;340(6):409–17.

22. Peake SL, Delaney A, Bailey M, et al. Goal-directed resuscitation for patients with early septic shock. N Engl J Med 2014;371(16):1496–506.

23. Mouncey PR, Osborn TM, Power GS, et al. Trial of early, goal-directed resuscitation for septic shock. N Engl J Med 2015;372(14):1301–11.

24. Yealy DM, Kellum JA, Huang DT, et al. A randomized trial of protocol-based care for early septic shock. N Engl J Med 2014;370(18):1683–93.

25. Lam C, Tyml K, Martin C, et al. Microvascular perfusion is impaired in a rat model of normotensive sepsis. J Clin Invest 1994;94(5):2077–83.

26. Lee WL, Slutsky AS. Sepsis and endothelial permeability. N Engl J Med 2010;363(7):689–91.

27. Opal SM, van der Poll T. Endothelial barrier dysfunction in septic shock. J Intern Med 2015; 277(3):277–93.

28. Schmidt EP, Yang Y, Janssen WJ, et al. The pulmonary endothelial glycocalyx regulates neutrophil adhesion and lung injury during experimental sepsis. Nat Med 2012;18(8):1217–23.

29. de Stoppelaar SF, van 't Veer C, van der Poll T. The role of platelets in sepsis. Thromb Haemost 2014; 112(4):666–77.

30. Tyml K. Role of connexins in microvascular dysfunction during inflammation. Can J Physiol Pharmacol 2011;89(1):1–12.

31. Matthay MA, Ware LB, Zimmerman GA. The acute respiratory distress syndrome. J Clin Invest 2012; 122(8):2731–40.

32. Prowle JR, Bellomo R. Sepsis-associated acute kidney injury: macrohemodynamic and microhemodynamic alterations in the renal circulation. Semin Nephrol 2015;35(1):64–74.

33. Taccone FS, Su F, De Deyne C, et al. Sepsis is associated with altered cerebral microcirculation and tissue hypoxia in experimental peritonitis. Crit Care Med 2014;42(2):e114–22.

34. Page AV, Liles WC. Biomarkers of endothelial activation/dysfunction in infectious diseases. Virulence 2013;4(6):507–16.

35. Klijn E, Den Uil CA, Bakker J, et al. The heterogeneity of the microcirculation in critical illness. Clin Chest Med 2008;29(4):643–54, viii.

36. De Backer D, Hollenberg S, Boerma C, et al. How to evaluate the microcirculation: report of a round table conference. Crit Care 2007;11(5):R101.

37. Arnold RC, Parrillo JE, Phillip Dellinger R, et al. Point-of-care assessment of microvascular blood flow in critically ill patients. Intensive Care Med 2009;35(10):1761–6.

38. Boerma EC, Mathura KR, van der Voort PH, et al. Quantifying bedside-derived imaging of microcirculatory abnormalities in septic patients: a prospective validation study. Crit Care 2005;9(6): R601–6.

39. Sallisalmi M, Oksala N, Pettila V, et al. Evaluation of sublingual microcirculatory blood flow in the critically ill. Acta Anaesthesiol Scand 2012;56(3): 298–306.

40. Vellinga NA, Boerma EC, Koopmans M, et al. International study on microcirculatory shock occurrence in acutely ill patients. Crit Care Med 2015; 43(1):48–56.

41. Boerma EC, van der Voort PH, Spronk PE, et al. Relationship between sublingual and intestinal microcirculatory perfusion in patients with abdominal sepsis. Crit Care Med 2007;35(4):1055–60.

42. De Backer D, Creteur J, Preiser JC, et al. Microvascular blood flow is altered in patients with sepsis. Am J Respir Crit Care Med 2002;166(1):98–104.

43. Sakr Y, Dubois MJ, De Backer D, et al. Persistent microcirculatory alterations are associated with organ failure and death in patients with septic shock. Crit Care Med 2004;32(9):1825–31.

44. Trzeciak S, Dellinger RP, Parrillo JE, et al. Early microcirculatory perfusion derangements in patients with severe sepsis and septic shock: relationship to hemodynamics, oxygen transport, and survival. Ann Emerg Med 2007;49(1):88–98, 98. e81–2.

45. Edul VS, Enrico C, Laviolle B, et al. Quantitative assessment of the microcirculation in healthy volunteers and in patients with septic shock. Crit Care Med 2012;40(5):1443–8.

46. Paize F, Sarginson R, Makwana N, et al. Changes in the sublingual microcirculation and endothelial adhesion molecules during the course of severe meningococcal disease treated in the paediatric intensive care unit. Intensive Care Med 2012;38(5):863–71.

47. Creteur J, De Backer D, Sakr Y, et al. Sublingual capnometry tracks microcirculatory changes in septic patients. Intensive Care Med 2006;32(4): 516–23.

48. Cohen J. The immunopathogenesis of sepsis. Nature 2002;420(6917):885–91.

49. Natanson C, Esposito CJ, Banks SM. The sirens' songs of confirmatory sepsis trials: selection bias

and sampling error. Crit Care Med 1998;26(12): 1927–31.

50. Opal SM, Laterre PF, Francois B, et al. Effect of eritoran, an antagonist of MD2-TLR4, on mortality in patients with severe sepsis: the ACCESS randomized trial. JAMA 2013;309(11):1154–62.

51. Rice TW, Wheeler AP, Bernard GR, et al. A randomized, double-blind, placebo-controlled trial of TAK-242 for the treatment of severe sepsis. Crit Care Med 2010;38(8):1685–94.

52. Hotchkiss RS, Monneret G, Payen D. Sepsis-induced immunosuppression: from cellular dysfunctions to immunotherapy. Nat Rev Immunol 2013;13(12):862–74.

53. De Backer D, Creteur J, Dubois MJ, et al. The effects of dobutamine on microcirculatory alterations in patients with septic shock are independent of its systemic effects. Crit Care Med 2006;34(2):403–8.

54. Schmidt EP, Damarla M, Rentsendorj O, et al. Soluble guanylyl cyclase contributes to ventilator-induced lung injury in mice. Am J Physiol Lung Cell Mol Physiol 2008;295(6):L1056–65.

55. Forstermann U. Janus-faced role of endothelial NO synthase in vascular disease: uncoupling of oxygen reduction from NO synthesis and its pharmacological reversal. Biol Chem 2006;387(12):1521–33.

56. Kuebler WM. The Janus-faced regulation of endothelial permeability by cyclic GMP. Am J Physiol Lung Cell Mol Physiol 2011;301(2):L157–60.

57. Boerma EC, Koopmans M, Konijn A, et al. Effects of nitroglycerin on sublingual microcirculatory blood flow in patients with severe sepsis/septic shock after a strict resuscitation protocol: a double-blind randomized placebo controlled trial. Crit Care Med 2010;38(1):93–100.

58. Trzeciak S, Glaspey LJ, Dellinger RP, et al. Randomized controlled trial of inhaled nitric oxide for the treatment of microcirculatory dysfunction in patients with sepsis. Crit Care Med 2014;42(12): 2482–92.

59. Vincent JL, Zhang H, Szabo C, et al. Effects of nitric oxide in septic shock. Am J Respir Crit Care Med 2000;161(6):1781–5.

60. Trzeciak S, Cinel I, Phillip Dellinger R, et al. Resuscitating the microcirculation in sepsis: the central role of nitric oxide, emerging concepts for novel therapies, and challenges for clinical trials. Acad Emerg Med 2008;15(5):399–413.

61. Yang Y, Schmidt EP. The endothelial glycocalyx: an important regulator of the pulmonary vascular barrier. Tissue Barriers 2013;1(1):e23494.

62. Luft JH. Fine structures of capillary and endocapillary layer as revealed by ruthenium red. Fed Proc 1966;25(6):1773–83.

63. Potter DR, Damiano ER. The hydrodynamically relevant endothelial cell glycocalyx observed in vivo is absent in vitro. Circ Res 2008;102(7):770–6.

64. Chappell D, Jacob M, Paul O, et al. The glycocalyx of the human umbilical vein endothelial cell: an impressive structure ex vivo but not in culture. Circ Res 2009;104(11):1313–7.

65. Ebong EE, Macaluso FP, Spray DC, et al. Imaging the endothelial glycocalyx in vitro by rapid freezing/ freeze substitution transmission electron microscopy. Arterioscler Thromb Vasc Biol 2011;31(8): 1908–15.

66. Wiesinger A, Peters W, Chappell D, et al. Nanomechanics of the endothelial glycocalyx in experimental sepsis. PLoS One 2013;8(11):e80905.

67. Curry FE, Adamson RH. Endothelial glycocalyx: permeability barrier and mechanosensor. Ann Biomed Eng 2012;40(4):828–39.

68. Florian JA, Kosky JR, Ainslie K, et al. Heparan sulfate proteoglycan is a mechanosensor on endothelial cells. Circ Res 2003;93(10):e136–42.

69. Mulivor AW, Lipowsky HH. Inhibition of glycan shedding and leukocyte-endothelial adhesion in postcapillary venules by suppression of matrixmetalloprotease activity with doxycycline. Microcirculation 2009;16(8):657–66.

70. Cabrales P, Vazquez BY, Tsai AG, et al. Microvascular and capillary perfusion following glycocalyx degradation. J Appl Physiol (1985) 2007;102(6):2251–9.

71. Zuurbier CJ, Demirci C, Koeman A, et al. Short-term hyperglycemia increases endothelial glycocalyx permeability and acutely decreases lineal density of capillaries with flowing red blood cells. J Appl Physiol (1985) 2005;99(4):1471–6.

72. Lygizos MI, Yang Y, Altmann CJ, et al. Heparanase mediates renal dysfunction during early sepsis in mice. Physiol Rep 2013;1(6):e00153.

73. Marechal X, Favory R, Joulin O, et al. Endothelial glycocalyx damage during endotoxemia coincides with microcirculatory dysfunction and vascular oxidative stress. Shock 2008;29(5):572–6.

74. Nieuwdorp M, Meuwese MC, Mooij HL, et al. Tumor necrosis factor-alpha inhibition protects against endotoxin-induced endothelial glycocalyx perturbation. Atherosclerosis 2009;202(1):296–303.

75. Nelson A, Berkestedt I, Schmidtchen A, et al. Increased levels of glycosaminoglycans during septic shock: relation to mortality and the antibacterial actions of plasma. Shock 2008;30(6):623–7.

76. Sallisalmi M, Tenhunen J, Yang R, et al. Vascular adhesion protein-1 and syndecan-1 in septic shock. Acta Anaesthesiol Scand 2012;56(3):316–22.

77. Ostrowski SR, Berg RMG, Windeløv NA, et al. Coagulopathy, catecholamines, and biomarkers of endothelial damage in experimental human endotoxemia and in patients with severe sepsis: a prospective study. J Crit Care 2013;28(5):586–96.

78. Schmidt EP, Li G, Li L, et al. The circulating glycosaminoglycan signature of respiratory failure in critically ill adults. J Biol Chem 2014;289(12):8194–202.

79. Nelson A, Berkestedt I, Bodelsson M. Circulating glycosaminoglycan species in septic shock. Acta Anaesthesiol Scand 2014;58(1):36–43.

80. Berg S, Brodin B, Hesselvik F, et al. Elevated levels of plasma hyaluronan in septicaemia. Scand J Clin Lab Invest 1988;48(8):727–32.

81. Steppan J, Hofer S, Funke B, et al. Sepsis and major abdominal surgery lead to flaking of the endothelial glycocalix. J Surg Res 2011;165(1):136–41.

82. Yagmur E, Koch A, Haumann M, et al. Hyaluronan serum concentrations are elevated in critically ill patients and associated with disease severity. Clin Biochem 2012;45(1–2):82–7.

83. Oragui EE, Nadel S, Kyd P, et al. Increased excretion of urinary glycosaminoglycans in meningococcal septicemia and their relationship to proteinuria. Crit Care Med 2000;28(8):3002–8.

84. Sun X, Li L, Overdier KH, et al. Analysis of total human urinary glycosaminoglycan disaccharides by liquid chromatography–tandem mass spectrometry. Anal Chem 2015;87(12):6220–7.

85. Ostrowski SR, Johansson PI. Endothelial glycocalyx degradation induces endogenous heparinization in patients with severe injury and early traumatic coagulopathy. J Trauma Acute Care Surg 2012;73(1):60–6.

86. Nieuwdorp M, Meuwese MC, Mooij HL, et al. Measuring endothelial glycocalyx dimensions in humans: a potential novel tool to monitor vascular vulnerability. J Appl Physiol (1985) 2008;104(3): 845–52.

87. Michel CC, Curry FR. Glycocalyx volume: a critical review of tracer dilution methods for its measurement. Microcirculation 2009;16(3):213–9.

88. Donati A, Damiani E, Domizi R, et al. Alteration of the sublingual microvascular glycocalyx in critically ill patients. Microvasc Res 2013;90:86–9.

89. Shapiro NI, Angus DC. A review of therapeutic attempts to recruit the microcirculation in patients with sepsis. Minerva Anestesiol 2014;80(2):225–35.

90. De Backer D, Verdant C, Chierego M, et al. Effects of drotrecogin alfa activated on microcirculatory alterations in patients with severe sepsis. Crit Care Med 2006;34(7):1918–24.

91. Bernard GR, Vincent JL, Laterre PF, et al. Efficacy and safety of recombinant human activated protein C for severe sepsis. N Engl J Med 2001;344(10): 699–709.

92. Abraham E, Laterre PF, Garg R, et al. Drotrecogin alfa (activated) for adults with severe sepsis and a low risk of death. N Engl J Med 2005;353(13): 1332–41.

93. Thooft A, Favory R, Salgado DR, et al. Effects of changes in arterial pressure on organ perfusion during septic shock. Crit Care 2011;15(5):R222.

94. Dubin A, Pozo MO, Casabella CA, et al. Increasing arterial blood pressure with norepinephrine does not improve microcirculatory blood flow: a prospective study. Crit Care 2009;13(3):R92.

95. Asfar P, Meziani F, Hamel JF, et al. High versus low blood-pressure target in patients with septic shock. N Engl J Med 2014;370(17):1583–93.

96. Russell JA. Adding fuel to the fire–the supranormal oxygen delivery trials controversy. Crit Care Med 1998;26(6):981–3.

97. Buchele GL, Silva E, Ospina-Tascon GA, et al. Effects of hydrocortisone on microcirculatory alterations in patients with septic shock. Crit Care Med 2009;37(4):1341–7.

98. Sprung CL, Caralis PV, Marcial EH, et al. The effects of high-dose corticosteroids in patients with septic shock. A prospective, controlled study. N Engl J Med 1984;311(18):1137–43.

99. Veterans Administration Systemic Sepsis Cooperative Study Group. Effect of high-dose glucocorticoid therapy on mortality in patients with clinical signs of systemic sepsis. N Engl J Med 1987; 317(11):659–65.

100. Cronin L, Cook DJ, Carlet J, et al. Corticosteroid treatment for sepsis: a critical appraisal and meta-analysis of the literature. Crit Care Med 1995;23(8):1430–9.

101. Sprung CL, Annane D, Keh D, et al. Hydrocortisone therapy for patients with septic shock. N Engl J Med 2008;358(2):111–24.

102. Berlot G, Bianco N, Tomasini A, et al. Changes in microvascular blood flow during coupled plasma filtration and adsorption. Anaesth Intensive Care 2011;39(4):687–9.

103. Ruiz C, Hernandez G, Godoy C, et al. Sublingual microcirculatory changes during high-volume hemofiltration in hyperdynamic septic shock patients. Crit Care 2010;14(5):R170.

104. Cruz DN, Antonelli M, Fumagalli R, et al. Early use of polymyxin B hemoperfusion in abdominal septic shock: the EUPHAS randomized controlled trial. JAMA 2009;301(23):2445–52.

105. Ospina-Tascon G, Neves AP, Occhipinti G, et al. Effects of fluids on microvascular perfusion in patients with severe sepsis. Intensive Care Med 2010;36(6):949–55.

106. Dubin A, Pozo MO, Casabella CA, et al. Comparison of 6% hydroxyethyl starch 130/0.4 and saline solution for resuscitation of the microcirculation during the early goal-directed therapy of septic patients. J Crit Care 2010;25(4):659.e651–8.

107. Finfer S, McEvoy S, Bellomo R, et al. Impact of albumin compared to saline on organ function and mortality of patients with severe sepsis. Intensive Care Med 2011;37(1):86–96.

108. Brunkhorst FM, Engel C, Bloos F, et al. Intensive insulin therapy and pentastarch resuscitation in severe sepsis. N Engl J Med 2008; 358(2):125–39.

109. Myburgh JA, Finfer S, Bellomo R, et al. Hydroxyethyl starch or saline for fluid resuscitation in intensive care. N Engl J Med 2012;367(20):1901–11.

110. Perner A, Haase N, Guttormsen AB, et al. Hydroxyethyl starch 130/0.42 versus Ringer's acetate in severe sepsis. N Engl J Med 2012;367(2):124–34.

111. Zarychanski R, Abou-Setta AM, Kanji S, et al. The efficacy and safety of heparin in patients with sepsis: a systematic review and metaanalysis. Crit Care Med 2015;43(3).511–8.

112. Levi M, Levy M, Williams MD, et al. Prophylactic heparin in patients with severe sepsis treated with drotrecogin alfa (activated). Am J Respir Crit Care Med 2007;176(5):483–90.

113. Wang L, Fuster M, Sriramarao P, et al. Endothelial heparan sulfate deficiency impairs L-selectin- and chemokine-mediated neutrophil trafficking during inflammatory responses. Nat Immunol 2005;6(9): 902–10.

114. Goetz R, Mohammadi M. Exploring mechanisms of FGF signalling through the lens of structural biology. Nat Rev Mol Cell Biol 2013;14(3):166–80.

115. Al-Banna NA, Pavlovic D, Bac VH, et al. Acute administration of antibiotics modulates intestinal capillary perfusion and leukocyte adherence during experimental sepsis. Int J Antimicrob Agents 2013;41(6):536–43.

116. Becker BF, Jacob M, Leipert S, et al. Degradation of the endothelial glycocalyx in clinical settings: searching for the sheddases. Br J Clin Pharmacol 2015;80(3):389–402.

117. Zeng Y, Adamson RH, Curry FR, et al. Sphingosine-1-phosphate protects endothelial glycocalyx by inhibiting syndecan-1 shedding. Am J Physiol Heart Circ Physiol 2014;306(3):H363–72.

118. Meuwese MC, Mooij HL, Nieuwdorp M, et al. Partial recovery of the endothelial glycocalyx upon rosuvastatin therapy in patients with heterozygous familial hypercholesterolemia. J Lipid Res 2009; 50(1):148–53.

119. Kruger P, Bailey M, Bellomo R, et al. A multicenter randomized trial of atorvastatin therapy in intensive care patients with severe sepsis. Am J Respir Crit Care Med 2013;187(7):743–50.

120. Blum CA, Nigro N, Briel M, et al. Adjunct prednisone therapy for patients with community-acquired pneumonia: a multicentre, double-blind, randomised, placebo-controlled trial. Lancet 2015;385(9977):1511–8.

121. Torres A, Sibila O, Ferrer M, et al. Effect of corticosteroids on treatment failure among hospitalized patients with severe community-acquired pneumonia and high inflammatory response: a randomized clinical trial. JAMA 2015;313(7):677–86.

# Management of Acute Kidney Injury and Acid-Base Balance in the Septic Patient

 CrossMark

Paul D. Weyker, MD[a], Xosé L. Pérez, MD[b], Kathleen D. Liu, MD, PhD, MAS[c,*]

## KEYWORDS

- Acute kidney injury • Acute renal failure • Sepsis • Acid-base • Biomarkers
- Renal replacement therapy

## KEY POINTS

- Acute kidney injury (AKI) is an abrupt decrease in kidney function that takes place over hours to days that is associated with increased morbidity and mortality in sepsis.
- Many trials have studied pharmacotherapies to prevent or treat AKI, with disappointing results.
- Management strategies for septic AKI should focus around treatment of underlying sepsis, maintaining adequate intravascular volume and avoiding fluid overload, maintaining adequate mean arterial pressure for renal perfusion, and avoidance of nephrotoxic agents.
- The mainstay of current treatment for septic AKI is renal replacement therapy, which can be delivered either intermittently or continuously.

## INTRODUCTION

### Definitions

Broadly speaking, acute kidney injury (AKI, also known as acute renal failure) is an abrupt decrease in kidney function that occurs over hours to days. This is in contradistinction to chronic kidney disease (CKD), where renal function declines over the course of months to years. In 2004, the Acute Dialysis Quality Initiative (ADQI) published the first AKI consensus definition, with the goal of standardizing disease recognition and endpoints for clinicians as well as for research studies, including clinical trials.[1] The RIFLE criteria (an acronym that stands for risk, injury, failure, loss, and end-stage renal disease [ESRD]) use acute changes in serum creatinine and urine output, 2 readily available measurements, to define 3 progressive levels of renal dysfunction (R, I, and F) and 2 clinical outcomes (L, E). These criteria were subsequently refined by the Acute Kidney Injury Network (AKIN) and then by the Kidney Disease Improving Global Outcomes (KDIGO) group (**Table 1**).[2,3] The association of AKI defined by these criteria with adverse outcomes has now been validated in a large number of clinical studies.[4–8]

### Epidemiology

These consensus definitions for AKI have greatly facilitated large epidemiologic studies examining the incidence and outcomes of AKI. Using RIFLE

K.D. Liu adjudicated clinical outcomes for clinical trials by Astute. The other authors have nothing to disclose.
[a] Division of Critical Care, Department of Anesthesia, Columbia University, 630 West, 160th Street, New York, NY 10032, USA; [b] Intensive Care Medicine, Bellvitge University Hospital, L'Hospitalet de Llobregat, Barcelona 08907, Spain; [c] Division of Critical Care Medicine, Department of Anesthesia, University of California, San Francisco, 533 Parnassus Avenue, San Francisco, CA 94143, USA
* Corresponding author. Division of Nephrology, Department of Medicine, University of California, San Francisco, Box 0532, San Francisco, CA 94143-0532.
E-mail address: Kathleen.liu@ucsf.edu

Clin Chest Med 37 (2016) 277–288
http://dx.doi.org/10.1016/j.ccm.2016.01.012
0272-5231/16/$ – see front matter © 2016 Elsevier Inc. All rights reserved.

**Table 1**
**Comparison of creatinine-based consensus definitions for acute kidney injury**

|  | RIFLE Criteria |  | AKIN Criteria | KDIGO Criteria |
|---|---|---|---|---|
| R(isk) | SCr ≥150% baseline within 7 d, OR >25% decrease in eGFR | Stage 1 | SCr ≥150% baseline, OR SCr ≥0.3 mg/L increase within 48 h | SCr ≥150% baseline within 7 d, OR SCr ≥0.3 mg/L increase within 48 h |
| I(njury) | SCr ≥200% baseline, OR >50% decrease in eGFR | Stage 2 | SCr ≥200% baseline | SCr ≥200% baseline |
| F(ailure) | SCr ≥300% baseline OR SCr >4 mg/dL with acute rise >0.5 mg/dL, OR >75% decrease in eGFR | Stage 3 | SCr ≥300% baseline, OR SCr ≥4 mg/dL with acute rise of ≥0.5 mg/dL, OR initiation of RRT | SCr ≥300% baseline, OR SCr ≥4 mg/dL,[a] OR Initiation of RRT, OR If <18 y, eGFR <35 mL/min/1.73m2 |
| L(oss) | Persistent loss for >4 wk | — | — | — |
| E(nd-stage kidney disease) | ESRD >3 mo | — | — | — |

Urine output criteria are the same for all 3 staging systems and are as follows: stage 1: <0.5 ml/kg per hour for 6 to 12 hours; stage 2: <0.5 ml/kg per hour for ≥12 hours; stage 3 <0.3 ml/kg per hour for ≥24 hours OR anuria ≥12 hours.
*Abbreviations:* AKIN, Acute Kidney Injury Network; eGFR, estimated glomerular filtration rate; ESRD, end-stage renal disease; KDIGO, Kidney Disease Improving Global Outcomes; RRT, renal replacement therapy.
[a] Must meet criteria for stage 1 as well.

criteria to define AKI, numerous large studies have found that the incidence of AKI during an admission to the intensive care unit (ICU) is often greater than 60%, although this rate will vary depending on the ICU population (medical ICU vs neurosurgery ICU, for example).[4,9–11] Other studies have found that sepsis contributes in 33% to 50% of all cases of AKI, making sepsis the leading cause of AKI.[5,12,13] Along the same lines, sepsis studies have found that AKI develops in 40% to 60% of these patients.[14–19] Not surprisingly, sepsis that is complicated by AKI has a higher mortality rate than sepsis alone, and the severity of sepsis correlates with the severity of AKI.[16,20] Mortality rates of patients with AKI needing renal replacement therapy (RRT) are approximately 35% to 50%, although again will vary based on the population.[21,22]

## Pathophysiology

Septic AKI was classically thought to be caused by an ischemic "pre-renal" etiology, attributed to hypoperfusion due to decreased renal blood flow in the setting of leaky vasculature and systemic vasodilation leading to decreased preload. However, several studies have disputed this notion, and research studies are ongoing. For example, arguing against a central role for hypoperfusion per se, a large cohort study found that 25% of hospitalized patients with community-acquired pneumonia who never developed shock or required ICU admission developed AKI.[23]

A major insight in the pathophysiology of sepsis-induced AKI came from an autopsy series of 44 patients who died of sepsis, which found that the degree of renal tubular cell injury in most patients was regional within the kidney, not severe enough to explain the AKI, and most tubular cells appeared relatively normal by electron microscopy.[24] Furthermore, it is unclear if renal blood flow uniformly decreases during sepsis in humans. A systematic review on this topic concluded that cardiac output is the major determinant of renal blood flow, and because cardiac output is typically increased in sepsis, consequently global renal blood flow may therefore be unchanged or even increased.[25] However, the glomerular filtration rate (GFR) may still be reduced in the face of normal or supranormal blood flow due to changes in afferent and efferent arteriole vasoconstriction.

Thus, it is thought that a large component of septic AKI is due to functional rather than structural or ischemic injury per se.[26] This is supported by histopathology from large animal models.[27] These effects may be mediated by proinflammatory cytokines and other plasma mediators. For example, plasma from patients with septic AKI can induce changes in polarity in podocytes and renal tubular epithelial cells in *in vitro* cell culture.[28] Recently, Gomez and colleagues[29] proposed a "unifying theory" of septic AKI. In this analysis, the decrease in GFR is in part an adaptive response to inflammatory mediators such as cytokines and lipopolysaccharide (LPS) in which renal tubular cells downregulate metabolic function to use energy toward cell survival.[29] There is also microvascular blood flow dysregulation within the kidneys, which may act to further enhance this adaptive downregulation of cellular metabolism or contribute to regional cellular dysfunction.[29] Furthermore, it has been proposed that both the afferent and efferent arterioles vasodilate, with the efferent arteriole preferentially dilating more.[30] This leads to decreased glomerular capillary pressure and thus decreased GFR.[30] In support of this theory, in animal models of sepsis, use of a selective efferent arteriole vasoconstrictor, angiotensin II, has been shown to increase GFR and urine output.[30]

In sum, at this time the exact mechanism of septic AKI is not fully elucidated. Nonetheless, it seems clear that the primary mechanism is not isolated hypoperfusion. As research in this arena continues, hopefully we will find clinically relevant targets to mitigate the deleterious effects of sepsis on the kidney. As an example, catalytic iron (iron that is not bound to transferrin or protein and is released during tissue injury and during hemolysis) has been proposed to be injurious to the kidney.[31] At least one source of catalytic iron is plasma-free hemoglobin, which can derive from hemolysis or red blood cell transfusions. Furthermore, it is thought that plasma-free hemoglobin itself may cause cell damage through oxidation of lipid membranes.[32] A small single-center, randomized, double-blind, placebo-controlled trial compared 3 days of enteral acetaminophen with placebo in reducing oxidative injury in patients with severe sepsis and detectable plasma cell–free hemoglobin.[32] The proposed mechanism is the ability of acetaminophen to reduce the ferryl radical in the free hemoglobin and thus prevent lipid peroxidation. In this small study, acetaminophen improved renal function during and after the study.[32] Although there are many limitations to generalizability, this finding warrants further investigation in larger trials and highlights the importance of further studies focused on the pathogenesis of septic AKI.

## Risk Factors

Many studies have examined clinical risk factors for AKI; however, relatively few studies have specifically focused on patients presenting with sepsis. In a large prospective cohort study of 390 patients who presented in septic shock without preexisting ESRD or AKI, 237 (61%) developed AKI.[15] Delay in antibiotic administration, intra-abdominal sepsis, use of blood products, angiotensin-converting enzyme (ACE)-inhibitor/angiotensin receptor blocker (ARB) use, and elevated body mass index were independently associated with development of septic AKI.[15] Higher baseline GFR and successful early goal-directed resuscitation were associated with better renal outcomes.[15] In a large retrospective study of nearly 1000 patients presenting with sepsis,[19] increasing age, CKD, ACE-inhibitor/ARB use, shock, positive blood cultures, and lower white blood cell or platelet counts were all independently associated with development of septic AKI.[19] Although studies like these are important to elucidate potential targets for clinical intervention, unfortunately a number of risk factors (age, CKD) are not modifiable, and some targets represent "best clinical practice" for sepsis. For example, early antibiotic administration has been shown to decrease mortality in sepsis and is a cornerstone of sepsis management, and may also help mitigate septic AKI.

## MANAGEMENT GOALS

At present, no specific treatments exist for either the prevention or treatment of septic AKI, with the exception of supportive care for established AKI with RRT. The optimal care of patients at risk for septic AKI or with established AKI is supportive care and avoidance of nephrotoxins. Fluid management in patients with sepsis is discussed extensively in other sections of this issue, so we focus on issues related specifically to patients with established AKI in this article.

### "Euvolemia"

As discussed earlier, septic AKI is much more complex than decreased renal perfusion; however, improving renal perfusion in the setting of hypotension may help mitigate some of the harmful effects of septic AKI. Renal blood flow can be estimated as follows: Renal Blood Flow = (Mean Arterial Pressure – Renal Venous Pressure)/Renal Vascular Resistance. Although this is probably an oversimplification of actual renal blood flow, it conceptualizes the importance of attempting to find the "sweet spot" of "euvolemia" when resuscitating a septic patient; by this, we mean a fluid state in which intravascular volume is optimized with minimal fluid overload. We can see that renal blood flow can be affected by mean arterial pressure (MAP), renal venous pressure, and renal vascular resistance. It has long been known that hypovolemia produces "pre-renal" ischemic AKI, and the treatment is fluid administration to improve cardiac output and thus oxygen delivery to the kidneys; however, it has become increasingly clear that overzealous fluid administration can cause AKI as well.[33–35] If the renal venous pressure increases, as it often does when large amounts of fluid are administered, it can lead to decreased renal blood flow and decreased GFR.[35] The combination of low MAP and intra-abdominal hypertension (which increases renal venous pressure), which are often seen in sepsis, may contribute to AKI. In the surgical literature there is some evidence that goal-directed therapy, which is a protocol that tries to maximize cardiac output through fluid and inotrope administration, may decrease incidence of AKI.[33] However, 3 recent large sepsis trials found no benefit with early goal-directed therapy compared with usual care with regard to mortality or kidney outcomes.[36–38] A small retrospective study looking specifically at the development of AKI in a cohort of patients treated with early goal-directed therapy versus those treated with usual care found no difference in development of AKI (46% vs 51%, respectively).[17]

The ADQI had a recent consensus conference on fluid therapy.[39] As part of this conference, a conceptual framework for fluid management was proposed (**Fig. 1**) that highlights the importance of individualizing fluid resuscitation and the fact that the goals of fluid therapy may vary over the course of disease.[40] Early on, during the "rescue" phase of resuscitation, fluids are needed to improve circulation, as described previously. This is followed by "optimization" and "stabilization" phases in which fluid therapy is titrated to the individual patients. Finally, during the recovery phase, "deescalation" of fluid therapy, which may include diuretics to enhance fluid mobilization, is needed to avoid the sequelae of volume overload. In this context, it should be noted that retrospective studies of clinical trials of fluid management have suggested that positive fluid balance, but not diuretic administration, is associated with increased mortality in patients with the acute respiratory distress syndrome and early AKI.[41]

## Mean Arterial Pressure Goals

Autoregulation is the ability of an organ to maintain a relatively constant blood flow across a wide range of MAPs. In a patient who is normotensive, renal autoregulation is intact between MAPs of between approximately 60 to 160 mm Hg. Below 60 mm Hg, renal blood flow decreases and thus GFR decreases. A recent study by Asfar and colleagues[42] looking at blood-pressure targets in patients with septic shock found no mortality benefit of targeting a higher MAP (80–85 mm Hg) versus a lower MAP (65–70 mm Hg). However, in patients with chronic hypertension, a decreased incidence of AKI and lower need for RRT was observed in the higher MAP group.[42] In hypotensive patients with vasodilatory shock refractory to adequate volume resuscitation, judicious use of vasopressors to restore MAP to a level above the lower limit of autoregulation will likely improve renal blood flow and thus GFR.[35] Of course, vasopressors should be used cautiously in cardiogenic shock and only after volume resuscitation in hypovolemic shock.

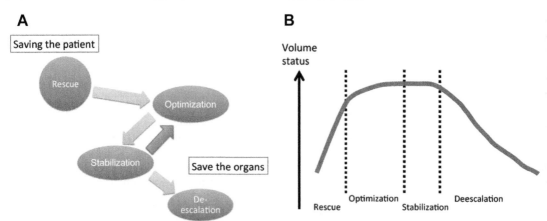

**Fig. 1.** Conceptual model of fluid management proposed by the ADQI. (A) In the critically ill patient, fluid management is proposed to follow 4 stages: rescue, optimization, stabilization and deescalation. (B) Fluid balance during the 4 stages of fluid management. The rescue phase is characterized by positive fluid balance; during the optimization and stabilization phases fluid balance is the most positive and the goal of these phases is to optimize effective circulating volume. Finally, during the deescalation phase, diuretics or RRT may be needed to resolve fluid overload, while maintaining an effective intravascular volume. (*Courtesy of* Acute Dialysis Quality Initiative. Available at: www.adqi.org.)

The choice of vasopressor has been the subject of several large trials over the years. In recent years, it has become widely accepted that norepinephrine is the initial vasopressor of choice for septic shock.[43–46] However, there is growing interest in the use of vasopressin in vasodilatory septic shock. Vasopressin, an endogenous stress hormone, acts via the V1 receptor located on vascular smooth muscle to cause vasoconstriction.[47] Endogenous vasopressin levels, as well as vasopressin receptors, are decreased in septic shock.[47,48] Importantly for septic shock, the actions of vasopressin include efferent arteriole vasoconstriction (which increases GFR) and improvement in the sensitivity of other vasopressor agents at catecholamine receptors and have been shown in small clinical studies.[48–50] A much larger study comparing the use of norepinephrine and vasopressin in septic shock found possible mortality benefit in patients with less severe shock (as defined by norepinephrine infusion rates between 5 and 15 µg/min) but no mortality difference in patients with severe shock.[51] This has led some to advocate for vasopressin as a second choice vasopressor agent in septic shock when adequate MAP goals cannot be achieved with low-dose norepinephrine.[46,47] Finally, for completeness sake, we note that there are no data to support the use of dopamine to improve renal outcomes,[52–54] and given the increased rate of arrhythmias observed with dopamine compared with norepinephrine in clinical trials, in general, dopamine should be avoided.[43]

## Nephrotoxins

Although we have no effective treatments for septic AKI at present, avoidance of nephrotoxic agents is paramount. The list of agents known to be injurious to the kidneys is extensive; however, there are few agents worth special mention, as they are commonly used in treatment of septic patients. Hydroxyethyl starch is a colloid that was once commonly used in resuscitation for patients with septic shock. However, several large studies and systematic reviews have shown use of hydroxyethyl starch is associated with increased risk of AKI and RRT, and in some cases, with an increased risk of death.[55–58] Fluid selection in the setting of septic shock is more globally addressed in other articles in this issue.

A growing body of literature suggests that administration of large volumes of crystalloids with supraphysiologic concentrations of chloride (ie, normal saline) may be associated with poorer outcomes than more balanced crystalloid solutions (ie, Ringer Lactate and Plasmalyte).[59,60]

Proposed mechanisms include a renal vasoconstrictive effect of high concentrations of chloride, as well as a macula densa–mediated tubuloglomerular feedback mechanism, which triggers afferent arteriolar vasoconstriction, thus lowering the GFR.[59,61] A large recent study suggested no benefit to balanced salt solutions over normal saline in a large population of critically ill patients,[62] but more research is clearly needed. For example, only 4% of study subjects had a primary diagnosis of sepsis in this trial. Furthermore, in an observational study comparing normal saline and balanced salt solutions during open abdominal surgery,[63] fewer blood gas and lactate measurements were obtained in subjects who received balanced salt solution. Thus, in patients with sepsis who are at high risk of lactic acidosis, the use of balanced salt solutions may be prudent from a resource utilization perspective as well.

Several antimicrobial agents have been associated with kidney injury through a variety of mechanisms. Amphotericin, aminoglycosides, and colistin are associated with acute tubular necrosis.[64] Many antibiotics, and in particular the beta-lactams, can cause interstitial nephritis.[64] Given the high rates of AKI with aminoglycosides and amphotericin, the KDIGO guidelines make special note of these agents.[3] Specifically, the guidelines recommend that aminoglycosides should be used only if no other alternative is available; similarly, amphotericin should be used only when azole or echinocandins cannot be used, and lipid formulations, which are associated with lower rates of nephrotoxicity, should be used.[3]

One of the most commonly used antibiotics in the ICU, vancomycin, deserves special mention. Originally approved in the 1950s, vancomycin remains the antibiotic of choice for methicillin-resistant Staphylococcus aureus (MRSA) infection. In the early years of clinical use, vancomycin nephrotoxicity was attributed to impurities from the manufacturing process.[65] Although the manufacturing process has improved, there has been a reported increase in the rate of vancomycin-associated AKI in recent years where a target trough of 15 to 20 mg/dL has been recommended for MRSA infections.[65–68] However, whether or not this is a true condition or whether much of this represents confounding remains controversial.[65,67] Some studies have suggested that concomitant exposure to other nephrotoxic agents (specifically piperacillin-tazobactam) increases the incidence of vancomycin toxicity.[68] Regardless, close attention should be paid to vancomycin dosing in the setting of AKI, and frequent monitoring of vancomycin levels should be used to guide dosing.

Iodinated contrast agents are perhaps the most widely recognized nephrotoxin used in clinical practice, although newer low-osmolar contrast agents confer a lower risk of nephrotoxicity. Patients with CKD and those with sepsis are at a higher risk of developing AKI from iodinated contrast. Early recognition of AKI using the consensus definitions described previously is also important. In these patient groups (those with AKI or CKD and those with sepsis) it is important to balance the risks and benefits when deciding to obtain these studies. Discussion with a radiologist can help determine if there are alternative means of imaging that can avoid iodinated contrast agents. The use of bicarbonate and N-acetylcysteine to prevent contrast nephropathy is controversial and is the subject of large randomized clinical trials.[69] However, there is clear benefit to intravenous fluid administration, so it is critical to ensure patients are volume resuscitated before iodinated contrast administration.[70,71] Finally, gadolinium, the contrast material used in MRI, has been linked to nephrogenic systemic fibrosis in patients with both AKI and CKD.[72,73] Small studies have suggested an association between gadolinium and AKI in particular in the setting of sepsis, but this association remains controversial.[74]

## PHARMACOLOGIC STRATEGIES

Despite numerous studies, at present there are no pharmacotherapies to directly prevent or treat AKI. Although an exhaustive review of the literature as it pertains to these medications is beyond the scope of this review, many of these studies are reviewed in the KDIGO AKI guidelines.[3] Due to their anti-inflammatory properties, there has been significant recent interest in the use of statins (HMG-CoA reductase inhibitors) as a treatment for AKI in multiple settings, including sepsis. In the setting of sepsis, there have been no randomized clinical trials focused on AKI, but in a large prospective cohort study of patients hospitalized with pneumonia, statins were not found to reduce the risk of AKI, and in fact prehospital statin use was associated with a small increased risk of AKI, which was attributed to indication bias.[75] Furthermore, a meta-analysis of randomized clinical trials suggested that statins did not improve mortality in patients with sepsis.[76]

## NONPHARMACOLOGIC STRATEGIES
### Renal Replacement Therapy

The mainstay of treatment for septic AKI is RRT to treat and prevent complications associated with AKI. Several topics important to the critical care physician are discussed, namely timing of RRT initiation, choice of continuous versus intermittent modality, and dose of RRT.

### Indications
The classic indications for RRT in septic AKI are the same as for other critically ill patients: acidemia, volume overload, electrolyte abnormalities (hyperkalemia), and uremia (pericarditis, encephalopathy). In all cases, the risks of RRT (placement of a large-bore dialysis catheter), as well as blood loss and potential complications of RRT, such as electrolyte disturbances, hemodynamic compromise, air embolism, and worsening kidney injury,[77,78] must be weighed against potential benefits. Strategies to minimize risks and complications associated with RRT have been proposed, and may be of benefit.[79]

### Timing (early vs late)
Optimal timing of RRT initiation continues to be debated in the literature. Although aggregate studies have suggested that earlier initiation of RRT in critically ill patients may improve survival,[80,81] there is significant confounding given the heterogeneity of published studies. Specifically, "early" versus "late" have been variably defined; although blood urea nitrogen levels have most commonly been used as the cutoff, studies have also used serum creatinine, urine output, and RIFLE criteria.[81] Clearly, large, well-executed randomized clinical trials are needed, although the design of such studies is complex, as some patients may recover from AKI with supportive care alone. Although a pilot randomized clinical trial of accelerated versus standard initiation dialysis demonstrated that this approach was feasible, in the standard arm 13 (25%) of 51 subjects never required dialysis and had renal recovery; a large randomized clinical trial based on this pilot study has been initiated.[82]

### Modality (intermittent vs continuous)
The use of continuous RRT (CRRT) versus intermittent modalities (including conventional intermittent hemodialysis [IHD] and prolonged intermittent RRT [PIRRT]) also remains a subject of interest. Several randomized clinical trials and systematic reviews have found no differences in mortality or recovery of kidney function.[77] However, the entry criteria for many of the randomized clinical trials in this field required that an MAP greater than 70 mm Hg could be maintained (with or without vasopressors), which may not be possible in the setting of septic shock. Thus, the KDIGO guidelines, which recommend that use of CRRT and IHD be complementary, and that CRRT be

considered in hemodynamically unstable patients, seem measured and reasonable.[83] Because hypotension has been associated with prolonged renal recovery in animal models and because there are more episodes of hypotension (on average) with IHD than CRRT, there has been tremendous interest in the impact of modality on renal recovery. A recent retrospective cohort study of more than 4000 patients with AKI requiring some form of RRT found that CRRT was associated with a decreased risk of long-term dialysis.[84] This effect was more prominent in the patients with CKD.[84] It should be noted that the costs of CRRT are considerably more than IHD.[85] Finally, PIRRT (originally named sustained/slow low-efficiency dialysis or SLED), is an alternative for hemodynamically unstable patients in particular in centers without CRRT capability.[86] This modality of therapy is typically performed over 6 to 12 hours per day to allow for more gentle fluid removal and solute clearance than IHD. However, a particular concern for this modality is antibiotic dosing, because there is an extended period with increased clearance, followed by a long period of reduced clearance, by design.[87,88]

## Dose

The dose of dialysis has been the subject of a number of large randomized clinical trials. In CRRT, the dose is the sum of the ultrafiltrate plus dialysate (the effluent) normalized to body weight.[77] For IHD, dialysis adequacy is standardly measured as the Kt/V or urea reduction ratio. Although early studies suggested a benefit to higher doses of dialysis,[89,90] 2 large randomized clinical trials suggested no benefit to higher doses of RRT.[21,22] However, it is crucial to quantify dose of dialysis for patients with dialysis requiring AKI, as IHD treatments in particular may need to be optimized to achieve the target dose.[21,22]

## Antibiotic dosing during renal replacement therapy

A number of small studies have shown that it is not uncommon for patients on CRRT to not achieve adequate serum levels of antibiotics needed to optimally treat infections, a particular problem in the setting of septic AKI.[91–93] Dosing of antimicrobials may be even more problematic for PIRRT, in which an extended period of increased clearance is followed by a period of minimal clearance. Not only are there virtually no data to guide antimicrobial dosing, recommendations from expert pharmacists vary widely.[87,88]

For patients on CRRT where clearance is continuous, one general concept is that dosing of antibiotics that are concentration-dependent (fluoroquinolones, aminoglycosides, daptomycin, and amphotericin), should be adjusted by changing dosing interval, whereas the dosing interval of time-dependent antibiotics (beta-lactams and azoles) is constant, while actual dose is reduced.[94] Another important point is that in general initial dose of antibiotics should remain the same or slightly higher due to increased volume of distribution in patients with renal failure.[94,95] Antibiotics/ antifungals that are extremely nephrotoxic, such as aminoglycosides and amphotericin, are best avoided unless there no other suitable alternatives.[3] Finally, when drug levels can be measured, levels should be used to help guide dose and interval of administration.[95]

## Acid-Base Balance

### pH goal

The kidneys play a critical role in the maintenance of acid-base homeostasis. Severe sepsis is often associated with lactic acidosis that overwhelms the ability of the pulmonary system to maintain a normal pH through respiratory compensation. Along with the liver, the kidney plays an important role in lactate metabolism.[96] Furthermore, in the setting of AKI, renal acid excretion is impaired. Severe acidosis may have a number of adverse effects, including cardiac dysfunction, arrhythmias, and catecholamine refractory vasodilation. However, the optimal pH goal and management strategies for obtaining that goal are areas of intense debate. Specifically, the use of bicarbonate in lactic acidosis, which is the most commonly encountered acid-base disturbance in sepsis, is intensely debated.[97,98] The current Surviving Sepsis Guidelines do not recommend the use of bicarbonate for lactic acidosis unless the pH is lower than 7.15, and others have advocated for even lower pH targets.[98] However, not all acidosis is treated equal; for example, in the case of lactic acidosis associated with metformin use (which may be precipitated by sepsis), dialysis may be indicated to remove metformin as well as to stabilize pH.[99]

### Buffers

The treatment of patients with refractory acidemia (pH <7.15) is generally accomplished with either the use of dialysis (which removes metabolic acids and includes a buffer, typically bicarbonate) or a buffer alone. As mentioned previously, severe acidemia is considered an indication for RRT. The use of bicarbonate is quite common, although controversial and with many theoretic harmful effects, such as hypervolemia, hypernatremia, impaired oxygen delivery, and hypocalcemia.[100] An alternative to bicarbonate is tris-hydroxymethyl aminomethane (THAM), a weak base that is able to diffuse intracellularly, and bind carbon dioxide and metabolic acids.[101] Protonated THAM is then excreted through the kidneys.[101] Adverse effects of THAM include hyperkalemia, hypoglycemia, pseudohyponatremia, and increased osmolal gap in patients with renal dysfunction, so its use should be avoided in patients with AKI.[101]

### Avoidance of hyperchloremic solutions

As mentioned previously, the use of high chloride solutions is controversial at present because these solutions have been associated in some studies with increased rates of AKI and morbidity after abdominal surgery.[59,60] However, regardless of these effects, high chloride solutions are associated with a hyperchloremic metabolic acidosis, and in the setting of septic AKI, this acidosis may be exacerbated by concomitant lactic acidosis, respiratory acidosis in the setting of low tidal volume, lung protective ventilation, as well as the impaired ability of the kidney to excrete chloride. Thus, it is prudent to avoid large volume resuscitation with large volumes of 0.9% sodium chloride solution, and instead use balanced salt solutions.

## FUTURE DIRECTIONS

Consensus definitions for AKI have been critical to move the AKI clinical research field forward, but have significant limitations because they use creatinine and urine output for the detection of kidney injury. Creatinine is a marker of glomerular filtration and consequently is a late marker of kidney injury (eg, by the time creatinine rises, injury has long occurred), and it has been suggested that creatinine production may be affected by sepsis.[102] Urine output may reflect a number of states including AKI, such as volume depletion and dehydration.[103] Numerous studies have focused on identifying more sensitive and specific biomarkers of AKI to aid in earlier detection and better prognostication. These include urinary biomarkers of tubular injury such as kidney injury molecule-1 (KIM-1) and neutrophil gelatinase-associated lipocalin, as well as markers of glomerular filtration, such as cystatin C, which is less dependent on muscle mass than creatinine.[104] Recently, a novel biomarker panel has become available to identify patients at increased risk of AKI in the ICU; this test combines insulinlike growth factor-binding protein 7 (IGFBP7) and tissue inhibitor of metalloproteinases-2 (TIMP-2), inducers of cell cycle arrest.[105,106] However, further studies are needed to determine how to optimally use this test in clinical practice.

## SUMMARY

In summary, despite improving outcomes overall from sepsis, septic AKI remains associated with significant morbidity and mortality. At present, all care for septic AKI is supportive, and focused on best practices for patients with sepsis (early fluid resuscitation and antibiotics, as well as source control), minimizing fluid overload, consideration of higher MAP targets in patients with chronic hypertension, and avoidance of nephrotoxins. For patients with severe AKI, dialysis may be needed. In this context, IHD and PIRRT/CRRT can be considered complementary modalities, although a major concern for PIRRT in septic patients is the lack of data to guide antimicrobial dosing. With regard to acid-base balance, hyperchloremic solutions may exacerbate acidosis and should be avoided; other adverse consequences of these solutions remain controversial. Dialysis is often needed in patients with severe septic AKI for supportive management of acidosis.

## REFERENCES

1. Bellomo R, Ronco C, Kellum JA, et al. Acute renal failure - definition, outcome measures, animal models, fluid therapy and information technology needs: the Second International Consensus Conference of the Acute Dialysis Quality Initiative (ADQI) Group. Crit Care 2004;8(4):R204–12.
2. Mehta RL, Kellum JA, Shah SV, et al. Acute Kidney Injury Network: report of an initiative to improve outcomes in acute kidney injury. Crit Care 2007; 11(2):R31.
3. Kellum JA, Lameire N, KDIGO AKI Guideline Work Group. Diagnosis, evaluation, and management of acute kidney injury: a KDIGO summary (Part 1). Crit Care 2013;17(1):204.
4. Hoste EA, Clermont G, Kersten A, et al. RIFLE criteria for acute kidney injury are associated with hospital mortality in critically ill patients: a cohort analysis. Crit Care 2006;10(3):R73.
5. Uchino S, Kellum JA, Bellomo R, et al. Acute renal failure in critically ill patients: a multinational, multi-center study. JAMA 2005;294(7):813–8.
6. Lopes JA, Jorge S, Resina C, et al. Prognostic utility of RIFLE for acute renal failure in patients with sepsis. Crit Care 2007;11(2):408.
7. Thakar CV, Christianson A, Freyberg R, et al. Incidence and outcomes of acute kidney injury in intensive care units: a Veterans Administration study. Crit Care Med 2009;37(9):2552–8.
8. Joannidis M, Metnitz B, Bauer P, et al. Acute kidney injury in critically ill patients classified by AKIN versus RIFLE using the SAPS 3 database. Intensive Care Med 2009;35(10):1692–702.

9. Piccinni P, Cruz DN, Gramaticopolo S, et al. Prospective multicenter study on epidemiology of acute kidney injury in the ICU: a critical care nephrology Italian collaborative effort (NEFROINT). Minerva Anestesiol 2011;77(11):1072–83.

10. Kane-Gill SL, Sileanu FE, Murugan R, et al. Risk factors for acute kidney injury in older adults with critical illness: a retrospective cohort study. Am J Kidney Dis 2014;65(6):860–9.

11. Hoste EA, Bagshaw SM, Bellomo R, et al. Epidemiology of acute kidney injury in critically ill patients: the multinational AKI-EPI study. Intensive Care Med 2015;41(8):1411–23.

12. Ali T, Khan I, Simpson W, et al. Incidence and outcomes in acute kidney injury: a comprehensive population-based study. J Am Soc Nephrol 2007; 18(4):1292–8.

13. Bagshaw SM, Uchino S, Bellomo R, et al. Septic acute kidney injury in critically ill patients: clinical characteristics and outcomes. Clin J Am Soc Nephrol 2007;2(3):431–9.

14. Poukkanen M, Vaara ST, Pettila V, et al. Acute kidney injury in patients with severe sepsis in Finnish intensive care units. Acta Anaesthesiol Scand 2013;57(7):863–72.

15. Plataki M, Kashani K, Cabello-Garza J, et al. Predictors of acute kidney injury in septic shock patients: an observational cohort study. Clin J Am Soc Nephrol 2011;6(7):1744–51.

16. Rangel-Frausto MS, Pittet D, Costigan M, et al. The natural history of the systemic inflammatory response syndrome (SIRS). A prospective study. JAMA 1995;273(2):117–23.

17. Ahmed W, Memon AI, Rehmani R, et al. Outcome of patients with acute kidney injury in severe sepsis and septic shock treated with early goal-directed therapy in an intensive care unit. Saudi J Kidney Dis Transpl 2014;25(3):544–51.

18. Bagshaw SM, George C, Bellomo R, et al. Early acute kidney injury and sepsis: a multicentre evaluation. Crit Care 2008;12(2):R47.

19. Suh SH, Kim CS, Choi JS, et al. Acute kidney injury in patients with sepsis and septic shock: risk factors and clinical outcomes. Yonsei Med J 2013;54(4):965–72.

20. Lopes JA, Jorge S, Resina C, et al. Acute renal failure in patients with sepsis. Crit Care 2007;11(2):411.

21. Palevsky PM, Zhang JH, O'Connor TZ, et al, for the VA/NIH Acute Renal Failure Trials Network. Intensity of renal support in critically ill patients with acute kidney injury. N Engl J Med 2008; 359(1):7–20.

22. Bellomo R, Cass A, Cole L, et al, for the RENAL Replacement Therapy Study Investigators. Intensity of continuous renal-replacement therapy in critically ill patients. N Engl J Med 2009;361(17): 1627–38.

23. Murugan R, Karajala-Subramanyam V, Lee M, et al. Acute kidney injury in non-severe pneumonia is associated with an increased immune response and lower survival. Kidney Int 2010;77(6):527–35.

24. Takasu O, Gaut JP, Watanabe E, et al. Mechanisms of cardiac and renal dysfunction in patients dying of sepsis. Am J Respir Crit Care Med 2013; 187(5):509–17.

25. Langenberg C, Bellomo R, May C, et al. Renal blood flow in sepsis. Crit Care 2005;9(4):R363–74.

26. Morrell ED, Kellum JA, Pastor-Soler NM, et al. Septic acute kidney injury: molecular mechanisms and the importance of stratification and targeting therapy. Crit Care 2014;18(5):501.

27. Langenberg C, Gobe G, Hood S, et al. Renal histopathology during experimental septic acute kidney injury and recovery. Crit Care Med 2014; 42(1):e58–67.

28. Mariano F, Cantaluppi V, Stella M, et al. Circulating plasma factors induce tubular and glomerular alterations in septic burns patients. Crit Care 2008; 12(2):R42.

29. Gomez H, Ince C, De Backer D, et al. A unified theory of sepsis-induced acute kidney injury: inflammation, microcirculatory dysfunction, bioenergetics, and the tubular cell adaptation to injury. Shock 2014;41(1):3–11.

30. Bellomo R, Wan L, Langenberg C, et al. Septic acute kidney injury: the glomerular arterioles. Contrib Nephrol 2011;174:98–107.

31. Leaf DE, Rajapurkar M, Lele SS, et al. Plasma catalytic iron, AKI, and death among critically ill patients. Clin J Am Soc Nephrol 2014;9(11): 1849–56.

32. Janz DR, Bastarache JA, Rice TW, et al. Randomized, placebo-controlled trial of acetaminophen for the reduction of oxidative injury in severe sepsis: the acetaminophen for the reduction of oxidative injury in severe sepsis trial. Crit Care Med 2014;43(3):534–41.

33. Prowle JR, Chua HR, Bagshaw SM, et al. Clinical review: Volume of fluid resuscitation and the incidence of acute kidney injury - a systematic review. Crit Care 2012;16(4):230.

34. Legrand M, Dupuis C, Simon C, et al. Association between systemic hemodynamics and septic acute kidney injury in critically ill patients: a retrospective observational study. Crit Care 2013; 17(6):R278.

35. Prowle JR, Kirwan CJ, Bellomo R. Fluid management for the prevention and attenuation of acute kidney injury. Nat Rev Nephrol 2014; 10(1):37–47.

36. Investigators A, Group ACT, Peake SL, et al. Goal-directed resuscitation for patients with early septic shock. N Engl J Med 2014;371(16): 1496–506.

37. Pro CI, Yealy DM, Kellum JA, et al. A randomized trial of protocol-based care for early septic shock. N Engl J Med 2014;370(18):1683–93.

38. Mouncey PR, Osborn TM, Power GS, et al. Trial of early, goal-directed resuscitation for septic shock. N Engl J Med 2015;372(14):1301–11.

39. Kellum JA, Mythen MG, Shaw AD. The 12th consensus conference of the Acute Dialysis Quality Initiative (ADQI XII). Br J Anaesth 2014; 113(5):729–31.

40. Hoste EA, Maitland K, Brudney CS, et al. Four phases of intravenous fluid therapy: a conceptual model. Br J Anaesth 2014;113(5):740–7.

41. Grams ME, Estrella MM, Coresh J, et al. Fluid balance, diuretic use, and mortality in acute kidney injury. Clin J Am Soc Nephrol 2011;6(5):966–73.

42. Asfar P, Meziani F, Hamel JF, et al. High versus low blood-pressure target in patients with septic shock. N Engl J Med 2014;370(17):1583–93.

43. De Backer D, Biston P, Devriendt J, et al. Comparison of dopamine and norepinephrine in the treatment of shock. N Engl J Med 2010; 362(9):779–89.

44. De Backer D, Aldecoa C, Njimi H, et al. Dopamine versus norepinephrine in the treatment of septic shock: a meta-analysis*. Crit Care Med 2012; 40(3):725–30.

45. Vasu TS, Cavallazzi R, Hirani A, et al. Norepinephrine or dopamine for septic shock: systematic review of randomized clinical trials. J Intensive Care Med 2012;27(3):172–8.

46. Dellinger RP, Levy MM, Rhodes A, et al. Surviving sepsis campaign: international guidelines for management of severe sepsis and septic shock: 2012. Crit Care Med 2013;41(2):580–637.

47. Russell JA. Bench-to-bedside review: vasopressin in the management of septic shock. Crit Care 2011;15(4):226.

48. Holmes CL, Patel BM, Russell JA, et al. Physiology of vasopressin relevant to management of septic shock. Chest 2001;120(3):989–1002.

49. Tsuneyoshi I, Yamada H, Kakihana Y, et al. Hemodynamic and metabolic effects of low-dose vasopressin infusions in vasodilatory septic shock. Crit Care Med 2001;29(3):487–93.

50. Patel BM, Chittock DR, Russell JA, et al. Beneficial effects of short-term vasopressin infusion during severe septic shock. Anesthesiology 2002;96(3): 576–82.

51. Russell JA, Walley KR, Singer J, et al. Vasopressin versus norepinephrine infusion in patients with septic shock. N Engl J Med 2008;358(9):877–87.

52. Chertow GM, Sayegh MH, Allgren RL, et al. Is the administration of dopamine associated with adverse or favorable outcomes in acute renal failure? Auriculin Anaritide Acute Renal Failure Study Group. Am J Med 1996;101(1):49–53.

53. Bellomo R, Chapman M, Finfer S, et al. Low-dose dopamine in patients with early renal dysfunction: a placebo-controlled randomised trial. Australian and New Zealand Intensive Care Society (ANZICS) Clinical Trials Group. Lancet 2000; 356(9248):2139–43.

54. Jones D, Bellomo R. Renal-dose dopamine: from hypothesis to paradigm to dogma to myth and, finally, superstition? J Intensive Care Med 2005; 20(4):199–211.

55. Perner A, Haase N, Guttormsen AB, et al. Hydroxyethyl starch 130/0.42 versus Ringer's acetate in severe sepsis. N Engl J Med 2012;367(2):124–34.

56. Myburgh JA, Finfer S, Bellomo R, et al. Hydroxyethyl starch or saline for fluid resuscitation in intensive care. N Engl J Med 2012;367(20):1901–11.

57. Haase N, Perner A, Hennings LI, et al. Hydroxyethyl starch 130/0.38–0.45 versus crystalloid or albumin in patients with sepsis: systematic review with meta-analysis and trial sequential analysis. BMJ 2013;346:f839.

58. Zarychanski R, Abou-Setta AM, Turgeon AF, et al. Association of hydroxyethyl starch administration with mortality and acute kidney injury in critically ill patients requiring volume resuscitation: a systematic review and meta-analysis. JAMA 2013; 309(7):678–88.

59. Yunos NM, Bellomo R, Hegarty C, et al. Association between a chloride-liberal vs chloride-restrictive intravenous fluid administration strategy and kidney injury in critically ill adults. JAMA 2012; 308(15):1566–72.

60. Raghunathan K, Shaw A, Nathanson B, et al. Association between the choice of IV crystalloid and in-hospital mortality among critically ill adults with sepsis*. Crit Care Med 2014;42(7):1585–91.

61. Yunos NM, Bellomo R, Story D, et al. Bench-to-bedside review: chloride in critical illness. Crit Care 2010;14(4):226.

62. Young P, Bailey M, Beasley R, et al. Effect of a buffered crystalloid solution vs saline on acute kidney injury among patients in the intensive care unit: the split randomized clinical trial. JAMA 2015; 314(16):1701–10.

63. Shaw AD, Bagshaw SM, Goldstein SL, et al. Major complications, mortality, and resource utilization after open abdominal surgery: 0.9% saline compared to Plasma-Lyte. Ann Surg 2012;255(5): 821–9.

64. Eftekhari P. Evaluation of acute kidney injury in the hospital setting. Prim Care 2014;41(4):779–802.

65. Hazlewood KA, Brouse SD, Pitcher WD, et al. Vancomycin-associated nephrotoxicity: grave concern or death by character assassination? Am J Med 2010;123(2):182.e1–7.

66. Cano EL, Haque NZ, Welch VL, et al. Incidence of nephrotoxicity and association with vancomycin

use in intensive care unit patients with pneumonia: retrospective analysis of the IMPACT-HAP Database. Clin Ther 2012;34(1):149–57.

67. Elyasi S, Khalili H, Dashti-Khavidaki S, et al. Vancomycin-induced nephrotoxicity: mechanism, incidence, risk factors and special populations. A literature review. Eur J Clin Pharmacol 2012; 68(9):1243–55.

68. Meaney CJ, Hynicka LM, Tsoukleris MG. Vancomycin-associated nephrotoxicity in adult medicine patients: incidence, outcomes, and risk factors. Pharmacotherapy 2014;34(7):653–61.

69. Weisbord SD, Gallagher M, Kaufman J, et al. Prevention of contrast-induced AKI: a review of published trials and the design of the prevention of serious adverse events following angiography (PRESERVE) trial. Clin J Am Soc Nephrol 2013; 8(9):1618–31.

70. Mueller C. Prevention of contrast-induced nephropathy with volume supplementation. Kidney Int Suppl 2006;(100):S16–9.

71. Trivedi HS, Moore H, Nasr S, et al. A randomized prospective trial to assess the role of saline hydration on the development of contrast nephrotoxicity. Nephron Clin Pract 2003;93(1):C29–34.

72. Kallen AJ, Jhung MA, Cheng S, et al. Gadolinium-containing magnetic resonance imaging contrast and nephrogenic systemic fibrosis: a case-control study. Am J Kidney Dis 2008;51(6):966–75.

73. Zou Z, Zhang HL, Roditi GH, et al. Nephrogenic systemic fibrosis: review of 370 biopsy-confirmed cases. JACC Cardiovasc Imaging 2011;4(11):1206–16.

74. Chien CC, Wang HY, Wang JJ, et al. Risk of acute kidney injury after exposure to gadolinium-based contrast in patients with renal impairment. Ren Fail 2011;33(8):758–64.

75. Murugan R, Weissfeld L, Yende S, et al. Association of statin use with risk and outcome of acute kidney injury in community-acquired pneumonia. Clin J Am Soc Nephrol 2012;7(6):895–905.

76. Deshpande A, Pasupuleti V, Rothberg MB. Statin therapy and mortality from sepsis: a meta-analysis of randomized trials. Am J Med 2015; 128(4):410–7.e1.

77. Palevsky PM. Renal replacement therapy in acute kidney injury. Adv Chronic Kidney Dis 2013;20(1): 76–84.

78. Palevsky PM, Baldwin I, Davenport A, et al. Renal replacement therapy and the kidney: minimizing the impact of renal replacement therapy on recovery of acute renal failure. Curr Opin Crit Care 2005; 11(6):548–54.

79. Maynar Moliner J, Honore PM, Sanchez-Izquierdo Riera JA, et al. Handling continuous renal replacement therapy-related adverse effects in intensive care unit patients: the daily trauma concept. Blood Purif 2012;34(2):177–85.

80. Liu KD, Himmelfarb J, Paganini E, et al. Timing of initiation of dialysis in critically ill patients with acute kidney injury. Clin J Am Soc Nephrol 2006;1(5): 915–9.

81. Karvellas CJ, Farhat MR, Sajjad I, et al. A comparison of early versus late initiation of renal replacement therapy in critically ill patients with acute kidney injury: a systematic review and meta-analysis. Crit Care 2011;15(1):R72.

82. Wald R, Adhikari NK, Smith OM, et al. Comparison of standard and accelerated initiation of renal replacement therapy in acute kidney injury. Kidney Int 2015;88(4):897–904.

83. Lameire N, Kellum JA, KDIGO AKI Guideline Work Group. Contrast-induced acute kidney injury and renal support for acute kidney injury: a KDIGO summary (Part 2). Crit Care 2013;17(1):205.

84. Wald R, Shariff SZ, Adhikari NK, et al. The association between renal replacement therapy modality and long-term outcomes among critically ill adults with acute kidney injury: a retrospective cohort study*. Crit Care Med 2014;42(4):868–77.

85. Rewa O, Bagshaw SM. Acute kidney injury-epidemiology, outcomes and economics. Nat Rev Nephrol 2014;10(4):193–207.

86. Fieghen HE, Friedrich JO, Burns KE, et al. The hemodynamic tolerability and feasibility of sustained low efficiency dialysis in the management of critically ill patients with acute kidney injury. BMC Nephrol 2010;11:32.

87. Harris LE, Reaves AB, Krauss AG, et al. Evaluation of antibiotic prescribing patterns in patients receiving sustained low-efficiency dialysis: opportunities for pharmacists. Int J Pharm Pract 2013; 21(1):55–61.

88. Mei JP, Ali-Moghaddam A, Mueller BA. Survey of pharmacists' antibiotic dosing recommendations for sustained low-efficiency dialysis. Int J Clin Pharm 2015. [Epub ahead of print].

89. Ronco C, Bellomo R, Homel P, et al. Effects of different doses in continuous veno-venous haemofiltration on outcomes of acute renal failure: a prospective randomized trial. Lancet 2000;356:26–30.

90. Schiffl H, Lang S, Fischer R. Daily hemodialysis and the outcome of acute renal failure. N Engl J Med 2002;346:305–10.

91. Roberts DM, Roberts JA, Roberts MS, et al. Variability of antibiotic concentrations in critically ill patients receiving continuous renal replacement therapy: a multicentre pharmacokinetic study. Crit Care Med 2012;40(5):1523–8.

92. Seyler L, Cotton F, Taccone FS, et al. Recommended beta-lactam regimens are inadequate in septic patients treated with continuous renal replacement therapy. Crit Care 2011;15(3):R137.

93. Bauer SR, Salem C, Connor MJ Jr, et al. Pharmacokinetics and pharmacodynamics of

piperacillin-tazobactam in 42 patients treated with concomitant CRRT. Clin J Am Soc Nephrol 2012;7(3):452–7.

94. Fissell WH. Antimicrobial dosing in acute renal replacement. Adv Chronic Kidney Dis 2013;20(1): 85–93.

95. Jamal JA, Economou CJ, Lipman J, et al. Improving antibiotic dosing in special situations in the ICU: burns, renal replacement therapy and extracorporeal membrane oxygenation. Curr Opin Crit Care 2012;18(5):460–71.

96. Bellomo R. Bench-to-bedside review: lactate and the kidney. Crit Care 2002;6(4):322–6.

97. Forsythe SM, Schmidt GA. Sodium bicarbonate for the treatment of lactic acidosis. Chest 2000;117(1): 260–7.

98. Boyd JH, Walley KR. Is there a role for sodium bicarbonate in treating lactic acidosis from shock? Curr Opin Crit Care 2008;14(4):379–83.

99. Calello DP, Liu KD, Wiegand TJ, et al. Extracorporeal treatment for metformin poisoning: systematic review and recommendations from the extracorporeal treatments in poisoning workgroup. Crit Care Med 2015;43(8):1716–30.

100. Kraut JA, Madias NE. Lactic acidosis. N Engl J Med 2014;371(24):2309–19.

101. Hoste EA, Colpaert K, Vanholder RC, et al. Sodium bicarbonate versus THAM in ICU patients with mild metabolic acidosis. J Nephrol 2005;18(3):303–7.

102. Doi K, Yuen PS, Eisner C, et al. Reduced production of creatinine limits its use as marker of kidney injury in sepsis. J Am Soc Nephrol 2009;20(6): 1217–21.

103. Solomon AW, Kirwan CJ, Alexander ND, et al. Urine output on an intensive care unit: case-control study. BMJ 2010;341:c6761.

104. Delanaye P, Cavalier E, Morel J, et al. Detection of decreased glomerular filtration rate in intensive care units: serum cystatin C versus serum creatinine. BMC Nephrol 2014;15:9.

105. Bihorac A, Chawla LS, Shaw AD, et al. Validation of cell-cycle arrest biomarkers for acute kidney injury using clinical adjudication. Am J Respir Crit Care Med 2014;189(8):932–9.

106. Kashani K, Al-Khafaji A, Ardiles T, et al. Discovery and validation of cell cycle arrest biomarkers in human acute kidney injury. Crit Care 2013; 17(1):R25.

# Cardiac Function and Dysfunction in Sepsis

Kimberly E. Fenton, MD, FAAP*, Margaret M. Parker, MD, MCCM

## KEYWORDS

• Cardiac dysfunction • Sepsis • Ventricular function • Hemodynamics • Echocardiography
• Troponin

## KEY POINTS

• Cardiac function and dysfunction are important in the clinical outcomes of sepsis and septic shock.
• Cardiac dysfunction results from a variety of pathophysiologic, metabolic microvascular, functional, and anatomic derangements.
• Intrinsic cardiac function is greatly affected by extrinsic factors such as preload, afterload, and neurohumoral responses to sepsis.

## INTRODUCTION

Cardiac dysfunction plays a pivotal role in the clinical outcomes of severe sepsis and septic shock. Myocardial depression was first described in 1984, and since then numerous studies have focused on further elucidating the mechanisms causing myocardial depression.[1,2] Although much remains unknown, cardiac dysfunction is not a single clinical entity but is a broad spectrum of syndromes with a multitude of pathophysiologic, metabolic, microvascular, functional, and anatomic derangements. The term septic cardiomyopathy has evolved to describe many of these conditions.[3,4] Further elucidation of the underlying pathophysiology has focused primarily on functional disturbances of the myocardium rather than anatomic abnormalities. However, recent evidence from both human studies and experimental models of sepsis shows that structural changes occur as well.[5–7] In addition, cardiac dysfunction in sepsis is a principal cause of morbidity and mortality in severe sepsis and septic shock; many therapies have focused on treating functional abnormalities, with only limited success. Furthermore, although the heart is the central component of the cardiovascular system, it is also affected by perturbations of the peripheral vascular system during sepsis. These changes in the peripheral vascular system have direct and indirect effects on the loading conditions of the myocardium. The cardiac response to alterations in preload, afterload, and the neurohumoral response during sepsis may be clinically indistinguishable from direct septic cardiotoxicity, which makes accurate diagnosis and treatment of cardiovascular failure during sepsis a highly complex task.

## PATHOPHYSIOLOGY
### Functional Abnormalities

The underlying pathophysiology of cardiac dysfunction in sepsis is caused by a myriad of genetic, molecular, metabolic, and structural mechanisms that are highly complex and may have both stand-alone unique contributions as well as highly complex intricate influences on each other. Although much is known, many of the pathophysiologic mechanisms are proposed and the full influence of each is yet to be elucidated.

Disclosures: The authors have nothing to disclose.
Department of Pediatrics, Stony Brook University School of Medicine, Stony Brook, NY 11794-8111, USA
* Corresponding author. Health Sciences Center, T11 Room 040, Stony Brook, NY 11790-8111.
E-mail address: kimberly.fenton@stonybrookmedicine.edu

Clin Chest Med 37 (2016) 289–298
http://dx.doi.org/10.1016/j.ccm.2016.01.014
0272-5231/16/$ – see front matter © 2016 Elsevier Inc. All rights reserved.

## Genetics

The Human Genome Project and many others have sought to elucidate the genetic expression of specific diseases and syndromes. However, these important links exist only in animal models of sepsis in which there is a suggestion that inducible nitric oxide synthase (iNOS) deficiency may be cardioprotective.[8] Further research must be done to identify the linkage between genomics and sepsis-induced cardiac dysfunction.

## Molecular

- Cytokines: activation of the immune system plays a key role in the pathogenesis of sepsis. The innate immune system essentially goes into overdrive with a production of proinflammatory mediators. Tumor necrosis factor alpha, interleukin (IL)-1beta, and IL-6 are considered to be the main mediators that cause cardiac dysfunction in sepsis and are considered to be direct myocardial depressants.[2]
- Nitric oxide (NO) is a widely recognized contributor in sepsis and causes the following:
  - Vasodilation, which in turn causes reduced preload, afterload, and cardiac perfusion. It may also serve as a myocardial depressant.[8,9]
  - Glutathione depletion, which leads to oxidative stress and mitochondrial dysfunction.[10]
- Calcium: intracellular calcium is a potent inotrope. Experimental models suggest calcium channel alterations, which reduce intracellular calcium and ultimately cause myocardial depression[11] (**Fig. 1**).
- Toll-like receptors (TLRs): critical to the initiation of the innate inflammatory response. TLRs recognize specific pathogen-associated patterns of bacterial and viral structures and nucleic acid composition.
- Endothelin-1 (ET-1) is known to play a role in myocardial contractility. In sepsis, ET-1 levels are increased in both the blood and myocardium. There is a suggestion that increased levels are associated with myocardial dysfunction.[12]

## Metabolic

- Neurohumoral: early sepsis causes a catecholamine surge from the autonomic nervous system, gut, white blood cells, and macrophages, resulting in massive sympathetic response and stimulation of alpha-adrenergic and beta-adrenergic receptors. This adrenergic stimulation leads to a downregulation of catecholamine receptors, and ultimately catecholamine resistance.[13,14] Autonomic dysfunction is further exacerbated by glial and neuronal apoptosis in cardiovascular autonomic centers.[15]
- Mitochondrial dysfunction[9]: adequate ATP and oxygen delivery is essential for cardiac function. Several mitochondrial disturbances are proposed to play a significant role in cardiac dysfunction during sepsis:
  - Edema of the mitochondrial matrix, which may lead to functional impairment of cardiac myocytes.
  - Oxidative stress: increased superoxide ($O_2^-$) and NO production can cause direct oxidative damage or inhibition of oxidative phosphorylation, decreased mitochondrial membrane potential, and ultimately decreased oxygen consumption.
  - Altered membrane permeability: affecting the electron transport chain and impaired mitochondrial calcium handling, which may lead to mitochondrial calcium overload and impaired membrane permeability, which in turn, may contribute to cardiac mitochondrial contractile dysfunction.[16]
  - Mitochondrial uncoupling: ATP synthesis may be physiologically uncoupled from oxygen consumption whereby ATP is not synthesized in response to cardiac oxygen consumption.
  - Mitochondrial biogenesis: the process of mitochondrial growth and division may be impaired by a variety of mechanisms (eg, NO, oxidative stress) that occur during sepsis. Mitochondrial biogenesis is thought to be responsible for the reversal of organ damage in sepsis. However, it is possible that mitochondrial biogenesis may not be sufficient or that, alternatively, the newly produced mitochondria are dysfunctional.
  - Mitophagy: the removal of dysfunctional mitochondria via autophagy is important for organ recovery. Ideally, mitophagy and mitochondrial biogenesis should be balanced; however, mitophagy has been shown to be increased in various organs in sepsis (which is proposed to occur in the heart as well). However, decreased mitochondrial mass may occur if mitophagy exceeds mitochondrial biogenesis.

## Structural Abnormalities

In addition to functional derangements, recent evidence suggests that structural abnormalities may play a role in the pathophysiology of cardiac dysfunction of sepsis. Increased serum levels of

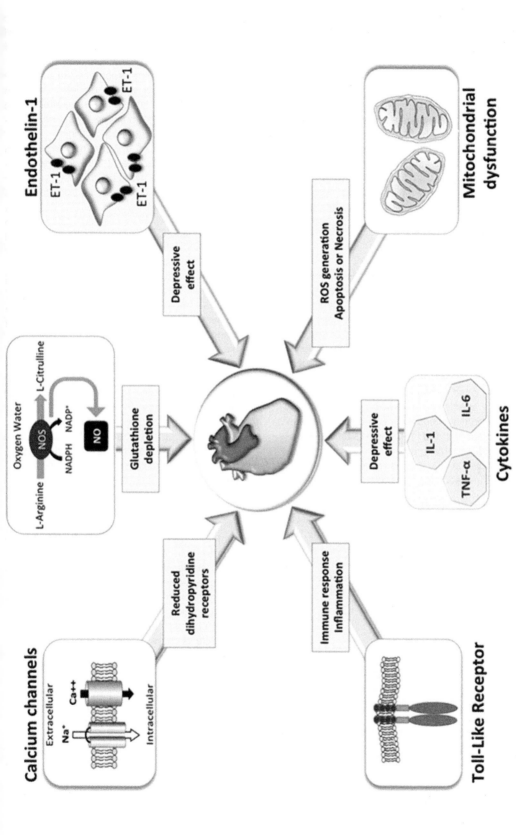

**Fig. 1.** Molecular factors involved in myocardial depression. ET, endothelin-1; NOS, nitric oxide synthase; ROS, reactive oxygen species; TNF-$\alpha$, tumor necrosis factor alpha. (*From* Antonucci E, Fiaccadori E, Donadello K, et al. Myocardial depression in sepsis: from pathogenesis to clinical manifestations and treatment. J Crit Care 20:4;29:502; with permission.)

cardiac troponins T and I in sepsis suggest that there has been myocardial injury but do not define whether there is necrosis versus a troponin leakage caused by reversible cell membrane disruption. Necrosis and apoptosis cause cell death, which implies an irreversible process in the septic heart; however, myocardial dysfunction is well known clinically to be a reversible process.[1] Necrosis has been identified in autopsies from septic human hearts, whereas apoptosis has only been identified in experimental models of sepsis.[6] Autopsies from human hearts show myocardial infiltration by white blood cells and macrophages, disruption of the contractile apparatus, increased collagen, and damaged mitochrondria.[7,17]

### Necrosis and apoptosis

Myocardial cell apoptosis has not been found in human autopsy specimens but is described experimentally in models of sepsis.[6] Focal myocardial necrosis and subendocardial necrosis have been identified in experimental models of sepsis, and myocardial contraction band necrosis was identified by Schmittinger and colleagues[7] in a prospective histologic autopsy study in 20 human hearts. Contraction band necrosis was found in 95% of the autopsy specimens and was generalized and distributed homogeneously in all heart cross sections. Contraction band necrosis has been experimentally induced by infusion of catecholamines and is observed in diseases associated with adrenergic overstimulation (eg, pheochromocytoma).[7]

### Myocardial infiltration

Inflammatory cardiomyopathy is a hallmark histologic finding in the septic human heart characterized by interstitial infiltration by neutrophils and monocytes/macrophages.[5,7] The inflammation is also concomitantly associated with interstitial myocardial edema, fibrosis, and thrombi in the vasculature.

### Hemodynamic Abnormalities

#### Contractile dysfunction

Impaired cardiac contractility is the hallmark of severe sepsis and involves biventricular dysfunction characterized by cardiac dilatation and decreased stroke volume.[1] Because patients with septic shock typically present with a hyperdynamic hemodynamic state, myocardial depression may not be readily apparent.[18] Both radionuclide imaging and, more recently, increasingly sophisticated echocardiographic techniques have shown that either systolic or diastolic dysfunction, or both, is commonly present.[1,19–22] Systolic dysfunction occurs in 30% to 60% of patients, and is not clearly associated with mortality.[19,20] Diastolic dysfunction is reported in nearly half of patients with sepsis and is strongly associated with mortality.[21,22] Left ventricular systolic dysfunction has been the most studied and well characterized in the literature and is highly dependent on left ventricular afterload (discussed later).[1,23] When afterload is reduced, cardiac function may seem normal or increased despite reduced intrinsic cardiac contractility. Aside from imaging techniques, this may not be clinically apparent until impaired afterload is corrected, and it can be challenging to clinically separate reduced afterload from impaired cardiac performance.[20]

- Left ventricular diastolic dysfunction: tachycardia and left ventricular dilatation resulting in an increased left ventricular end-diastolic volume may contribute to impaired ventricular relaxation during diastole. Diastolic dysfunction has been shown to occur independently of systolic dysfunction[24,25] and is primarily diagnosed by echocardiography. Clinically, diastolic dysfunction may affect fluid management, requiring a more conservative approach. In addition, diastolic dysfunction is an independent risk factor for mortality even when APACHE-II (Acute Physiology and Chronic Health Evaluation) score is adjusted.[25]
- Right ventricular function may be caused by a reduced preload causing decreased right ventricular ejection fraction but is primarily characterized by increased right atrial pressure and decreased systemic venous return. It may occur alone or in association with left ventricular systolic dysfunction.[20] Similarly to the left ventricle, right ventricular systolic function is affected by afterload; however, right ventricular afterload is usually increased /because of acute respiratory distress syndrome.[3,26,27] Unlike the left ventricle, the right ventricle is unable to anatomically and physiologically adapt to rapid increases in afterload, therefore the right ventricle is more prone to early dysfunction. Recent data suggest increased mortality with early right ventricular dysfunction.[3,28,29]

Although biventricular cardiac dysfunction may occur independently, cardiac function overall is extremely dependent on loading conditions (ie, preload and afterload); alterations of either or both produce direct cardiac and hemodynamic consequences[26,30] and the clinical management of sepsis must take these loading conditions into account.

- Impaired preload: absolute or relative hypovolemia is frequently observed in sepsis. In addition, maldistribution of blood flow (ie, venous pooling and capillary leak) occurs and further exacerbates a reduction in intravascular volume.[26] These findings are observed clinically in humans and in experimental models of sepsis.

- Impaired afterload: decreased afterload is frequently observed in adults with septic shock.[18,23] Children frequently have increased afterload in sepsis.[30] Alterations in afterload are caused by reduced vascular tone (ie, systemic vascular resistance), which may in turn help preserve systolic cardiac function in early shock, allowing a hyperdynamic state. However, as contractility worsens and afterload decreases, cardiac function may seem grossly normal, but be severely impaired.[26] Furthermore, impaired contractility and afterload-related cardiac performance correlate with a worse prognosis.[4,26] The cause of afterload abnormalities is multifactorial but includes a vasodilatory response to cytokines, autonomic dysregulation, and NO abnormalities.[26,27] Wilhelm and colleagues[31] used afterload-related cardiac performance (ACP) to determine whether the cardiac output in patients with sepsis was appropriate for the patient's systemic vascular resistance. ACP is calculated as follows:

$$ACP\ (\%) = 100 \times CO/[560.68 \times ((MAP - CVP) \times 80/CO)^{-0.645}]$$

The denominator is based on the predicted normal cardiac output (CO) calculated from the given systemic vascular resistance SVR. A normal ACP is greater than 80%.[31]

ACP was predictive of mortality at the time of admission to the emergency department and a decreased ACP indicated reduced cardiac function. These investigators further reported that ACP correlated significantly with troponin and with brain natriuretic peptide levels. Cardiac index was not associated with severity of sepsis, mortality, or biomarker levels.

- Microcirculatory dysfunction: perfusion abnormalities in the microcirculation occur during sepsis whereby there is thrombin deposition, increased inflammatory cell migration, and altered endothelial permeability leading to a decreased perfusion, increased viscosity, and an impaired endothelial response to vasoconstriction and vasodilation.[26,27,32]

## MECHANISMS OF CARDIAC DYSFUNCTION

Experimental models of sepsis suggest that impaired loading conditions of the heart caused by altered vascular tone, and microcirculatory dysfunction frequently lead to a reduced oxygen extraction even in the presence of normal oxygen delivery. Clinically this may translate to an increased central venous oxygen saturation in the presence of severe cardiac dysfunction[26,33] (Fig. 2).

### Impact of Chronic Heart Disease on Acute Hemodynamics

In a recent study by Ouellette and Shah,[34] patients with preexisting left ventricular dysfunction were not shown to have different clinical outcomes compared with patients with no underlying cardiac disease. Although, in the first 24 hours, patients with underlying cardiac dysfunction received similar amounts of fluid resuscitation as the control group, there was no difference in respiratory measures at 24 hours or other clinical outcomes, suggesting that volume resuscitation in early sepsis is appropriate for those patients with underlying cardiac dysfunction. For patients with preexisting left ventricular dysfunction, low central venous oxygen saturation was an independent risk factor for mortality, which it was not in the control patients.

In summary, the hemodynamic responses of patients with sepsis may be heterogeneous and are likely influenced by the patient's underlying cardiovascular status and by acute changes in preload and afterload that accompany sepsis.

### Laboratory Studies

- Troponin: many studies have reported that an increased cardiac troponin level is common in patients with sepsis, in both adults and children, and is associated with a worse prognosis.[35–38] Landesberg and colleagues[39] performed advanced echocardiography as well as troponin-T measurements in 106 patients with severe sepsis or septic shock. Left ventricular diastolic dysfunction and right ventricular end-systolic volume were associated with in-hospital mortality and troponin-T concentrations. Left ventricular systolic dysfunction did not correlate with troponin-T concentration. The cause of myocardial dysfunction in sepsis, and of troponin level increases, remains unclear. Troponin may be released by damaged myocardial cells from sepsis-induced myocardial injury, or possibly by myocardial cells that are put under increased demand in critically ill patients.

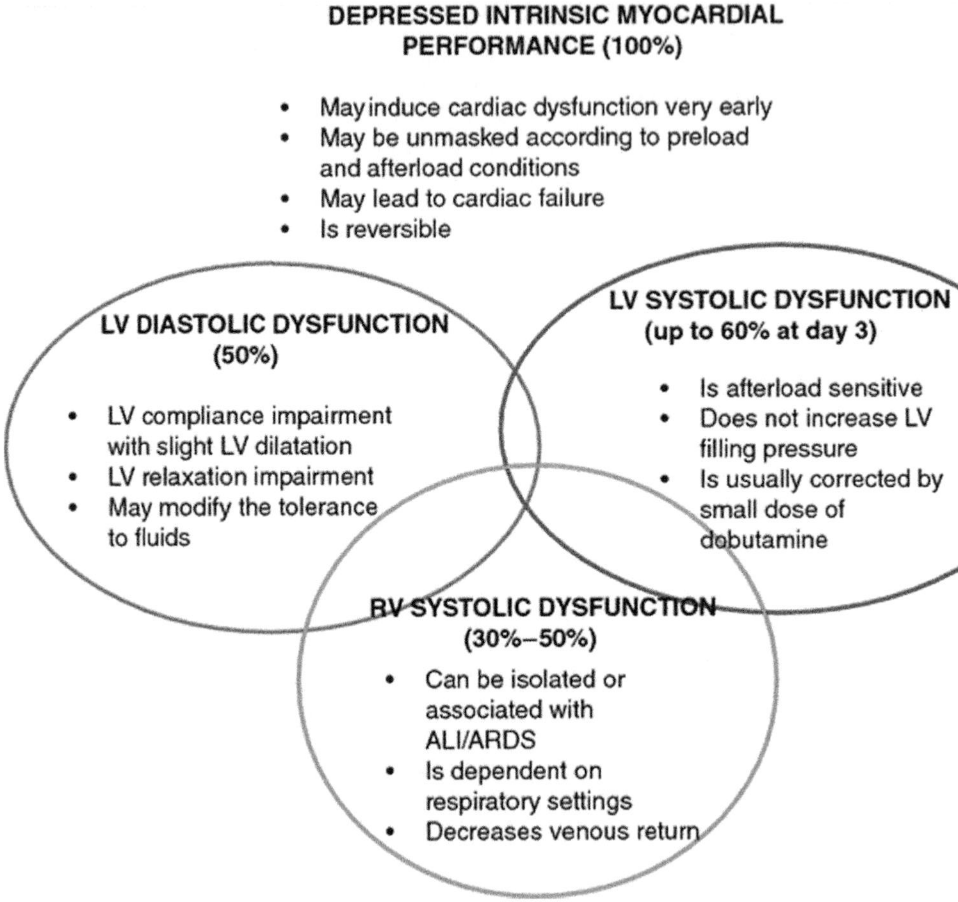

**DEPRESSED INTRINSIC MYOCARDIAL
PERFORMANCE (100%)**

- May induce cardiac dysfunction very early
- May be unmasked according to preload
  and afterload conditions
- May lead to cardiac failure
- Is reversible

**LV DIASTOLIC DYSFUNCTION
(50%)**

- LV compliance impairment
  with slight LV dilatation
- LV relaxation impairment
- May modify the tolerance
  to fluids

**LV SYSTOLIC DYSFUNCTION
(up to 60% at day 3)**

- Is afterload sensitive
- Does not increase LV
  filling pressure
- Is usually corrected by
  small dose of
  dobutamine

**RV SYSTOLIC DYSFUNCTION
(30%–50%)**

- Can be isolated or
  associated with
  ALI/ARDS
- Is dependent on
  respiratory settings
- Decreases venous return

**Fig. 2.** Main mechanisms of cardiac dysfunction, their consequences, and their incidences (in brackets) in severe sepsis and septic shock. ALI, acute lung injury; ARDS, acute respiratory distress syndrome; LV, left ventricular; RV, right ventricular. (*From* Vieillard-Baron A, Cecconi M. Understanding cardiac failure in sepsis. Intensive Care Med 2014;40:1561; with permission.)

Although the association of increased troponin-T level and myocardial dysfunction is clearly present, it is unclear whether more aggressive treatment approaches would improve mortality in these patients.

- B-type natriuretic peptide (BNP): increased BNP level has been described as a marker for myocardial dysfunction, as well as a prognostic indicator, in patients with sepsis.[40,41] Daily BNP levels and echocardiographic and hemodynamic measurements were evaluated by Papanikolaou and colleagues[42] in a prospective observational study of 42 patients with severe sepsis or septic shock. Patients with septic shock had markedly increased BNP levels, which correlated with right and left ventricular ejection fraction on univariate analysis but were not independently associated on multivariate analysis. Severity of illness as defined by APACHE-II or maximum SOFA (Sepsis-

related Organ Failure Assessment) scores were independently associated with BNP levels, and BNP level on day 1 was an independent predictor of 28-day mortality. These investigators concluded that it is the severity of illness rather than cardiac dysfunction that explains the increase in BNP levels in patients with severe sepsis or septic shock. Failure of the BNP level to decrease rapidly over the first few days was associated with mortality. Trends in BNP levels may be helpful in assessing response to therapy and prognosis.

- Cytokines: in vitro studies have suggested that inflammatory cytokines may cause myocardial dysfunction in sepsis.[2] Landesberg and colleagues[43] measured inflammatory cytokines, troponin-T, and BNP levels in 105 patients with severe sepsis and septic shock. They evaluated myocardial function by echocardiography, including tissue

Doppler imaging. The cytokine levels predicted mortality, but did not correlate with systolic or diastolic left ventricular dysfunction. BNP and troponin-T levels did correlate with some measures of myocardial dysfunction in this study. Measurement of cytokine levels is not helpful in the evaluation or management of myocardial dysfunction in patients with septic shock.

## Imaging Studies

The initial studies reporting myocardial depression in septic shock used radionuclide gated blood pool scans to measure left and right ventricular ejection fraction.[1] Echocardiography is a useful and more easily available tool for evaluating myocardial function in critically ill patients with septic shock.

- Transthoracic echocardiography is a widely available tool but the quality of images in critically ill patients may be limited. In a retrospective study in 76 patients with septic shock who had a transthoracic echocardiogram, Beraud and colleagues[44] reported that the left ventricular ejection fraction could be calculated in 90% of patients and diastolic function in 74%, showing that transthoracic echocardiography may be a useful tool to evaluate cardiac function in patients with septic shock. Significant valvular disease was the most frequent impediment to evaluation of diastolic dysfunction. This study confirmed that myocardial dysfunction is common in patients with septic shock.
  - Speckle tracking echocardiography is a newer and more sensitive technique that may identify systolic or diastolic dysfunction not appreciated with conventional echocardiography.[45,46] In septic patients with a normal left ventricular ejection fraction, Dalla and colleagues[46] identified left ventricular strain in 50%. Strain echocardiography may be useful for early detection of myocardial dysfunction in sepsis. In addition, De Geer and colleagues[47] showed that global longitudinal peak strain remained reduced in patients with septic shock beyond 7 days, whereas the left ventricular ejection fraction and BNP level improved over that time.

## Management Goals and Treatment

Myocardial dysfunction can be readily identified in patients with severe sepsis and septic shock using echocardiography and measurement of the levels of biomarkers troponin-T and BNP. However,

there is no specific treatment of the myocardial depression that is commonly seen. Management is supportive, optimizing hemodynamic stability by ensuring adequate ventricular filling, inotropic support with dobutamine, and vasopressor support with norepinephrine, epinephrine, and/or vasopressin.[48]

- Early goal-directed therapy: specific therapeutic goals based on central venous pressure and central venous oxygen saturation were recommended by Rivers and colleagues[49] in 2001 but were subject to much controversy. However, 3 recent multicenter, randomized trials of goal-directed therapy compared with usual care failed to show an improvement in outcomes with goal-directed therapy.[50–52]
- Vasopressors: many studies have assessed vasopressor agents for their effectiveness in septic shock. Dopamine was for many years considered the agent of choice, but recent studies have refuted that thought. DeBacker and colleagues[53] performed a meta-analysis of dopamine versus norepinephrine for the treatment of septic shock, reviewing 5 observational and 6 randomized trials. They reported that dopamine administration was associated with an increase in mortality and more arrhythmias than norepinephrine. Dopamine is no longer recommended as a first-line agent for patients with septic shock.[54] Norepinephrine should be the first-choice vasopressor, with epinephrine or vasopressin as options if additional agents are needed. Low-dose vasopressin as an adjunct to patients receiving norepinephrine is as effective as norepinephrine alone but does not reduce mortality compared with norepinephrine in patients with septic shock receiving catecholamine vasopressors.[55]
- Dobutamine or milrinone may be considered when there is evidence of cardiac dysfunction and/or hypoperfusion despite adequate intravascular volume resuscitation and adequate mean arterial blood pressure.[54] Dobutamine may be titrated up to 20 μg/kg/min or milrinone may be added at 0.25 to 0.75 μg/kg/min. Dobutamine use is cautioned in patients with risks of tachyarrhythmias or absolute or relative bradycardia and may lead to hypotension given its vasodilatory affects. Milrinone increases inotropy but has little effect on the heart rate; however, given its long half-life, it may lead to a prolonged episode of vasodilatory hypotension. Milrinone has been used primarily in pediatric septic shock.[54]

- β-Blocker therapy: the use of β-blocker therapy for heart rate control has recently been proposed for patients with septic shock. Although perhaps counterintuitive, there may be some benefit in controlling heart rate and countering the deleterious effects of beta-adrenergic receptor stimulation. Morelli and colleagues[56] randomized 77 patients with septic shock who were tachycardic and required high-dose norepinephrine to esmolol to maintain a heart rate between 80 and 94 beats/min and 77 patients to standard treatment in an open-label study. Mortality was significantly lower in the esmolol group than in the control group. This intriguing study suggests that β-blocker therapy for heart rate control deserves further study. If confirmed, there may be an additional treatment designed to improve cardiac support for patients with septic shock.
- Goal-directed oxygen delivery: based on the available evidence, there are no specific targets for optimal oxygen delivery. Instead, clinicians should clinically target both global and organ-specific markers of perfusion both at the bedside and in the laboratory.
- Hypertonic saline: another study of a mechanism-directed therapy was an animal study by Wang and colleagues.[57] They studied hypertonic saline as a potentially cardioprotective agent for the treatment of sepsis in a rat model. Following endotoxin challenge, hypertonic saline prevented hypotension and improved cardiac function. The mechanisms were thought to be improved intracellular calcium handling and inhibitory effects on neutrophil infiltration. Such mechanistic studies can lead to further understanding of myocardial dysfunction in sepsis and have the potential to lead to new therapies.

## SUMMARY

Cardiac dysfunction in sepsis continues to be an important cause of morbidity and mortality from sepsis and is caused by a series of functional as well as structural aberrations in the heart that are clinically manifested by biventricular systolic and diastolic cardiac dysfunction. Intrinsic cardiac function is greatly affected by extrinsic factors such as preload, afterload, and neurohumoral responses to sepsis. Biomarkers such as troponin and BNP are useful tools in conjunction with bedside echocardiography techniques and allow more specific sophisticated techniques to define diastolic dysfunction. Therapy remains largely supportive, and is intended to correct the underlying abnormalities. Future research must focus on targeted therapies designed to treat specific pathophysiologic abnormalities.

## REFERENCES

1. Parker MM, Shelhamer JH, Bacharach SL, et al. Profound but reversible myocardial depression in patients with septic shock. Ann Intern Med 1984;100:483–90.
2. Kumar A, Thota V, Dee L, et al. Tumor necrosis factor alpha and interleukin 1 beta are responsible for in vitro myocardial cell depression induced by human septic shock serum. J Exp Med 1996;183:949–58.
3. Viellard-Baron A, Cecconi M. Understanding cardiac failure in sepsis. Intensive Care Med 2014;4:1560–3.
4. Werdan K, Oelke A, Hettwer S, et al. Septic cardiomyopathy: hemodynamic quantification, occurrence, and prognostic implications. Clin Res Cardiol 2011;100:661–8.
5. Celes MRN, Prado CM, Rossi MA. Sepsis: going to the heart of the matter. Pathobiology 2013;80:70–86.
6. Smeding L, Plotz FB, Groeneveld ABJ, et al. Structural changes of the heart during severe sepsis or septic shock. Shock 2012;37:449–56.
7. Schmittinger CA, Dunser MW, Torgersen C, et al. Histologic pathologies of the myocardium in septic shock: a prospective observational study. Shock 2013;39:329–35.
8. Dos Santos CC, Gattas DJ, Tsoporis JN, et al. Sepsis-induced myocardial depression is associated with transcriptional changes in energy metabolism and contractile related genes: a physiological and gene expression based approach. Crit Care Med 2010;38:894–902.
9. Cimolai MC, Alvarez S, Bode C, et al. Mitochondrial mechanisms in septic cardiomyopathy. Int J Mol Sci 2015;16:17763–78.
10. Brealey D, Karyampudi S, Jacques TS, et al. Mitochondrial dysfunction in a long-term rodent model of sepsis and organ failure. Am J Physiol Regul Integr Comp Physiol 2004;286:491–7.
11. Stengl M, Bargak F, Sykora R, et al. Reduced L-type calcium current in ventricular myocytes from pigs with hyperdynamic septic shock. Crit Care Med 2010;38:580–7.
12. Sharma AC, Motew SJ, Farias S, et al. Sepsis alters myocardial and plasma concentrations of endothelin and nitric oxide in rats. J Mol Cell Cardiol 1997;29:1469–77.
13. Silverman HJ, Penaranda R, Orens JB, et al. Impaired beta-adrenergic receptor stimulation of cyclic adenosine monophosphate in human septic shock: association with myocardial hyporesponsiveness to catecholamines. Crit Care Med 1993;21:31–9.

14. Norbury WB, Jeschke JMG, Hernan DN. Metabolism modulators in sepsis: propranolol. Crit Care Med 2007;35:S616–20.

15. Sharshar T, Gray F, de la Grandmaison L, et al. Apoptosis of neurons in cardiovascular autonomic centres triggered by inducible nitric oxide synthase after death from septic shock. Lancet 2003;362: 1799–805.

16. Costa AD, Quinlan CL, Andrukhiv A, et al. The direct physiological effects of mitoK(ATP) opening on heart mitochondria. Am J Physiol Heart Circ Physiol 2006; 290:H406–15.

17. Soriano FG, Nogueira AC, Caldini EG. Potential role of poly (adenosine 5'-diphosphate-ribose) polymer- ase activation in the pathogenesis of myocardial contractile dysfunction associated with human sep- tic shock. Crit Care Med 2006;34(4):1073–9.

18. Parker MM, Shelhamer JH, Natanson C, et al. Serial cardiovascular patterns in survivors and nonsurvi- vors of human septic shock: heart rate as an early predictor of prognosis. Crit Care Med 1987;15: 923–9.

19. Berrios RAS, O'Horo JC, Velagapudi V, et al. Corre- lation of left ventricular systolic dysfunction deter- mined by low ejection fraction and 30-day mortality in patients with severe sepsis and septic shock: a systematic review and meta-analysis. J Crit Care 2014;29:495–9.

20. Vieillard-Baron A, Caille V, Charron C, et al. Actual incidence of global left ventricular hypokinesia in adult septic shock. Crit Care Med 2008;36:1701–6.

21. Sanfilippo F, Corredor C, Fletcher N, et al. Diastolic dysfunction and mortality in septic patients: a sys- tematic review and meta-analysis. Intensive Care Med 2015;41:1004–13.

22. Mourad M, Chow-Chine L, Faucher M, et al. Early diastolic dysfunction is associated with intensive care unit mortality in cancer patients presenting with septic shock. Br J Anaesth 2014;112:102–9.

23. Suffredini AF, Fromm RE, Parker MM, et al. The car- diovascular response of normal humans to the administration of endotoxin. N Engl J Med 1989; 321(5):280–7.

24. Bouhemad B, Nicolas-Robin A, Arbelot C, et al. Iso- lated and reversible impairment of ventricular relax- ation in patients with septic shock. Crit Care Med 2008;36:766–74.

25. Landesberg G, Gilon D, Meroz Y, et al. Diastolic dysfunction and mortality in severe sepsis and sep- tic shock. Eur Heart J 2012;33:895–903.

26. Antonucci E, Fiaccadori E, Donadello K, et al. Myocardial depression in sepsis: from pathogenesis to clinical manifestations and treatment. J Crit Care 2014;29:500–11.

27. Romero-Bermejo FJ, Ruiz-Bailen M, Gil-Cebrian J, et al. Sepsis-induced cardiomyopathy. Curr Cardiol Rev 2011;7:163–83.

28. Harmankaya A, Akilli H, Gul M, et al. Assessment of right ventricular functions in patients with sepsis, se- vere sepsis and septic shock and its prognostic importance: a tissue Doppler study. J Crit Care 2013;28:1111.e7–11.

29. Furian T, Aguiar C, Prado K, et al. Ventricular dysfunction and dilation in severe sepsis and septic shock: relation to endothelial function and mortality. J Crit Care 2012;27(3):319.e9–15.

30. Feltes TF, Pyinatelli R, Kleinert S, et al. Quantitated left ventricular systolic mechanics in children with septic shock utilizing noninvasive wall-stress anal- ysis. Crit Care Med 1994;22(10):1647–58.

31. Wilhelm J, Hettwer S, Schuermann M, et al. Severity of cardiac impairment in the early stage of community-acquired sepsis determines worse prog- nosis. Clin Res Cardiol 2013;102:735–44.

32. Aird WC. The hematologic system as a marker of or- gan dysfunction in sepsis. Mayo Clin Proc 2003; 78(7):869–81.

33. Bouferrache K, Amiel JB, Chimot L, et al. Initial resuscitation guided by the Surviving Sepsis Campaign recommendations and early echocardio- graphic assessment of hemodynamics in intensive care unit septic patients: a pilot study. Crit Care Med 2012;40:2821–7.

34. Ouellette DR, Shah SZ. Comparison of outcomes from sepsis between patients with and without pre- existing left ventricular dysfunction: a case-control analysis. Crit Care 2014;18:R79.

35. Turner A, Tsamitros M, Bellomo R. Myocardial cell injury in septic shock. Crit Care Med 1999;27: 1775–80.

36. Ver Elst K, Spapen H, Nguyen D, et al. Cardiac tro- ponins I and T are biological markers of left ventric- ular dysfunction in septic shock. Clin Chem 2001;46: 650–7.

37. Fenton KE, Sable CA, Bell MJ, et al. Increases in serum levels of troponin I are associated with car- diac dysfunction and disease severity in pediatric patients with septic shock. Pediatr Crit Care Med 2004;5:533–8.

38. Sheyin O, Davies O, Duan W, et al. The prognostic significance of troponin elevation in patients with sepsis: a meta-analysis. Heart Lung 2015;44:75–81.

39. Landesberg G, Jaffe AS, Gilon D, et al. Troponin elevation in severe sepsis and septic shock: the role of left ventricular diastolic dysfunction and right ven- tricular dilatation. Crit Care Med 2014;42:790–800.

40. Post F, Weilemann LS, Messow CM, et al. B-type natriuretic peptide as a marker for sepsis-induced myocardial depression in intensive care patients. Crit Care Med 2008;36:3030–7.

41. Charpentier J, Luyt CE, Fulla Y, et al. Brain natriuretic peptide: a marker of myocardial dysfunction and prognosis during severe sepsis. Crit Care Med 2004;32:660–5.

42. Papanikolaou J, Makris D, Mpaka M, et al. New insights into the mechanisms involved in B-type natriuretic peptide elevation and its prognostic value in septic patients. Crit Care 2014;18:R94.

43. Landesberg G, Levin PD, Gilon D, et al. Myocardial dysfunction in severe sepsis and septic shock: no correlation with inflammatory cytokines in real-life clinical setting. Chest 2015;148:93–102.

44. Beraud AS, Guillamet CV, Hammes JL, et al. Efficacy of transthoracic echocardiography for diagnosis heart failure in septic shock. Am J Med Sci 2014; 347:295–8.

45. Orde SR, Pulido JN, Masaki M, et al. Outcome prediction in sepsis: speckle tracking echocardiography based assessment of myocardial function. Crit Care 2014;18:R149.

46. Dalla K, Hallman C, Bech-Hanssen O, et al. Strain echocardiography identifies impaired longitudinal systolic function in patients with septic shock and preserved ejection fraction. Cardiovasc Ultrasound 2015;13:30.

47. De Geer L, Engvall J, Oscarsson A. Strain echocardiography in septic shock – a comparison with systolic and diastolic function parameters, cardiac biomarkers and outcome. Crit Care 2015;19:122.

48. Jozwiak M, Persichini R, Monnet X, et al. Management of myocardial dysfunction in severe sepsis. Semin Respir Crit Care Med 2011;32:206–14.

49. Rivers E, Nguyen B, Havstad S, et al. Early goal-directed therapy in the treatment of severe sepsis and septic shock. N Engl J Med 2001;345:1368–77.

50. The ProCESS Investigators. A randomized trial of protocol-based care for early septic shock. N Engl J Med 2014;370:1683–93.

51. The ARISE Investigators, ANZICS Clinical Trials Group. Goal-directed resuscitation for patients with early septic shock. N Engl J Med 2014;371:1496–506.

52. Mouncey PR, Osborn TM, Power GS, et al. Trial of early goal-directed resuscitation for septic shock. N Engl J Med 2015;372:1301–11.

53. DeBacker D, Aldecoa C, Njimi H, et al. Dopamine versus norepinephrine in the treatment of septic shock: a meta-analysis. Crit Care Med 2012;40: 725–30.

54. Dellinger RP, Levy MM, Rhodes A, et al. Surviving sepsis campaign: international guidelines for management of severe sepsis and septic shock. Crit Care Med 2013;41(2):580–637.

55. Russell JA, Walley KR, Singer J, et al. Vasopressin versus norepinephrine infusion in patients with septic shock. N Engl J Med 2008;358:877–87.

56. Morelli A, Ertmer C, Westphal M, et al. Effect of heart rate control with esmolol on hemodynamic and clinical outcomes in patients with septic shock: a randomized clinical trial. JAMA 2013;310:1683–91.

57. Wang YL, Lam KK, Cheng PY, et al. The cardioprotective effect of hypertonic saline is associated with inhibitory effect on macrophage migration inhibitory factor in sepsis. Biomed Res Int 2013;2013: 201614.

# The Use of Ultrasound in Caring for Patients with Sepsis

Laurent Guérin, MD[a,b],
Antoine Vieillard-Baron, MD, PhD[a,b,c],*

## KEYWORDS

- Critical care echocardiography • Hemodynamic monitoring • Septic shock
- Septic cardiomyopathy

## KEY POINTS

- Echocardiography is essential for hemodynamic management of patients with septic shock.
- Echocardiography provides an independent evaluation of every mechanism involved in sepsis: hypovolemia, right and left cardiac dysfunction, and persistent vasoplegia.
- Septic cardiomyopathy is a constant phenomenon during septic shock, but may be masked by profound vasoplegia. Repeated echocardiography could unmask left ventricular (LV) systolic failure caused by sepsis after correction of LV afterload by norepinephrine.
- Dobutamine is the first-line therapy in septic cardiomyopathy when LV systolic dysfunction is associated with clinical and biochemical markers of uncontrolled shock.
- Fluid responsiveness can be predicted by respiratory variation in the collapsibility index of the superior vena cava in patients fully adapted to mechanical ventilation by transesophageal echocardiography.

## INTRODUCTION

Echocardiography has been developed over the last 30 or more years and is now considered as the first-line noninvasive investigation in the hemodynamic assessment of circulatory failure in the intensive care unit. Explaining circulatory failure in septic shock is a challenge because it results from intricate mechanisms, such as hypovolemia, vasoplegia, and cardiac dysfunction of both ventricles, which is also called septic cardiomyopathy.[1,2] These mechanisms can occur throughout the process of sepsis, evolving quickly from one status to another or even being associated (**Fig. 1**). Through its ability to assess these mechanisms independently at the bedside, echocardiography is perfectly adapted to hemodynamic assessment in septic shock. It allows clinicians to understand the hemodynamic situation and then to propose appropriate therapy.

This article focuses on echocardiography, whereas lung or abdominal ultrasonography has also been described as useful for intensivists, such as in diagnosing the origin of infection.[3,4]

Conflicts of Interest: None.
[a] Intensive Care Unit, Section Thorax-Vascular Diseases-Abdomen-Metabolism, Hôpital Ambroise Paré, AP-HP, University Hospital Ambroise Paré, 9 Avenue Charles de Gaulle, Boulogne Billancourt 92104, France; [b] Faculté de Médecine Paris Ile de France Ouest, Université de Versailles Saint Quentin en Yvelines, Versailles 78000, France; [c] INSERM U-1018, CESP, Team 5 (EpReC, Renal and Cardiovascular Epidemiology), UVSQ, Villejuif 94807, France
* Corresponding author. Intensive Care Unit, Hôpital Ambroise Paré, AP-HP, 9 Avenue Charles de Gaulle, Boulogne Billancourt 92104, France.
E-mail address: antoine.vieillard-baron@apr.aphp.fr

Clin Chest Med 37 (2016) 299–307
http://dx.doi.org/10.1016/j.ccm.2016.01.005

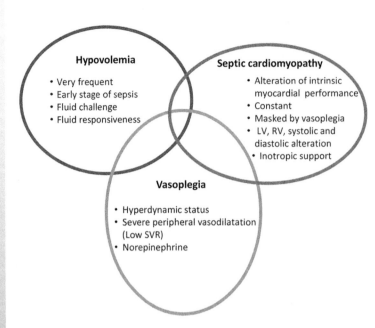

**Fig. 1.** Main mechanisms of hemo dynamic failure in septic shock, their characteristics, and therapeutics. LV, left ventricle; RV, right ventricle SVR, systemic vascular resistance.

First, we summarize the different echocardiographic views and parameters that are useful. Second, we discuss the different hemodynamic profiles that can be detected when performing echocardiography. Finally, we consider the practical use and impact on management of echocardiography. All are discussed in terms of the echocardiography skills of intensivists.

## KEYS TO LEARNING AND UNDERSTANDING CRITICAL CARE ULTRASOUND

Recently, critical care echocardiography (CCE) has been defined and developed to promote echocardiography in the intensive care unit. It has been separated into two different skill levels, basic and advanced.[3,5] The approach to evaluating hemodynamics in septic shock clearly differs according to these skill levels.

### Basic Critical Care Echocardiography

Basic CCE is exclusively based on a transthoracic approach and mainly uses the two-dimensional mode. It was initially proposed for use in patients with shock or respiratory failure to identify quickly and safely gross hemodynamic abnormalities, such as acute cor pulmonale (ACP), marked hypovolemia, or severe left ventricular (LV) systolic dysfunction.[6] This approach is therefore limited and only provides a snapshot of the hemodynamic situation and not really full hemodynamic monitoring. However, it is perfectly suitable for intensivists without special skills and with limited training

in CCE, and the interpretation of echocardiography is more dependent on the quality of image acquisition than on cognitive skills. Competence in basic CCE is recommended for inclusion in the curriculum of all intensivists.[5] It requires short training comprising 10 hours of theory and 30 fully supervised transthoracic echocardiography (TTE) examinations.[5] Basic CCE has to be used in association with other hemodynamic monitoring devices in patients with severe sepsis or septic shock. It has several limitations. TTE may be difficult, especially in mechanically ventilated patients with sepsis, or in patients with acute respiratory distress syndrome or chronic respiratory disease. As a consequence, it is much more operator-dependent, less reproducible, and therefore less accurate than transesophageal echocardiography (TEE).[7] Moreover, it is proposed only to detect gross abnormalities and so complicated situations with associated mechanisms of shock (eg, hypovolemia and septic cardiomyopathy) may be hard to diagnose.

### Advanced Critical Care Echocardiography

In contrast, advanced CCE is mainly, but not exclusively, based on TEE and uses all modes of echocardiography, including Doppler for cardiac output measurement or LV diastolic function evaluation. Advanced CCE allows the intensivist to achieve full hemodynamic monitoring and to diagnose the most complicated situations where the different mechanisms of circulatory failure are intricate. We previously summarized and illustrated this approach.[8] TEE is a minimally invasive and safe procedure provided patients are ventilated and contraindications respected. A 2.6% incidence of complications has been reported, most being considered as minor and occurring in spontaneously breathing patients.[9] For adequate training in advanced CCE, a recent international consensus considered 40 hours of theory, at least 100 full TTE studies, and 35 full TEE studies.[5] We have reported that such skills can be acquired after 6 months of active training.[10,11] This consensus also recommends a certification process. The European Society of Intensive Care Medicine is starting a diploma for intensivists in advanced CCE.

## Main Views and Echocardiographic Parameters Useful for Hemodynamic Evaluation

Only three main views are necessary for the "goal-directed examination" of basic CCE: (1) the apical four-chamber view, (2) the parasternal short-axis view, and (3) the subcostal view at the inferior vena cava (IVC). Basic images that can be obtained by TTE are represented in **Fig. 2**. Marked hypovolemia is suspected if a small and virtual IVC is associated with a hyperkinetic left ventricle, and sometimes LV systolic exclusion. LV systolic dysfunction is indicated by global LV hypokinesia on the short axis at the level of the papillary muscles, whereas ACP is indicated by the association of right ventricular (RV) dilatation on the four-chamber view with paradoxic septal motion on the short axis.[6,12]

As for TTE, limited views in multiplane TEE are also required to monitor hemodynamics in ventilated patients. Examination begins with the transverse (0°) mid-esophageal four-chamber view. From this view, rotating the ultrasound beam by around 120° visualizes the LV outflow tract. The second view is the transgastric short-axis view at the papillary muscles, which is observed by moving the probe down to the stomach and tilting its tip upward. From this view, rotating the ultrasound beam by around 100° to 110° visualizes the LV outflow tract in a good alignment for the use of Doppler. Finally, the examination concludes with the transverse upper esophageal view, the great vessel view. From this view, rotating the ultrasound beam by 90° visualizes a longitudinal view of the superior vena cava (SVC). LV systolic dysfunction and ACP are diagnosed as reported

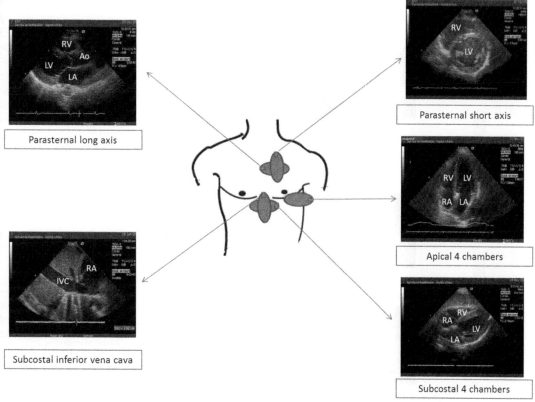

**Fig. 2.** Main views and images acquired during TTE examination. Ao, ascendant aorta; LA, left atrial; RA, right atrial; RV, right ventricle.

with TTE using the midesophageal and transgastric views. Fluid responsiveness status is defined using the SVC collapsibility index, representing diameter variations of the vessel during tidal ventilation.[13] Cardiac output is measured using the midesophageal view at 120° to measure the LV outflow tract diameter and the transgastric view at 110° to measure the velocity time integral in the LV outflow tract (**Fig. 3**).

## DIFFERENT HEMODYNAMIC PROFILES DETECTED BY ECHOCARDIOGRAPHY
### Hypovolemia or Fluid Responsiveness Status

These are clearly different. When hypovolemia has been corrected, fluid responsiveness is the only information available to intensivists and may be tolerated providing that tissue perfusion is adequately corrected. In the early stage of septic shock, hypovolemia (relative and absolute) is frequent[14] because of venous vasodilation, massive capillary leakage, reduction of central blood volume, and potential abdominal fluid effusion.[15] As a consequence, fluid infusion is always the first-line therapy in these patients and does not require any echocardiographic evaluation.

After initial resuscitation, echocardiography identifies patients with persistent hypovolemia or fluid responsiveness, and so helps to optimize volume status and to avoid fluid overload responsible for pulmonary edema, prolonged mechanical ventilation, and finally increased mortality.[16,17] A first way to assess fluid responsiveness by echocardiography is to evaluate changes in cardiac preload induced by tidal ventilation. The greater these changes, the higher the probability that patients are fluid-responsive. Different echocardiography parameters have been proposed, such as respiratory variations of the subaortic blood flow,[18] of the IVC at TTE, called IVC distensibility index,[19] or of the SVC diameter at TEE, called SVC collapsibility index.[13] However, these parameters have only been validated in a small selected population of patients with septic shock and have never been compared. A formal and prospective validation of their accuracy, utility, and impact on prognosis is clearly needed to increase their popularity and use among intensivists, who currently use them very little.[20] From a practical point of view, fluid infusion could be considered when the SVC collapsibility index is greater than 36%,[13] the IVC distensibility index is greater than 18%[19]

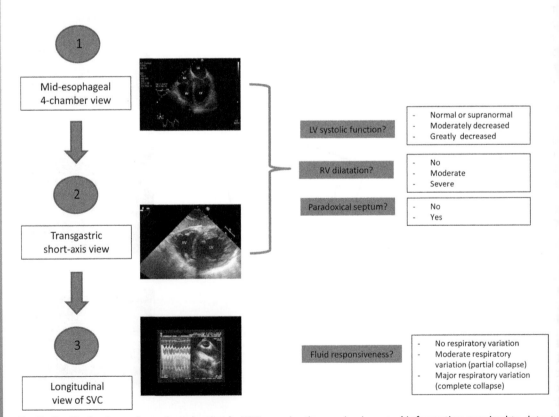

**Fig. 3.** Qualitative hemodynamic evaluation by TEE examination: main views and information required to detect hypovolemia, cardiac dysfunction, right ventricular failure, and vasoplegia.

r 12% according to the proposed formula, and ariation of subaortic blood flow is greater than 2%.[18] These cutoff values are not a magic number below or above which fluid expansion can or cannot be proposed. In real life there is frequently a gray zone[21] and fluid management must also be based on associated clinical and biochemical parameters.

However, more and more patients are less sedated and breathe spontaneously, thus limiting the accuracy of such indices.[22,23] In these patients, an alternative method has been proposed, which is the evaluation by echocardiography of the effect of passive leg raising on LV stroke volume.[24] This method requires measurement of LV stroke volume before and 1 minute after passive leg raising.[25] A 10% variation of stroke volume or more is predictive of fluid responsiveness. Another limitation of the parameters of fluid responsiveness is linked to the conditions of mechanical ventilation. In the case of low tidal volume, variations in intrathoracic pressure might be too small and thus not sufficient to result in significant preload variation, even in the case of preload responsiveness. This limitation is particularly significant in acute respiratory distress syndrome, in which low compliance and low tidal volume coexist.[26] It remains to be seen how fluid responsiveness can be detected with lower cutoff values. Finally, respiratory variation of subaortic Doppler flow is obviously limited in patients with cardiac arrhythmias, which induce variations of stroke volume unrelated to preload dependency.[24]

Whereas "dynamic" echocardiography parameters have been proposed to detect fluid responsiveness, as described previously, "static" parameters, such as Doppler evaluation of LV filling pressure, may be used to evaluate tolerance of volume expansion by focusing on the potential elevation of pressure after fluid expansion.[12]

## Cardiac Failure, Also Called Septic Cardiomyopathy

Septic cardiomyopathy is an acute and reversible myocardial depression induced by sepsis. It may present with different isolated or associated features, such as LV systolic or diastolic dysfunction and RV systolic dysfunction or failure (see Fig. 1).[27,28]

### Left ventricular systolic dysfunction

Depression of intrinsic contractility is constant in all animal models of septic shock.[29] Classic hemodynamic evaluation by pulmonary artery catheterization frequently prevents diagnosis of LV systolic dysfunction, because low cardiac output is not associated with elevated LV filling pressure in

this situation.[1,2] Echocardiography is therefore crucial to detection of such dysfunction. In human studies, LV systolic dysfunction has been defined on a short-axis view as an LV fractional area contraction, a surrogate of LV ejection fraction (LVEF), below 45%. However, its incidence has been reported to vary greatly depending on the time of evaluation, from 18% after 6 hours of resuscitation[30] to 60% after 3 days.[31] Indeed, LVEF depends on LV contractility and also on LV afterload. During the early stage of septic shock, defined by a markedly depressed LV afterload, echocardiography usually shows a hyperkinetic LV, a preserved or high cardiac output, and low LV filling pressure.[8] Restoring systemic vascular resistance by norepinephrine may unmask intrinsic myocardial depression of the left ventricle. These results emphasize that LVEF obtained by echocardiography is more a reflection of arterial tone than intrinsic LV contractility and that preserved LV systolic function following afterload correction could reflect persistent vasoplegia, leading to increased mortality.[2,32] In this specific situation, some authors have reported a dynamic LV obstruction.[33] A recent study by Weng and colleagues[34] showed that high peak systolic velocity measured at the mitral annulus by tissue Doppler imaging might be associated with mortality in patients with septic shock.

### Left ventricular diastolic dysfunction

LV compliance is usually altered during septic shock. In the past, because of the absence of a suitable device to evaluate LV diastolic function at the bedside, it was only detected by observing in diastole the abnormal relationship between LV volume and LV pressure during a fluid challenge.[35] Previous echocardiography studies suggested an increase in LV compliance by reporting a slight increase in LV size associated with a nonelevated filling pressure in patients with decreased LVEF.[36,37] Since the development of new technologies, and especially tissue Doppler, it is now easy to evaluate LV relaxation at the bedside. A maximal velocity of the tissue at the mitral annulus less than 8 cm/s at early diastole (E' wave) is highly suggestive of relaxation impairment.[38] Landesberg and colleagues[39] reported that half of their 262 patients with septic shock or severe sepsis had relaxation impairment. In another study, Bouhemad and colleagues[37] found an incidence of 40%. Interestingly, in the study by Landesberg and colleagues,[39] LV relaxation impairment was independently associated with a worse prognosis. The reason, which has yet to be confirmed, could be poor tolerance of fluids in these patients.

### Right ventricular dysfunction

RV dysfunction/failure is also frequent in sepsis or septic shock, either alone or in association with LV systolic dysfunction. Almost 30% of patients with sepsis have RV dysfunction attested by the presence of RV dilatation on TEE.[30] RV dysfunction may occur in relation to associated acute lung injury/acute respiratory distress syndrome in half of patients or only because of depressed RV contractility as described on the left side in the other half.[40] Whatever the cause, a pattern of ACP is not unusual because most patients are ventilated and positive pressure ventilation is known to induce uncoupling between the right ventricle and the pulmonary circulation, especially in this situation where RV contractility is depressed.[41] This hemodynamic profile has to be looked for systematically, because RV failure limits the efficacy of fluid expansion[42] and may also induce significant pulse pressure variations.

## IN PRACTICE

Many studies report a significant therapeutic impact of echocardiography when adequate images are obtained,[7,43] although no study has yet reported an impact of echocardiography on prognosis. A preliminary study performed in a series of 220 patients with "subacute shock," in addition to sepsis, has suggested a decrease in mortality in the limited echocardiography-guided therapy group compared with the control group.[44] The main difference in management between the two groups was principally related to management of fluids. This remains to be confirmed.

Different profiles can be associated, such as LV systolic dysfunction plus hypovolemia, and echocardiography is probably the only method able to detect both independently. In a given patient, different hemodynamic profiles may occur during disease progression or according to the treatment (eg, before or after norepinephrine infusion), so it is important to repeat the echocardiography evaluation. We recently published our protocol on adapting treatment in septic shock based on TEE if shock persists after initial resuscitation: more fluids in the case of partial or complete SVC collapse during tidal ventilation, dobutamine infusion in the case of depressed LVEF, increased norepinephrine when neither of these occurs, and adaptation of the respiratory settings in the case of ACP.[45] Although this protocol remains to be validated in

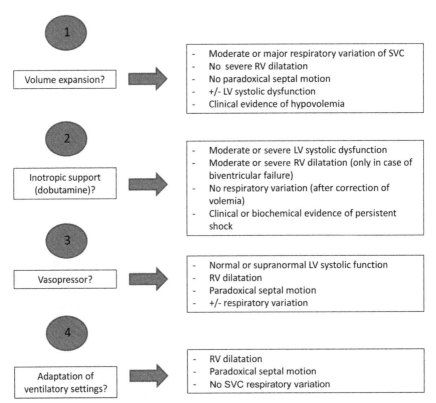

**Fig. 4.** Therapeutic interventions according to qualitative echocardiographic hemodynamic monitoring, based on our own protocol.[45] Readers should be aware that this protocol is a proposal based on our experience and studies, but has not been evaluated for its potential impact on prognosis.

terms of improved prognosis, it is at least interesting to note that we reported in this study a huge discrepancy with the proposed treatment based on the Surviving Sepsis Campaign protocol.[46]

Following our experience and research in the field, we promote a qualitative approach to echocardiographic evaluation, to avoid mistakes caused by measurements or calculations. This is perfectly adapted to the recently developed concept of functional hemodynamic monitoring (Fig. 4).[47] We reported in patients with septic shock that qualitative evaluation of LVEF, RV size, and SVC respiratory variations accurately classifies patients in the right hemodynamic profile, thus enabling appropriate treatment (see Fig. 4).[48] Recently, Haydar and colleagues[43] found that qualitative TTE helped diagnosis and changed hemodynamic treatment. Finally, we recently tested a small TEE probe that can be left in place for 3 days in patients with shock, caused mostly by sepsis.[49] This could be of value, especially in patients with sepsis requiring serial TEE evaluation.

## SUMMARY

CCE is absolutely mandatory for intensivists caring for patients with sepsis. At a basic level, it allows quick and accurate detection of gross abnormalities. At an advanced level, it allows full hemodynamic evaluation: by permitting inspection of the SVC and the right and LV cavities, echocardiography provides important information on mechanisms involved in hemodynamic instability, such as hypovolemia and cardiac dysfunction. Repeated bedside real-time echocardiography allows timely administration of appropriate hemodynamic treatment, which may be fluid infusion, inotropes, or vasopressors or a combination thereof. Echocardiography thus offers real "semicontinuous" and "personalized" hemodynamic monitoring. Acquisition of skills in basic or advanced CCE should be a priority for intensivists to improve intraobserver and interobserver variability and reproducibility and to make echocardiography a routine part of critical care practice, especially in patients with sepsis.

## REFERENCES

1. Jardin F, Brun-Ney D, Auvert B, et al. Sepsis-related cardiogenic shock. Crit Care Med 1990;18(10): 1055–60.
2. Parker MM, Shelhamer JH, Bacharach SL, et al. Profound but reversible myocardial depression in patients with septic shock. Ann Intern Med 1984; 100(4):483–90.
3. Mayo PH, Beaulieu Y, Doelken P, et al. American College of Chest Physicians/La Société de Réanimation de Langue Française statement on competence in critical care ultrasonography. Chest 2009;135(4): 1050–60.
4. Expert Round Table on Ultrasound in ICU. International expert statement on training standards for critical care ultrasonography. Intensive Care Med 2011; 37(7):1077–83.
5. Expert Round Table on Echocardiography in ICU. International consensus statement on training standards for advanced critical care echocardiography. Intensive Care Med 2014;40(5):654–66.
6. Repessé X, Charron C, Vieillard-Baron A. Intensive care ultrasound: V. Goal-directed echocardiography. Ann Am Thorac Soc 2014;11(1):122–8.
7. Charron C, Repessé X, Bodson L, et al. Ten good reasons why everybody can and should perform cardiac ultrasound in the ICU. Anaesthesiol Intensive Ther 2014;46(5):319–22.
8. Vieillard-Baron A, Prin S, Chergui K, et al. Hemodynamic instability in sepsis: bedside assessment by Doppler echocardiography. Am J Respir Crit Care Med 2003;168(11):1270–6.
9. Hüttemann E, Schelenz C, Kara F, et al. The use and safety of transoesophageal echocardiography in the general ICU: a minireview. Acta Anaesthesiol Scand 2004;48(7):827–36.
10. Charron C, Vignon P, Prat G, et al. Number of supervised studies required to reach competence in advanced critical care transesophageal echocardiography. Intensive Care Med 2013;39(6):1019–24.
11. Charron C, Prat G, Caille V, et al. Validation of a skills assessment scoring system for transesophageal echocardiographic monitoring of hemodynamics. Intensive Care Med 2007;33(10):1712–8.
12. Au S-M, Vieillard-Baron A. Bedside echocardiography in critically ill patients: a true hemodynamic monitoring tool. J Clin Monit Comput 2012;26(5): 355–60.
13. Vieillard-Baron A, Chergui K, Rabiller A, et al. Superior vena caval collapsibility as a gauge of volume status in ventilated septic patients. Intensive Care Med 2004;30(9):1734–9.
14. Rackow EC, Astiz ME. Mechanisms and management of septic shock. Crit Care Clin 1993;9(2): 219–37.
15. Dellinger RP. Cardiovascular management of septic shock. Crit Care Med 2003;31(3):946–55.
16. Vincent J-L, Sakr Y, Sprung CL, et al. Sepsis in European intensive care units: results of the SOAP study. Crit Care Med 2006;34(2):344–53.
17. Boyd JH, Forbes J, Nakada T, et al. Fluid resuscitation in septic shock: a positive fluid balance and elevated central venous pressure are associated with increased mortality. Crit Care Med 2011;39(2): 259–65.

18. Feissel M, Michard F, Mangin I, et al. Respiratory changes in aortic blood velocity as an indicator of fluid responsiveness in ventilated patients with septic shock. Chest 2001;119(3):867–73.

19. Barbier C, Loubières Y, Schmit C, et al. Respiratory changes in inferior vena cava diameter are helpful in predicting fluid responsiveness in ventilated septic patients. Intensive Care Med 2004;30(9):1740–6.

20. Cecconi M, Hofer C, Teboul J-L, et al. Fluid challenges in intensive care: the FENICE study: a global inception cohort study. Intensive Care Med 2015; 41(9):1529–37.

21. Cannesson M, Le Manach Y, Hofer CK, et al. Assessing the diagnostic accuracy of pulse pressure variations for the prediction of fluid responsiveness: a "gray zone" approach. Anesthesiology 2011; 115(2):231–41.

22. Repessé X, Bodson L, Vieillard-Baron A. Doppler echocardiography in shocked patients. Curr Opin Crit Care 2013;19(3):221–7.

23. Teboul J-L, Monnet X. Prediction of volume responsiveness in critically ill patients with spontaneous breathing activity. Curr Opin Crit Care 2008;14(3): 334–9.

24. Guerin L, Monnet X, Teboul J-L. Monitoring volume and fluid responsiveness: from static to dynamic indicators. Best Pract Res Clin Anaesthesiol 2013; 27(2):177–85.

25. Lamia B, Ochagavia A, Monnet X, et al. Echocardiographic prediction of volume responsiveness in critically ill patients with spontaneously breathing activity. Intensive Care Med 2007;33(7):1125–32.

26. De Backer D, Heenen S, Piagnerelli M, et al. Pulse pressure variations to predict fluid responsiveness: influence of tidal volume. Intensive Care Med 2005;31(4):517–23.

27. Vieillard-Baron A, Cecconi M. Understanding cardiac failure in sepsis. Intensive Care Med 2014; 40(10):1560–3.

28. Vieillard-Baron A. Septic cardiomyopathy. Ann Intensive Care 2011;1(1):6.

29. Barraud D, Faivre V, Damy T, et al. Levosimendan restores both systolic and diastolic cardiac performance in lipopolysaccharide-treated rabbits: comparison with dobutamine and milrinone. Crit Care Med 2007;35(5):1376–82.

30. Vieillard Baron A, Schmitt JM, Beauchet A, et al. Early preload adaptation in septic shock? A transesophageal echocardiographic study. Anesthesiology 2001;94(3):400–6.

31. Vieillard-Baron A, Caille V, Charron C, et al. Actual incidence of global left ventricular hypokinesia in adult septic shock. Crit Care Med 2008;36(6):1701–6.

32. Repessé X, Charron C, Vieillard-Baron A. Evaluation of left ventricular systolic function revisited in septic shock. Crit Care 2013;17(4):164.

33. Chauvet J-L, El-Dash S, Delastre O, et al. Early dynamic left intraventricular obstruction is associated with hypovolemia and high mortality in septic shock patients. Crit Care 2015;19:262.

34. Weng L, Liu Y, Du B, et al. The prognostic value of left ventricular systolic function measured by tissue Doppler imaging in septic shock. Crit Care 2012; 16(3):R71.

35. Ognibene FP, Parker MM, Natanson C, et al. Depressed left ventricular performance. Response to volume infusion in patients with sepsis and septic shock. Chest 1988;93(5):903–10.

36. Jardin F, Fourme T, Page B, et al. Persistent preload defect in severe sepsis despite fluid loading: a longitudinal echocardiographic study in patients with septic shock. Chest 1999;116(5): 1354–9.

37. Bouhemad B, Nicolas-Robin A, Arbelot C, et al. Acute left ventricular dilatation and shock-induced myocardial dysfunction. Crit Care Med 2009;37(2): 441–7.

38. Nagueh SF, Middleton KJ, Kopelen HA, et al. Doppler tissue imaging: a noninvasive technique for evaluation of left ventricular relaxation and estimation of filling pressures. J Am Coll Cardiol 1997; 30(6):1527–33.

39. Landesberg G, Gilon D, Meroz Y, et al. Diastolic dysfunction and mortality in severe sepsis and septic shock. Eur Heart J 2012;33(7):895–903.

40. Kimchi A, Ellrodt AG, Berman DS, et al. Right ventricular performance in septic shock: a combined radionuclide and hemodynamic study. J Am Coll Cardiol 1984;4(5):945–51.

41. Repessé X, Charron C, Vieillard-Baron A. Acute cor pulmonale in ARDS: rationale for protecting the right ventricle. Chest 2015;147(1):259–65.

42. Schneider AJ, Teule GJ, Groeneveld AB, et al. Biventricular performance during volume loading in patients with early septic shock, with emphasis on the right ventricle: a combined hemodynamic and radionuclide study. Am Heart J 1988;116(1 Pt 1): 103–12.

43. Haydar SA, Moore ET, Higgins GL, et al. Effect of bedside ultrasonography on the certainty of physician clinical decision making for septic patients in the emergency department. Ann Emerg Med 2012; 60(3):346–58.e4.

44. Kanji HD, McCallum J, Sirounis D, et al. Limited echocardiography-guided therapy in subacute shock is associated with change in management and improved outcomes. J Crit Care 2014;29(5): 700–5.

45. Bouferrache K, Amiel J-B, Chimot L, et al. Initial resuscitation guided by the Surviving Sepsis Campaign recommendations and early echocardiographic assessment of hemodynamics in intensive

care unit septic patients: a pilot study. Crit Care Med 2012;40(10):2821–7.

6. Dellinger RP, Levy MM, Carlet JM, et al. Surviving Sepsis Campaign: international guidelines for management of severe sepsis and septic shock: 2008. Crit Care Med 2008;36(1):296–327.

7. Pinsky MR, Payen D. Functional hemodynamic monitoring. Crit Care 2005;9(6):566–72.

48. Vieillard-Baron A, Charron C, Chergui K, et al. Bedside echocardiographic evaluation of hemodynamics in sepsis: is a qualitative evaluation sufficient? Intensive Care Med 2006;32(10):1547–52.

49. Vieillard-Baron A, Slama M, Mayo P, et al. A pilot study on safety and clinical utility of a single-use 72-hour indwelling transesophageal echocardiography probe. Intensive Care Med 2013;39(4):629–35.

# Dysglycemia and Glucose Control During Sepsis

Mark P. Plummer, MBBS[a,b,*], Adam M. Deane, PhD[a,b]

## KEYWORDS

- Sepsis • Hyperglycemia • Hypoglycemia • Glycemic variability

## KEY POINTS

- The 3 domains of sepsis-induced dysglycemia, hyperglycemia, hypoglycemia, and glycemic variability, occur frequently in patients with sepsis and are associated with increased mortality.
- Dysglycemia may not represent the same insult to all septic patients and may be altered by patients' long-term blood glucose control.
- Future randomized controlled trials should consider all 3 domains of dysglycemia as important outcomes with variable associations with mortality based on premorbid glycemic control.

## INTRODUCTION

The physiologic stress of sepsis results in marked disturbances in metabolism and glucose regulation. Disordered metabolism can be divided into 3 separate but interrelated categories, otherwise known as 3 domains of critical illness dysglycemia, which are hyperglycemia, hypoglycemia, and glycemic variability.[1–3] These dysglycemic states occur frequently, with the prevalence of hypoglycemia and hyperglycemia increasing along the continuum from sepsis through severe sepsis and septic shock.[4] Although hyperglycemia, hypoglycemia, and glycemic variability are all associated with increased mortality,[2,3,5] the management goals of patients with sepsis and hyperglycemia remain contentious. This review focuses on the relevance of the 3 domains of dysglycemia in septic patients, with particular emphasis on a rational approach to blood glucose management.

## DEFINITIONS, PREVALENCE, AND PATHOGENESIS

Hyperglycemia occurs frequently in patients who are critically ill due to sepsis and is a marker of illness severity.[6] Many of these patients have previously been diagnosed with diabetes mellitus. A smaller proportion of patients may have diabetes that was unrecognized before the onset of sepsis. Furthermore, patients may have hyperglycemia in the absence of preexisting glucose intolerance (whether diagnosed or not), so-called stress hyperglycemia. The distinction between these clinical entities is important as recent retrospective and prospective observational data indicate that the association between hyperglycemia and mortality may be modulated by patients' chronic glycemic state.[7–10]

### Stress Hyperglycemia

In the critically ill, the precise threshold blood glucose concentration that causes harm and, therefore, constitutes pathologic hyperglycemia remains controversial. The American Diabetes Association (ADA) Diabetes in Hospitals Writing Committee's guidelines recommend thresholds of fasting glucose greater than 6.9 mmol/L, 124 mg/dL or random glucose greater than 11 mmol/L, and 198 mg/dL[11] as identifying disordered glucose metabolism; but these are based on pathologic thresholds in health.[12] Although these values facilitate standardization in the

Conflicts of Interest: M.P. Plummer and A.M. Deane have no duality of interest to declare.
[a] Discipline of Acute Care Medicine, University of Adelaide, North Terrace, Adelaide 5000, Australia;
[b] Department of Critical Care Services, Royal Adelaide Hospital, North Terrace, Adelaide 5000, Australia
* Corresponding author. Level 4 Intensive Care Research Unit, Royal Adelaide Hospital, Emergency Block, North Terrace, Adelaide 5000, Australia.
E-mail address: mark.philip.plummer@gmail.com

Clin Chest Med 37 (2016) 309–319
http://dx.doi.org/10.1016/j.ccm.2016.01.010
0272-5231/16/$ – see front matter © 2016 Elsevier Inc. All rights reserved.

critically ill, the blood glucose thresholds that cause harm are likely more complex in patients with sepsis and may fluctuate throughout an individual patient's illness. Regardless of definitive values, it seems that hyperglycemia occurs frequently in critically ill patients with sepsis, even in those who did not previously have diabetes. The authors prospectively studied 1000 consecutively admitted patients and classified them as having recognized diabetes, unrecognized diabetes, stress hyperglycemia, or normal glucose according to their past medical history, glycated hemoglobin ($HbA_{1c}$) obtained on admission, and peak blood glucose in the first 48 hours.[10] Patients were deemed to have stress hyperglycemia if their blood glucose exceeded the aforementioned ADA thresholds and $HbA_{1c}$ was less than 6.5% (47.5 mmol/mol). Of the 1000 patients, 67 were admitted with a primary diagnosis of sepsis; in this subgroup, preexisting diabetes (recognized or not) occurred in approximately 45% and stress hyperglycemia in approximately 40% of patients (**Fig. 1**), consistent with the concept that disordered glucose metabolism occurs frequently during sepsis.

### Mechanism of Stress-Induced Hyperglycemia

Sepsis-induced hyperglycemia is initiated by the overwhelming activation of proinflammatory mediators and the release of counter-regulatory hormones leading to excessive hepatic gluconeogenesis and peripheral insulin resistance.[13] Cortisol, catecholamines, interleukin-6, tumor necrosis factor-$\alpha$, and glucagon independently and synergistically stimulate hepatic glucose production with hyperglucagonemia seeming to be of pivotal importance.[13–15]

Peripheral insulin resistance is directly proportional to the severity of the stress response[16] and results from defects in postreceptor insulin signaling, with subsequent downregulation of insulin-mediated GLUT-4 glucose transporters.[17] The exact mechanisms whereby sepsis induces defective translocation of GLUT-4 transporters is unclear; however, data from animal studies implicate cortisol,[18] catecholamines,[19] growth hormone,[20] and tumor necrosis factor-$\alpha$[21] as particularly important. The hyperglycemia attributed to these metabolic derangements is further exacerbated by therapeutic interventions, such as administration of catecholamines, dextrose, corticosteroids, and nutrition.

### Harm Secondary to Hyperglycemia

Acute hyperglycemia has been recognized as a marker of the severity of illness.[6,22,23] Moreover, various investigators have repeatedly reported that the magnitude of hyperglycemia is associated with increased mortality, even after adjusting for illness severity scores, suggesting that at some threshold hyperglycemia is harmful in patients with sepsis.[6,22,23] However, recent data from Kaukonen and colleagues[24] suggest the relationship between hyperglycemia and harm may be more complex and the variables used in previous studies to adjust for risk may have been imprecise. In a retrospective observational study of patients' concurrent glucose and lactate samples (n = 7925 critically ill patients), they used multivariable analysis and reported no association between hyperglycemia and mortality once lactate levels were incorporated into the model.[24] These data challenge the causal relationship of hyperglycemia with mortality within the spectrum of moderate-glucose

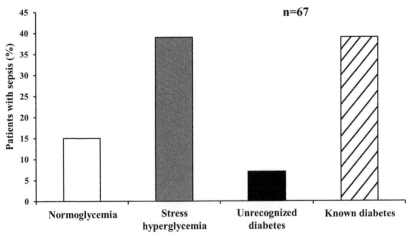

**Fig. 1.** Glycemic category in critically ill patients with a primary diagnosis of sepsis. In a population of 1000 consecutively admitted patients, there were 67 admitted with a primary diagnosis of sepsis. Most septic patients had preexisting diabetes or stress hyperglycemia.

ontrol targets. It should be highlighted, however, hat these patients had well-controlled glycemia with the mean (standard deviation) blood glucose during intensive care unit (ICU) stay reported as .6 (2.1) mmol/L, 137 (38.0) mg/dL in survivors and 8.1 (2.5) mmol/L, 146 (45.0) mg/dL in nonsurvivors.[24] It is plausible that extremes of hyperglycemia have increased toxicity and at higher levels may be independently associated with mortality.

Although the degree of hyperglycemia required for harm and the association between hyperglycemia and mortality remain uncertain, in vivo and n vitro studies have highlighted several putative pathophysiologic consequences of acute hyperglycemia. Glucose has been shown to be a powerful proinflammatory mediator stimulating cytokine production and exacerbating the oxidative stress response, thereby setting up a cycle whereby hyperglycemia leads to further hyperglycemia.[25] In human clinical trials, hyperglycemia has also been shown to exert prothrombotic effects,[26] reduce endothelial vascular reactivity,[27] and impair neutrophil chemotaxis and phagocytosis.[28]

## Diabetes and the Impact of Chronic Hyperglycemia

The relative risk of sepsis in patients with diabetes is 2- to 6-fold greater than in normal age-matched persons without diabetes.[29,30] It is, therefore, unsurprising that diabetes is a common comorbid illness in the septic critically ill population, with a reported prevalence between 17% and 45%.[1,10,22,23] However, somewhat counterintuitively, the diagnosis of diabetes does not identify critically ill patients at risk of dying in the ICU. Indeed outcomes in patients presenting with sepsis seem comparable despite patients with diabetes being older, sicker, and having higher blood glucose concentrations than patients without diabetes.[22,23,31] In the largest epidemiologic study to date into the effect of premorbid diabetes status on outcomes in sepsis, Esper and colleagues[23] analyzed data from 12.5 million acute-care admissions, of which 17% (2,070,459) were identified as having diabetes mellitus. Compared with patients with severe sepsis who were not known to have diabetes, patients with diabetes had a lesser case-fatality rate (18.5% vs 20.6% [$P<.05$]), shorter length of hospital stay, and were less likely to develop acute respiratory failure and acute respiratory distress syndrome (9% vs 14%).[23] Furthermore, although there is a strong association between the magnitude of hyperglycemia and mortality in the nondiabetic septic population (as described earlier), the strength of

this association is either markedly reduced or absent in studies that have adjusted for patients with recognized diabetes.[22]

A limitation of these epidemiologic studies is that patients with unrecognized diabetes have not been identified; more importantly, patients with diabetes have been viewed as a homogenous cohort irrespective of their premorbid glycemic control. This relatively crude approach is likely to be flawed, as it is increasingly recognized that chronic blood glucose control is important when evaluating associations between acute hyperglycemia and outcomes in the general intensive care population.[3,8–10,32] In the study the authors recently undertook to evaluate the prevalence of unrecognized diabetes, they concurrently evaluated the interaction between preexisting chronic hyperglycemia, acute glycemia, and mortality.[10] Using admission $HbA_{1c}$ as a measure of chronic glycemic control, the authors observed that acute hyperglycemia (glucose >11 mmol/L; 198 mg/dL) was associated with increased mortality in patients without diabetes and in those with adequately controlled diabetes ($HbA_{1c}$ <7%; 53 mmol/mol). However, there was no association between acute glycemia and mortality in patients with insufficiently controlled diabetes ($HbA_{1c}$ ≥7%), that is, those with chronic hyperglycemia such that blood glucose concentrations in excess of 15 mmol/L (270 mg/dL) were well tolerated (Fig. 2).[10] These prospective data support previous retrospective studies that indicated the benefit in treating hyperglycemia during critical illness may be diminished in patients with known diabetes.[3,7,8,31,33,34] Even more startling are observations from Egi and colleagues[8] who conducted a retrospective observational study and stratified patients with diabetes according to premorbid blood glucose control. Using this approach, higher blood glucose concentrations were associated with a reduction in mortality in patients with insufficiently controlled diabetes, suggesting that treating hyperglycemia in this population may actually be harmful.[8]

The mechanisms governing the interaction between acute hyperglycemia during sepsis and outcome in patients with poorly controlled diabetes and chronic hyperglycemia remain poorly understood. The effect of diabetes on the immune system has been hypothesized to play a role, possibly through impaired neutrophil function blunting the exaggerated inflammatory response.[23,35] Conditioning to chronic hyperglycemia has also been proposed to cause cellular adaptation with preferential downregulation of insulin-independent GLUT-1 and GLUT-3 glucose transporters preventing intracellular glucotoxicity.[32] Prospective studies classifying

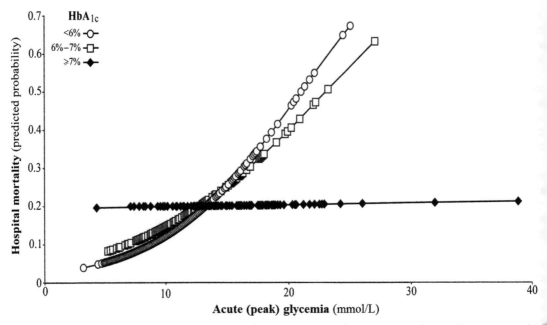

**Fig. 2.** Relationship between hospital mortality and acute glycemia when categorized according to premorbid glycemia (HbA$_{1c}$). In patients without diabetes and those with stringently controlled (*open circles*, HbA$_{1c}$ <6% [42 mmol/mol], n = 672, odds ratio = 1.20 [95% CI 1.12, 1.28]; *P*<.001) and adequately controlled diabetes (*open squares*, 6 ≤ HbA$_{1c}$ <7% [53 mmol/mol], n = 199, odds ratio = 1.14 [95% 1.05, 1.25]; *P* = .003), increasing peak blood glucose concentrations was associated with increasing mortality. However, there was no association apparent in patients with insufficiently controlled diabetes (*filled diamonds*, HbA$_{1c}$ ≥7%, n = 129, odds ratio = 1.0 [95% CI = 0.92, 1.1]; *P* = .95). The model was an adequate fit according to the Hosmer-Lemeshow goodness-of-fit test. (*From* Plummer MP, Bellomo R, Cousins CE, et al. Dysglycaemia in the critically ill and the interaction of chronic and acute glycaemia with mortality. Intensive Care Med 2014;40(7):978; with permission.)

diabetic patients according to premorbid glycemic control are required to further delineate the importance of, and mechanisms for, the protective effect of chronic hyperglycemia in patients presenting with sepsis who have preexisting diabetes before their acute illness.[36]

A protective effect of oral hypoglycemic agents has also been proposed as a putative contributory factor explaining the paradox of improved outcome in septic patients with diabetes. There are recent data that suggest that metformin use before ICU admission may have a protective effect via an attenuation of the inflammatory response.[37] Preclinical studies have reported that metformin, when compared with placebo, reduces mortality in murine models of endotoxemia and acute lung injury via a reduction in proinflammatory cytokines and neutrophil activation.[38,39] In a parallel study of 40 nondiabetic mice using a lipopolysaccharide model of mouse sepsis, Tsoyi and colleagues[38] demonstrated a dramatic survival benefit in those mice pretreated with metformin (n = 20) compared with placebo (n = 20) (survival 75% vs 17%; *P*<.05). There are, however, limited data in

humans. In a retrospective observational study of 1284 patients with diabetes undergoing cardiac surgery, patients who were receiving metformin had fewer postoperative infections when compared with those patients not receiving metformin (0.7% in metformin users vs 3.2% in nonusers; odds ratio [OR] 0.2, 95% confidence interval [CI] 0.1, 0.7).[40] A retrospective, observational, multicenter study of 7404 critically ill adult patients with type 2 diabetes reported that users of metformin, both as monotherapy and in combination with other antidiabetic drugs, had less mortality at day 30 when compared with nonusers after adjustment for age, sex, diabetes duration, preadmission HbA$_{1c}$, preadmission morbidity, and use of concurrent cardiac medications (adjusted hazard ratio 0.84, 95% CI 0.75–0.94).[37] Metformin use was identified by data matching to a registry of filled prescriptions within 90 days before ICU admission, and medication compliance is unknown; however, any nonadherence would, if anything, bias estimates toward no association.[37]

Treatment with metformin during critical illness is contentious because of the risk of lactic acidosis n patients with shock and severe renal and liver and cardiac failure.[41] Only a single study has examined the effect of metformin use during critical illness.[42] In this small (n = 21) parallel randomized controlled trial of critically ill patients with a diagnosis of systemic inflammatory response syndrome and hyperglycemia, Ansari and colleagues[42] reported a nonsignificant reduction in proinflammatory cytokines at day 7 and a reduction in insulin requirement when metformin was compared with placebo in combination with intensive insulin therapy. However, interpretation of these results is limited considerably by a lack of clinical outcome data; further studies are required to assess the safety and efficacy of metformin use during critical illness.

Sulfonylurea drugs, such as glibenclamide, exert their glucose-lowering effect via blockade of the $K_{ATP}$ channel on pancreatic beta cells, triggering insulin release.[43] The $K_{ATP}$ channel is also present on vascular smooth muscle, the unchecked opening of which has been implicated in the pathogenesis of vasodilatory shock.[44] Several studies in animal model of septic shock have demonstrated improvement in vasopressor responsiveness after sulfonylurea administration via blockade of vascular smooth muscle $K_{ATP}$ channels.[45–47] In a small (n = 10) randomized double-blind crossover pilot study of sulfonylurea administration in human sepsis, Warrillow and colleagues[48] failed to demonstrate any difference in median norepinephrine requirement, hemodynamic parameters, or lactate concentration with sulfonylurea use and observed a concerning lowering of plasma glucose, confirming absorption of the drug. Thus, although animal data are encouraging, the $K_{ATP}$ channel may be a less important target in human vasodilatory shock; the side effect of hypoglycemia makes sulfonylureas a less attractive therapy for further evaluation in human sepsis.

### Unrecognized Diabetes

Given the association between chronic hyperglycemia and sepsis,[29,30] it is conceivable that unrecognized diabetes occurs frequently in this population; but there are insufficient data to be certain of this statement. The lack of information occurs because distinguishing acute stress hyperglycemia from unrecognized diabetes is problematic in critically ill patients with sepsis and hyperglycemia. Validated tests for the diagnosis of diabetes in the ambulant population, including fasting plasma glucose and the oral glucose tolerance test, are inaccurate or impractical during critical illness.[49] In health, an $HbA_{1c}$

greater than 6.5% (48 mmol/mol) has been endorsed as a suitable diagnostic criterion for the diagnosis of diabetes mellitus in both ambulant and inpatient populations.[49] The $HbA_{1c}$ may be less accurate in the critically ill than in outpatients, particularly if patients receive transfusions of erythrocytes or in other conditions that interfere with erythrocyte survival.[49] Despite these limitations, the $HbA_{1c}$ is the most robust test readily available for clinicians; a threshold of 6.5% (48 mmol/mol) seems reasonable. Using this cutoff, the authors reported the prevalence of undiagnosed diabetes in a sample population admitted to a general ICU as 5.5% and 7.4% in the subpopulation of critically ill patients admitted with a primary diagnosis of sepsis (see **Fig. 1**).[10]

### Hypoglycemia

Severe hypoglycemia, when defined as a blood glucose less than 2.2 mmol/L (40 mg/dL),[50] occurs relatively frequently in patients presenting with sepsis,[1,51] with the prevalence strongly associated with illness severity.[4] Waeschle and colleagues[4] analyzed hypoglycemia in a cohort of 191 critically ill septic patients treated with intensive insulin therapy (targeting 4.4–7.8 mmol/L; 80–140 mg/dL) and stratified patients according to illness severity. The percentage of patients with at least one episode of severe hypoglycemia was 2.1%, 6.0% and 11.5% for patients with sepsis, severe sepsis, and septic shock, respectively.[4] Intensive insulin therapy seems to be the most important risk factor for the development of hypoglycemia: the relationship between intensive insulin therapy and hypoglycemia has been consistently demonstrated in several large, prospective, randomized controlled trials.[1,51]

In unselected critically ill patients, there is a strong relationship between hypoglycemia and mortality.[1,50–53] Because hypoglycemia occurs in patients with greater severity of illness and, therefore, greater risk of death, several investigators have incorporated severity of illness as a variable in regression analyses. When this is done, in general, hypoglycemia seems to be independently associated with death.[3,52–54] Recent observational[3,53,54] and prospective[52] trial data suggest that even moderate hypoglycemia (blood glucose <3.9 mmol/L; 70 mg/dL) is associated with increased mortality, with the lower the nadir in glucose concentration, the stronger the association.[52] This point is evident even after a single episode of mild hypoglycemia, and the risk is apparent in both patients with and without preexisting diabetes.[3] The severity and duration of hypoglycemia required to cause harm remains uncertain, and the mechanisms by which hypoglycemia increases mortality in sepsis are yet to be fully elucidated. Neurons, as obligate users of glucose, have been purported to be at particular risk of damage in the setting of hypoglycemia; however, long-term neurocognitive outcome studies are lacking.[55]

It is important to recognize that pathologically low blood glucose also occurs secondary to impaired endogenous glucose production even in the absence of exogenous insulin. Accordingly, episodes of hypoglycemia are also a marker of illness severity; for example, a retrospective observational study of 102 critically ill patients with an episode of severe hypoglycemia reported that 27.5% had not received insulin within 12 hours of the hypoglycemic episode.[2]

### Glycemic Variability

Glycemic variability is a broad term describing marked fluctuations in blood glucose. There is a paucity of prevalence data on glycemic variability in sepsis, which may reflect the lack of standardization on the definition of variability, the thresholds at which swings in blood glucose become pathologic, and the metrics used to calculate it.[4,5,56,57] Nevertheless, there is evidence to suggest that fluctuations of blood glucose concentrations are associated with increased mortality in septic patients independent of hypoglycemic episodes and mean blood glucose.[4,5] Similar to hyperglycemia, patients with diabetes seem to be somewhat protected from the harmful effects of glycemic variability; the association between glycemic variability and mortality is reduced or absent in patients with diabetes.[3,58,59] However, none of these studies have assessed for interactions between chronic glycemia (HbA$_{1c}$), acute variability, and outcomes. Mechanistic studies into the effects of glycemic variability in sepsis are lacking; the causal link between glucose fluctuations and adverse outcomes have been drawn from studies in vitro and in patients with type 2 diabetes in the community, where marked acute fluctuations in blood glucose have been linked to oxidative stress–induced endothelial dysfunction and endothelial apoptosis.[60,61]

## GLUCOSE TARGETS

Until quite recently stress hyperglycemia was viewed as a normal physiologic response to critical illness and was, therefore, often tolerated.[62] However, in 2001 the landmark study from Van den Berghe and colleagues[50] caused a paradigm shift in the approach to blood glucose management in the critically ill. In this single-center open-label study from a surgical ICU in Leuven, Belgium, patients were randomized to intensive insulin therapy targeting 4.4 to 6.2 mmol/L, 80 to 110 mg/dL or to conventional therapy targeting 180 to 200 mg/dL, 10.0 to 11.1 mmol/L. The intervention caused a surprisingly large reduction in mortality (intensive care mortality: relative risk reduction of 43%, absolute risk reduction of 3.4%, and a number needed to treat with intensive insulin therapy to reduce one ICU death of 29 patients).[50] Although the number of patients with severe sepsis was not reported at baseline, intensive insulin therapy reduced episodes of nosocomial septicemia by 46% and reduced the proportion of patients requiring prolonged antibiotic therapy.[50] Given the sheer magnitude of the observed effect, it was essential to reproduce this study and determine external validity of the results.[63,64]

In 2006, the Leuven group performed a second randomized controlled trial of intensive insulin therapy using the same glucose targets and feeding regimen in medical ICU patients with an anticipated length of stay greater than 3 days.[65] In contrast to the initial study, there was no overall difference in mortality between intensive and conventional glycemic control.[65] Furthermore, there was no difference in the proportion of patients dying of therapy-resistant septic shock.[65] Analysis of the predefined subgroup of interest (patients admitted for >3 days) reported a more modest survival benefit from intensive insulin therapy; but this group experienced significantly more hypoglycemic episodes, with the prevalence of hypoglycemia more than 6-fold higher than in the original study.[50,64] The prevalence of hypoglycemia raised concerns for the use of intensive insulin therapy in patients with sepsis, particularly as post hoc analysis of pooled data from the two Leuven studies revealed an association between hypoglycemia and death that seemed to be independent.[66]

The Efficacy of Volume Substitution and Insulin Therapy in Severe Sepsis (VISEP) trial was the first to specifically examine the effect of intensive insulin therapy in patients with severe sepsis. This study, conducted in 18 ICUs in Germany, used a 2 × 2 factorial study design to compare intensive insulin therapy with conventional insulin therapy and resuscitation with intravenous hydroxyethyl starch to Ringer lactate.[1] At the planned interim analysis (n = 488 patients), the insulin comparative arm of the study was terminated by the data and safety monitoring board owing to a 6-fold increased risk of hypoglycemia.[3] There was no evidence of any beneficial effect of intensive insulin therapy.[27]

The Corticosteroid Treatment and Intensive Insulin Therapy for Septic Shock (COIITSS) trial was conducted to determine whether intensive glucose control would be beneficial in patients treated with corticosteroid for septic shock with a secondary objective to compare hydrocortisone plus fludrocortisone therapy with hydrocortisone therapy alone.[51] This 2 × 2 factorial study randomly assigned 509 patients with septic shock to either Leuven intensive insulin therapy or conventional blood glucose control. Patients treated with intensive glucose control had significantly more hypoglycemic episodes than the conventional arm; however, there was no difference in mortality, mechanical-ventilation-free days, or ICU and hospital length of stay.[51]

The NICE-SUGAR study provides data that are the most externally valid to inform blood glucose management during critical illness. Within this study, 6104 critically ill patients were randomly assigned to intensive therapy targeting 4.5 to 6.0 mmol/L, 81 to 108 mg/dL or conventional therapy targeting less than 10 mmol/L, 180 mg/dL and maintaining blood glucose between 8 and 10 mmol/L, 144 to 180 mg/dL.[67] Intensive therapy was associated with a markedly greater risk of severe hypoglycemia (OR 14.7; CI 9.0–25.9); in contradistinction to the Leuven trials, the NICE-SUGAR study reported that patients assigned to the intensive therapy had an increased risk of death (27.5% vs 24.9%, $P = .02$).[67] Severe sepsis was a predefined subgroup of interest, and outcomes were similar to the population as a whole.[67]

Although the NICE-SUGAR study is the only study to report increased mortality with intensive glucose control, several other randomized controlled trials in mixed populations of medical and surgical ICU patients have reported that intensive insulin therapy does not convey a survival benefit and is associated with a much higher incidence of severe hypoglycemia (**Table 1**).[68–70] Accordingly, the use of intensive insulin therapy should be avoided. However, it is now apparent that because diabetic status was considered a binary phenomenon (rather than a continuous variable) in these trials, the impact of chronic blood glucose control on acute hyperglycemia and outcome is uncertain. Future trials are warranted to further delineate this relationship and explore the concept of individualized blood glucose targets (**Fig. 3**).

**Table 1**
**Important randomized controlled trials of insulin therapy targeted to specific blood glucose concentrations in critically ill patients with sepsis**

| First Author, Year (Country) | Sites | N | N with Sepsis (%) | Glucose Goal (mmol/L) | Outcome of Intensive Therapy |
|---|---|---|---|---|---|
| Annane & Cariou,[51] 2010 (France) (COIITSS) | 8 | 509 | 509 (100) | IIT 4.4–6.1 Control 10.0–11.1 | No effect on hospital mortality ↑ Hypoglycemia |
| Arabi et al,[68] 2008 (Saudi Arabia) | 1 | 523 | 122 (24) | IIT 4.4–6.1 Control 10.0–11.1 | No effect on ICU or hospital mortality overall or in subgroup of patients with sepsis ↑ Hypoglycemia in all-comers |
| Brunkhorst et al,[1] 2008 (Germany) (VISEP) | 18 | 535 | 535 (100) | IIT 4.4–6.1 Control 10.0–11.1 | No effect on 90-d mortality ↑ Hypoglycemia led to early termination |
| Ellger et al,[72] 2008 (Belgium)[a] | 1 | 950 | 950 (100) | IIT 4.4–6.1 Control 10.0–11.1 | No effect on ICU or hospital mortality ↑ Hypoglycemia |
| Iapichino et al,[73] 2008 (Italy) | 3 | 72 | 72 (100) | IIT 4.4–6.1 Control 10.0–11.1 | No effect on ICU or 90-d mortality |
| Finfer & Chittock,[67] 2009 (Australia, New Zealand, Canada) (NICE-SUGAR) | 42 | 6104 | 1299 (21) | IIT 4.4–6.1 Control <10.0 | ↑ 90-d Mortality overall No effect on 90-d mortality in sepsis ↑ Hypoglycemia overall and in patients with sepsis |
| Savioli et al,[74] 2009 (Italy) | 3 | 90 | 90 (100) | IIT 4.4–6.1 Control 10.0–11.1 | No effect on 90-d mortality ↑ Hypoglycemia |

Abbreviation: IIT, intensive insulin therapy.
[a] Patients classified post hoc to severe sepsis from 2 larger randomized controlled trials in surgical[50] and medical ICUs.[65]

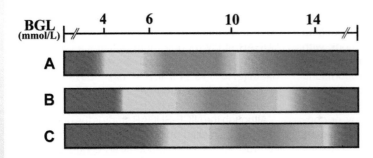

**Fig. 3.** The proposed model of personalized and dynamic optimal glucose targets (*green zone*). (*A*) Targeting a blood glucose less than 10 mmol/L while avoiding hypoglycemia may be appropriate for patients with normal glucose tolerance and those with well-controlled diabetes in the recovery phase from a septic insult. (*B*) Patients with inadequately controlled diabetes (ie, HbA$_{1c}$ >7%) who were chronically hyperglycemic before their septic episode may benefit from shifting the optimal glucose threshold to the right to avoid relative hyperglycemia. Such a shift in targets could theoretically also benefit those patients without preexisting diabetes who have severe septic shock and concurrent hypoxia. (*C*) Patients with poorly controlled diabetes who have developed cellular adaptation to chronic hyperglycemia may benefit from more liberal blood glucose targets and a further right shift in the optimal glucose range when critically ill to reflect the mean blood glucose level (BGL) before the onset of the acute illness.

## INTERPRETATION

The use of short-acting insulin administered intravenously with the dose based on protocols is currently the gold standard for the management of hyperglycemia during sepsis.[71] The results from the aforementioned large randomized controlled trials are somewhat contradictory, which has created uncertainty on the ideal glycemic range to target. The early termination of the VISEP study due to safety concerns of the increased incidence of severe hypoglycemia and the increased mortality demonstrated in the NICE-SUGAR study for patients randomized to intensive insulin therapy suggest that the ideal upper limit may be around 10 mmol/L, 180 mg/dL, particularly for patients with normal glucose tolerance. The current Surviving Sepsis guidelines do not distinguish stress hyperglycemia from hyperglycemia in patients with diabetes but strongly recommend threshold blood glucose concentrations of 10 mmol/L or less, 180 mg/dL.[71]

Although the Surviving Sepsis guidelines are written by expert clinicians, it may be that the one-size-fits-all strategy for the management of hyperglycemia in sepsis is inadequate, particularly given the dynamic course of diseases and the increasing appreciation of the role of chronic hyperglycemia in modifying the relationship between acute hyperglycemia and outcomes. To date, all studies to determine the optimal glycemic range in the critically ill have evaluated the effect of glucose targets that have been maintained for the duration of a patient's admission. However, stress hyperglycemia is by definition transient; the pathogenesis driving high blood glucose will be labile in response to changes in the course of the disease. It is intuitively plausible that the optimal blood glucose range fluctuates throughout the course of an individual patient's illness. Higher blood glucose concentrations may be tolerable, or even more desirable, for cellular function during the early phase of sepsis, particularly if concomitant hypoxia and hypotension are present, but less desirable as the insult resolves and patients improve, with the risk of infection from higher blood glucose concentrations outweighing any potential protection against cellular hypoglycemia. The authors also speculate that the ideal glycemic range will vary between patients with diabetes depending on their premorbid glycemic control (see **Fig. 3**). Patients with well-controlled diabetes, for example, HbA$_{1c}$ less than 7%, 53 mmol/mol, have a mean daily blood glucose of approximately 8 mmol/L, 144 mg/dL, whereas patients with poorly controlled diabetes and an HbA$_{1c}$ of 10%, 13.3 mmol/mol have a mean blood glucose of approximately 13 mmol/L, 234 mg/dL. The authors suggest that the metabolic milieu before the onset of sepsis will be different in such patients and will influence the optimal blood glucose range during critical illness. Accordingly, patients with chronic hyperglycemia may benefit from more liberal glucose targets. However, prospective randomized controlled studies are required to definitely determine the importance of dynamic glucose targets for stress hyperglycemia and individualized targets according to chronic glycemic control. In the interim, an intravenous insulin infusion protocol that targets an upper limit of 10 mmol/L, 180 mg/dL, avoids hypoglycemia, and minimizes glycemic variability seems to be a reasonable strategy.

## SUMMARY

Hyperglycemia, hypoglycemia, and glycemic variability occur frequently in patients with severe sepsis with and without preexisting diabetes. All 3 domains of sepsis-induced dysglycemia are associated with adverse outcomes in patients without diabetes, but current observational data indicate uncertainty as to whether hyperglycemia is harmful or protective in those with preexisting chronic hyperglycemia (HbA1c >7%). The current Surviving Sepsis Campaign recommendations for all patients with severe sepsis are for intravenous insulin therapy to be commenced when the blood glucose exceeds 10 mmol/L, 180 mg/dL, with the goal of maintaining blood glucose between approximately 8 and 10 mmol/L, 144 to 180 mg/dL. However, the authors remain cautious about the strength of the Surviving Sepsis guideline regarding glucose targets for patients with preexisting chronic hyperglycemia. The authors think further information is required in this subgroup because sepsis-induced dysglycemia seems to be a heterogeneous entity with unique pathophysiologic features that seem to be altered by long-term glycemia. It is also increasingly evident that strategies are required to minimize all 3 domains of sepsis-induced dysglycemia. The design of future randomized controlled trials should include consideration of hyperglycemia, hypoglycemia, and glycemic variability as important outcomes with variable associations with mortality based on premorbid glycemic control.

# REFERENCES

1. Brunkhorst FM, Engel C, Bloos F, et al. Intensive insulin therapy and pentastarch resuscitation in severe sepsis. N Engl J Med 2008;358(2):125–39.
2. Krinsley JS, Grover A. Severe hypoglycemia in critically ill patients: risk factors and outcomes. Crit Care Med 2007;35(10):2262–7.
3. Krinsley JS, Egi M, Kiss A, et al. Diabetic status and the relation of the three domains of glycemic control to mortality in critically ill patients: an international multicenter cohort study. Crit Care 2013;17(2):R37.
4. Waeschle RM, Moerer O, Hilgers R, et al. The impact of the severity of sepsis on the risk of hypoglycaemia and glycaemic variability. Crit Care 2008;12(5):R129.
5. Ali NA, O'Brien JM Jr, Dungan K, et al. Glucose variability and mortality in patients with sepsis. Crit Care Med 2008;36(8):2316–21.
6. Leonidou L, Michalaki M, Leonardou A, et al. Stress-induced hyperglycemia in patients with severe sepsis: a compromising factor for survival. Am J Med Sci 2008;336(6):467–71.
7. Rady MY, Johnson DJ, Patel BM, et al. Influence of individual characteristics on outcome of glycemic control in intensive care unit patients with or without diabetes mellitus. Mayo Clin Proc 2005;80(12): 1558–67.
8. Egi M, Bellomo R, Stachowski E, et al. Blood glucose concentration and outcome of critical illness: the impact of diabetes. Crit Care Med 2008;36(8):2249–55.
9. Egi M, Bellomo R, Stachowski E, et al. The interaction of chronic and acute glycemia with mortality in critically ill patients with diabetes. Crit Care Med 2011;39(1):105–11.
10. Plummer MP, Bellomo R, Cousins CE, et al. Dysglycaemia in the critically ill and the interaction of chronic and acute glycaemia with mortality. Intensive Care Med 2014;40(7):973–80.
11. Clement S, Braithwaite SS, Magee MF, et al, American Diabetes Association Diabetes in Hospitals Writing Committee. Management of diabetes and hyperglycemia in hospitals. Diabetes Care 2004; 27(2):553–91.
12. American Diabetes Association. Diagnosis and classification of diabetes mellitus. Diabetes Care 2007; 30(Suppl 1):S42–7.
13. Marik PE, Raghavan M. Stress-hyperglycemia, insulin and immunomodulation in sepsis. Intensive Care Med 2004;30(5):748–56.
14. Petit F, Bagby GJ, Lang CH. Tumor necrosis factor mediates zymosan-induced increase in glucose flux and insulin resistance. Am J Physiol 1995; 268(2 Pt 1):E219–28.
15. Siegel JH, Cerra FB, Coleman B, et al. Physiological and metabolic correlations in human sepsis. Invited commentary. Surgery 1979;86(2):163–93.
16. Mizock BA. Alterations in fuel metabolism in critical illness: hyperglycaemia. Best Pract Res Clin Endocrinol Metab 2001;15(4):533–51.
17. Lang CH, Dobrescu C, Meszaros K. Insulin-mediated glucose uptake by individual tissues during sepsis. Metab Clin Exp 1990;39(10):1096–107.
18. Dimitriadis G, Leighton B, Parry-Billings M, et al. Effects of glucocorticoid excess on the sensitivity of glucose transport and metabolism to insulin in rat skeletal muscle. Biochem J 1997;321(Pt 3):707–12.
19. Chiasson JL, Shikama H, Chu DT, et al. Inhibitory effect of epinephrine on insulin-stimulated glucose uptake by rat skeletal muscle. J Clin Invest 1981;68(3):706–13.
20. Smith TR, Elmendorf JS, David TS, et al. Growth hormone-induced insulin resistance: role of the insulin receptor, IRS-1, GLUT-1, and GLUT-4. Am J Physiol 1997;272(6 Pt 1):E1071–9.
21. Hotamisligil GS, Peraldi P, Budavari A, et al. IRS-1-mediated inhibition of insulin receptor tyrosine kinase activity in TNF-alpha- and obesity-induced insulin resistance. Science 1996;271(5249):665–8.
22. Stegenga ME, Vincent JL, Vail GM, et al. Diabetes does not alter mortality or hemostatic and inflammatory responses in patients with severe sepsis. Crit Care Med 2010;38(2):539–45.
23. Esper AM, Moss M, Martin GS. The effect of diabetes mellitus on organ dysfunction with sepsis: an epidemiological study. Crit Care 2009;13(1):R18.

24. Kaukonen KM, Bailey M, Egi M, et al. Stress hyper-lactatemia modifies the relationship between stress hyperglycemia and outcome: a retrospective obser-vational study. Crit Care Med 2014;42(6):1379–85.

25. Yu WK, Li WQ, Li N, et al. Influence of acute hyper-glycemia in human sepsis on inflammatory cytokine and counter-regulatory hormone concentrations. World J Gastroenterol 2003;9(8):1824–7.

26. Rao AK, Chouhan V, Chen X, et al. Activation of the tissue factor pathway of blood coagulation during prolonged hyperglycemia in young healthy men. Diabetes 1999;48(5):1156–61.

27. Giugliano D, Marfella R, Coppola L, et al. Vascular effects of acute hyperglycemia in humans are reversed by L-arginine. Evidence for reduced avail-ability of nitric oxide during hyperglycemia. Circula-tion 1997;95(7):1783–90.

28. Turina M, Fry DE, Polk HC Jr. Acute hyperglycemia and the innate immune system: clinical, cellular, and molecular aspects. Crit Care Med 2005;33(7): 1624–33.

29. Shah BR, Hux JE. Quantifying the risk of infectious diseases for people with diabetes. Diabetes Care 2003;26(2):510–3.

30. Laupland KB, Gregson DB, Zygun DA, et al. Severe bloodstream infections: a population-based assess-ment. Crit Care Med 2004;32(4):992–7.

31. Vincent JL, Preiser JC, Sprung CL, et al. Insulin-treated diabetes is not associated with increased mortality in critically ill patients. Crit Care 2010; 14(1):R12.

32. Dungan KM, Braithwaite SS, Preiser JC. Stress hy-perglycaemia. Lancet 2009;373(9677):1798–807.

33. Van den Berghe G, Wilmer A, Milants I, et al. Inten-sive insulin therapy in mixed medical/surgical inten-sive care units: benefit versus harm. Diabetes 2006; 55(11):3151–9.

34. Falciglia M, Freyberg RW, Almenoff PL, et al. Hyper-glycemia-related mortality in critically ill patients varies with admission diagnosis. Crit Care Med 2009;37(12):3001–9.

35. Frank JA, Nuckton TJ, Matthay MA. Diabetes melli-tus: a negative predictor for the development of acute respiratory distress syndrome from septic shock. Crit Care Med 2000;28(7):2645–6.

36. Kar P, Jones KL, Horowitz M, et al. Management of critically ill patients with type 2 diabetes: the need for personalised therapy. World J Diabetes 2015; 6(5):693–706.

37. Christiansen C, Johansen M, Christensen S, et al. Preadmission metformin use and mortality among intensive care patients with diabetes: a cohort study. Crit Care 2013;17(5):R192.

38. Tsoyi K, Jang HJ, Nizamutdinova IT, et al. Metformin inhibits HMGB1 release in LPS-treated RAW 264.7 cells and increases survival rate of endotoxaemic mice. Br J Pharmacol 2011;162(7):1498–508.

39. Zmijewski JW, Lorne E, Zhao X, et al. Mitochondrial respiratory complex I regulates neutrophil activation and severity of lung injury. Am J Respir Crit Care Med 2008;178(2):168–79.

40. Duncan AI, Koch CG, Xu M, et al. Recent metformin ingestion does not increase in-hospital morbidity or mortality after cardiac surgery. Anesth Analg 2007; 104(1):42–50.

41. American Diabetes Association. Standards of medi-cal care in diabetes–2013. Diabetes Care 2013; 36(Suppl 1):S11–66.

42. Ansari G, Mojtahedzadeh M, Kajbaf F, et al. How does blood glucose control with metformin influence intensive insulin protocols? Evidence for involve-ment of oxidative stress and inflammatory cytokines. Adv Ther 2008;25(7):681–702.

43. Gribble FM, Ashcroft FM. Sulfonylurea sensitivity of adenosine triphosphate-sensitive potassium chan-nels from beta cells and extrapancreatic tissues. Metabolism 2000;49(10 Suppl 2):3–6.

44. Landry DW, Oliver JA. The pathogenesis of vasodi-latory shock. N Engl J Med 2001;345(8):588–95.

45. Gardiner SM, Kemp PA, March JE, et al. Regional haemodynamic responses to infusion of lipopoly-saccharide in conscious rats: effects of pre- or post-treatment with glibenclamide. Br J Pharmacol 1999;128(8):1772–8.

46. Vanelli G, Hussain SN, Aguggini G. Glibenclamide, a blocker of ATP-sensitive potassium channels, re-verses endotoxin-induced hypotension in pig. Exp Physiol 1995;80(1):167–70.

47. Vanelli G, Hussain SN, Dimori M, et al. Cardiovascular responses to glibenclamide during endotoxaemia in the pig. Vet Res Commun 1997;21(3):187–200.

48. Warrillow S, Egi M, Bellomo R. Randomized, double-blind, placebo-controlled crossover pilot study of a potassium channel blocker in patients with septic shock. Crit Care Med 2006;34(4):980–5.

49. International Expert Committee. International Expert Committee report on the role of the A1C assay in the diagnosis of diabetes. Diabetes Care 2009;32(7): 1327–34.

50. van den Berghe G, Wouters P, Weekers F, et al. Intensive insulin therapy in critically ill patients. N Engl J Med 2001;345(19):1359–67.

51. COIITSS Study Investigators, Annane D, Cariou A, et al. Corticosteroid treatment and intensive insulin therapy for septic shock in adults: a randomized controlled trial. JAMA 2010;303(4):341–8.

52. NICE-SUGAR Study Investigators, Finfer S, Liu B, et al. Hypoglycemia and risk of death in critically ill patients. N Engl J Med 2012;367(12):1108–18.

53. Egi M, Bellomo R, Stachowski E, et al. Hypoglyce-mia and outcome in critically ill patients. Mayo Clin Proc 2010;85(3):217–24.

54. Krinsley JS, Schultz MJ, Spronk PE, et al. Mild hypoglycemia is independently associated with

increased mortality in the critically ill. Crit Care 2011; 15(4):R173.

5. Duning T, van den Heuvel I, Dickmann A, et al. Hypoglycemia aggravates critical illness-induced neurocognitive dysfunction. Diabetes Care 2010;33(3): 639–44.

6. Deane AM, Horowitz M. Dysglycaemia in the critically ill - significance and management. Diabetes Obes Metab 2013;15(9):792–801.

7. Mackenzie IM, Whitehouse T, Nightingale PG. The metrics of glycaemic control in critical care. Intensive Care Med 2011;37(3):435–43.

8. Krinsley JS. Glycemic variability and mortality in critically ill patients: the impact of diabetes. J Diabetes Sci Technol 2009;3(6):1292–301.

9. Lanspa MJ, Dickerson J, Morris AH, et al. Coefficient of glucose variation is independently associated with mortality in critically ill patients receiving intravenous insulin. Crit Care 2014;18(2):R86.

50. Quagliaro L, Piconi L, Assaloni R, et al. Intermittent high glucose enhances apoptosis related to oxidative stress in human umbilical vein endothelial cells: the role of protein kinase C and NAD(P)H-oxidase activation. Diabetes 2003;52(11):2795–804.

51. Ceriello A, Esposito K, Piconi L, et al. Oscillating glucose is more deleterious to endothelial function and oxidative stress than mean glucose in normal and type 2 diabetic patients. Diabetes 2008;57(5): 1349–54.

62. Finfer S. Clinical controversies in the management of critically ill patients with severe sepsis: resuscitation fluids and glucose control. Virulence 2014;5(1):200–5.

63. Bellomo R, Egi M. Glycemic control in the intensive care unit: why we should wait for NICE-SUGAR. Mayo Clin Proc 2005;80(12):1546–8.

64. Devos P, Preiser JC. Tight blood glucose control: a recommendation applicable to any critically ill patient? Crit Care 2004;8(6):427–9.

65. Van den Berghe G, Wilmer A, Hermans G, et al. Intensive insulin therapy in the medical ICU. N Engl J Med 2006;354(5):449–61.

66. Meyfroidt G, Keenan DM, Wang X, et al. Dynamic characteristics of blood glucose time series during the course of critical illness: effects of intensive insulin therapy and relative association with mortality. Crit Care Med 2010;38(4):1021–9.

67. NICE-SUGAR Study Investigators, Finfer S, Chittock DR, et al. Intensive versus conventional glucose control in critically ill patients. N Engl J Med 2009;360(13):1283–97.

68. Arabi YM, Dabbagh OC, Tamim HM, et al. Intensive versus conventional insulin therapy: a randomized controlled trial in medical and surgical critically ill patients. Crit Care Med 2008;36(12):3190–7.

69. De La Rosa Gdel C, Donado JH, Restrepo AH, et al. Strict glycaemic control in patients hospitalised in a mixed medical and surgical intensive care unit: a randomised clinical trial. Crit Care 2008;12(5):R120.

70. Preiser JC, Devos P, Ruiz-Santana S, et al. A prospective randomised multi-centre controlled trial on tight glucose control by intensive insulin therapy in adult intensive care units: the Glucontrol study. Intensive Care Med 2009;35(10):1738–48.

71. Dellinger RP, Levy MM, Rhodes A, et al. Surviving sepsis campaign: international guidelines for management of severe sepsis and septic shock: 2012. Crit Care Med 2013;41(2):580–637.

72. Ellger B, Westphal M, Stubbe HD, et al. Glycemic control in sepsis and septic shock: friend or foe? Anaesthesist 2008;57(1):43–8 [in German].

73. Iapichino G, Albicini M, Umbrello M, et al. Tight glycemic control does not affect asymmetric-dimethylarginine in septic patients. Intensive Care Med 2008;34(10):1843–50.

74. Savioli M, Cugno M, Polli F, et al. Tight glycemic control may favor fibrinolysis in patients with sepsis. Crit Care Med 2009;37(2):424–31.

# Metabolism, Metabolomics, and Nutritional Support of Patients with Sepsis

Joshua A. Englert, MD[a], Angela J. Rogers, MD, MPH[b],*

## KEYWORDS

- Sepsis • Metabolism • Metabolomics • Nutrition • ICU outcomes • Biomarker

## KEY POINTS

- Sepsis is characterized by profound metabolic derangements.
- Metabolic changes can serve as diagnostic and prognostic biomarkers for patients with sepsis. Lactate is already in widespread clinical use, but technological advances make broader metabolic profiling possible.
- Many large-scale clinical trials have been conducted to optimize nutrition in septic patients. Most failed to show a benefit to early full feeding or supplementation with specific nutrients or metabolites in patients with normal nutritional status at presentation.

## INTRODUCTION

Metabolism, derived from the Greek word "to change," refers to all chemical reactions required by cells. In the healthy state, human metabolism is characterized by synchronized catabolic and anabolic processes that not only allow cells to maintain homeostasis but also respond to their microenvironment. The main source of cellular energy is ATP from aerobic metabolism and nutritional needs are largely met through nutrient intake, not catabolism of endogenous lipid and protein stores.

This state of metabolic homeostasis is massively disrupted in sepsis. Sepsis is a syndrome characterized by a dysregulated inflammatory response leading to organ damage in following a microbial infection. Sepsis is associated with an overall catabolic state leading to the breakdown of carbohydrates, lipid, and protein stores.[1] Despite increased nutritional requirements, patients with sepsis are often unwilling (because of anorexia) or unable (because of encephalopathy, respiratory failure requiring mechanical ventilation, and so forth) to eat, which can lead to a large energy deficit and worse outcomes in critically ill patients.[2] This deficit, in turn, leads to profound skeletal muscle wasting and prolonged recovery.[3]

In this review, the authors highlight metabolic changes that occur in sepsis, including both the systemic and cellular alterations that lead to the dysregulation of normal human metabolism. The authors then review the use of metabolic changes as biomarkers for disease severity, with a focus first on lactate, the most widely used intensive care unit (ICU) biomarker, and then a broader discussion of metabolomics in general. Finally, given the marked changes in metabolism in sepsis and the association of worse short- and long-term prognosis in patients with severe metabolic derangements, the authors review the seminal trials conducted to optimize nutrition in the ICU.

[a] Division of Pulmonary, Allergy, Critical Care, and Sleep Medicine, The Ohio State University Wexner Medical Center, 473 West 12th Avenue, Columbus, OH 43210, USA; [b] Division of Pulmonary and Critical Care Medicine, Stanford University, 300 Pasteur Drive, H3143, Stanford, CA 94305-5236, USA
* Corresponding author.
E-mail address: ajrogers@stanford.edu

Clin Chest Med 37 (2016) 321–331
http://dx.doi.org/10.1016/j.ccm.2016.01.011
0272-5231/16/$ – see front matter © 2016 Elsevier Inc. All rights reserved.

## METABOLIC CHANGES IN SEPSIS
### Mediators of Altered Metabolism in Sepsis

The metabolic changes associated with sepsis are complex, with many of the key features highlighted in **Table 1**. Many of these metabolic derangements are mediated by changes in the endocrine and autonomic nervous systems. The activation of these two systems occurs simultaneously and, in general, increases energy consumption. Of note, neuroendocrine activation in sepsis is dynamic and can change frequently throughout a patient's course.

### Altered endocrine physiology
Acute illness, including sepsis, typically leads to activation of the hypothalamic-pituitary-adrenal (HPA) axis and increased cortisol release.[4] Increased circulating corticosteroid levels act to preserve vascular tone and reactivity in order to maintain perfusion of vital organs.[5] Although the normal response to stress is to increase adrenal corticosteroid secretion, there are many different factors that can lead to the impairment of adrenal function in septic patients. High levels of circulating cytokines can directly impair adrenal corticosteroid production,[6] and the use of medications that can impair adrenal function is common in septic patients.[5]

Although absolute adrenal insufficiency is rare in patients with sepsis, there has been substantial controversy surrounding the use of adjunctive corticosteroids to treat relative adrenal insufficiency in patients with septic shock. A randomized, multicenter, placebo-controlled trial of hydrocortisone in patients with septic shock did not decrease 28-day mortality regardless of whether an adrenocorticotropin hormone stimulation test was positive.[7] Patients treated with hydrocortisone did have a more rapid resolution of shock but also had an increased incidence of new infection.[7] In light of these results, debate persists among experts regarding the use of corticosteroids in sepsis and septic shock. In addition to the changes in the HPA axis with sepsis, altered function of other endocrine organs, such as the thyroid, can also lead to hormonal changes that alter metabolism.[8]

### Activation of the adrenergic nervous system
Activation of the adrenergic nervous system in septic patients leads to the release of endogenous catecholamines; in addition, patients with septic shock frequently require the administration of exogenous catecholamines for blood pressure support. The release or administration of epinephrine, norepinephrine, and dopamine can have profound effects on metabolism that increase catabolism of most macronutrients.[9] One of the main effects of catecholamine release is to increase the production of glucose by increasing hepatic glycogenolysis and gluconeogenesis.[10] Furthermore, the insulin resistance that occurs in sepsis is mediated, at least in part, by activation of the adrenergic system.[11] In addition to the effects of catecholamines on metabolic regulation, they also can affect immune function. Immune cells express adrenergic receptors[9] and catecholamines are known to affect cytokine production[12] and cell migration.[13] These effects have implications for the ability of patients to clear the inciting infection and return to a state of metabolic homeostasis.

### Metabolic effects of cytokine release
The inflammatory cytokines that mediate that pathogenesis of sepsis play a key role in the activation of the neuroendocrine system described earlier. In addition, these cytokines can also directly alter metabolism in septic patients. The role of cytokines in the pathogenesis of sepsis has been reviewed in detail by others.[14,15] Here the authors focus on the metabolic effects of some of the classic proinflammatory cytokines. Many years after its initial discovery, tumor necrosis factor alpha (TNFα) was reported to be the same substance as the hormone cachectin. Cachectin was initially described for its role in increasing catabolism by upregulating lipolysis in the setting of malignancy and chronic infection

**Table 1**
**Summary of major metabolic changes in sepsis**

| Physiologic Change in Sepsis | Metabolic Impact |
| --- | --- |
| ↑ Gluconeogenesis, glycolysis | Hyperglycemia |
| ↑ Protein catabolism | Altered circulating amino acids |
| ↑ Lipolysis | ↑ Triglycerides, ↓ lipoproteins |
| ↓ Micronutrients | ↑ Oxidative stress |
| ↑ Neuroendocrine activation | ↑ Catecholamines, ↑ counter-regulatory hormones |
| ↑ Cortisol | Hyperglycemia |
| ↑ Catecholamine release | ↑ Gluconeogenesis, ↑ glycolysis |
| ↑ Cytokine release | Hyperglycemia, insulin resistance |
| Impaired oxygen utilization | ↑ Reactive oxygen species |

before its description in the pathogenesis of shock and organ failure.[16] In experimental models, infusion of TNFα was also found to recapitulate the hyperglycemia and insulin resistance found in sepsis.[1]

TNFα is also a potent inducer of other cytokines that play a role in metabolism, such as interleukin-beta (IL-1β) and IL-6. Similar to TNFα, infusion of recombinant IL-1β is also able to induce a hypermetabolic state in preclinical models[17]; IL-6 seems to work synergistically with these other cytokines. Although there are extensive data regarding the key roles of these cytokines in the pathophysiology of sepsis, there have been more than 100 clinical trials in patients with sepsis targeted at these pathways that have failed to lead to the approval of novel therapies.[18] This failure is likely multifactorial because of the complex pathogenesis of sepsis, issues with some preclinical models, and substantial heterogeneity among septic patients.[18] It is also possible that an incomplete understanding of how cellular and systemic metabolism is altered in sepsis may be limiting progress in the development of novel therapeutics.

## Mechanisms of Altered Cellular Metabolism in Sepsis

It is well known that some patients with sepsis develop end organ failure despite appropriate therapy. Organ failure frequently develops in the later phases of sepsis following initial resuscitation, and the molecular mechanisms of multiorgan failure remain incompletely understood.[19] Given that sepsis is often accompanied by shock and lactic acidosis, it was initially thought that organ failure in sepsis was primarily due to tissue hypoxia from impaired oxygen delivery in the setting of increased microvascular permeability.[20]

Although this may be the case early in sepsis, in the later phases (that are characterized by organ failure), tissue oxygen delivery has been shown to be normal in animal models[21] and septic patients.[22,23] This finding led to the realization that sepsis is characterized by altered cellular metabolism and impaired oxygen utilization despite adequate oxygen delivery. This impairment in cellular respiration, termed *cytopathic hypoxia*, may be one of the mechanisms responsible for multiorgan failure in the setting of sepsis.[24] The concept of energetic dysfunction in sepsis was first proposed when abnormal swollen mitochondria were visualized in animal models of sepsis.[25] Since that time it has become clear that sepsis is characterized by impaired oxidative phosphorylation in multiple organs. This defect in the activity of the mitochondrial respiratory chain enzymes leads to a shift toward anaerobic ATP production and is accompanied by increased free radical generation.[26] In one small study, septic patients were found to have decreased tissue ATP and glutathione levels compared with nonseptic control subjects.[27] Interestingly, decreased tissue ATP levels were associated with worse outcomes in this group of patients.[27] Although it is known that cellular metabolism is altered in sepsis, a clear understanding of the exact metabolic derangements has been elusive because until recently the technology to simultaneously assess multiple metabolic pathways was not available.

## Macronutrients

The metabolism of all major types of macronutrients (carbohydrate, protein, and lipid) is dysregulated in sepsis. Hyperglycemia is one of the most common metabolic derangements in patients presenting with sepsis and results from altered glycogen metabolism and profound insulin resistance.[1,28] In late stages, sepsis can also be characterized by hypoglycemia due to multisystem organ failure. The molecular events leading to sepsis-induced hyperglycemia are complex and include the effects of inflammatory cytokines and alterations in the regulatory hormones that maintain normal glucose homeostasis, as discussed earlier.[28,29] Hyperglycemia impairs the function of innate immune system that further impairs the ability of the host to combat infection.[30] Given these effects, it is not surprising that hyperglycemia is an independent predictor of adverse outcomes in critically ill patients.[29,31]

In addition to abnormalities in carbohydrate metabolism, sepsis is also characterized by altered protein and lipid metabolism. Accelerated protein breakdown leads to a net negative nitrogen balance[1] that, in turn, leads to skeletal muscle wasting, deconditioning, and prolonged recovery for critically ill patients. In addition to generalized protein breakdown, sepsis is associated with altered concentrations of circulating amino acids.[32,33] In general, amino acids from the breakdown of peripheral tissues are shunted to the liver to support the synthesis of acute phase reactants.[1] One of the goals of supplemental nutrition in sepsis is to try to mitigate protein catabolism by providing adequate amino acids for protein synthesis, although controversy remains regarding the ideal strategy to prevent protein catabolism.

In addition to accelerated protein breakdown, sepsis is also characterized by increased lipolysis, as lipids are the primary source of energy in patients with infections.[1] Patients with sepsis have altered lipid metabolism characterized by increases in serum triglycerides and decreased levels circulating lipoproteins.[34] Furthermore, administration of certain antiinflammatory classes of lipid mediators has been shown to improve outcomes in patients with sepsis.[35]

## Micronutrients

In addition to changes in the metabolism of macronutrients, sepsis is also associated with changes in various micronutrients, including trace minerals and vitamins. Micronutrients play key roles in metabolism and cellular homeostasis, and evidence suggests that lower levels of micronutrients in critically ill patients are associated with a higher risk of death and multisystem organ failure.[36] Two of the most well-studied micronutrients in sepsis are selenium and zinc. Selenium is a trace mineral with antioxidant and anti-inflammatory properties that is deficient in patients with sepsis.[37] Low selenium levels are associated with poor outcomes in critically ill patients, and supplementation with selenium in critically ill patients has been shown to decrease mortality in some studies.[38,39] However, given methodological concerns with some of these studies, experts suggest additional studies are needed before the routine use of selenium can be recommended for septic patients.[40] Similarly, zinc is another essential micronutrient that plays a key role in cellular homeostasis, immune function, and response to stress.[41] Zinc deficiency increases mortality in preclinical models of sepsis,[42] and patients with sepsis have lower circulating zinc levels compared to nonseptic controls.[43] Although many agree that treatment with micronutrients may be beneficial in sepsis, controversy remains regarding patient selection, choice of specific micronutrients, and optimal dosing.[3,36]

## METABOLIC CHANGES AS BIOMARKERS IN SEPSIS
### Lactate: the Prototypical Biomarker for Sepsis Diagnosis and Prognosis

Human cells use ATP for energy. In the resting state, most glucose is metabolized through the aerobic pathway, with mitochondria processing pyruvate into carbon dioxide, water, and 38 ATP via the citric acid cycle. In times of stress, such as exercise or sepsis; however, high cellular ATP requirements coupled with mitochondrial dysfunction can outstrip the capacity of the cell for aerobic glycolysis, and the cell switches to less efficient anaerobic metabolism in which pyruvate is processed into 2 molecules of lactic acid and 2 ATP. This increase in lactate locally is a major reason for elevated plasma lactate levels, though additional mechanisms, including impaired lactate clearance in sepsis, may contribute.[44,45]

Lactic acid level is the most widely used biomarker used by clinicians caring for patients with severe sepsis today. The importance of lactic acid elevation has long been recognized.[46] Elevated lactate levels can occur because of impaired organ perfusion (type A lactic acidosis) or in the absence of tissue hypoperfusion (type B) due to malignancy, liver disease, or mitochondrial disorders. Despite this lack of specificity, an elevated lactate level has been validated in both sepsis diagnosis and prognosis; failure to normalize lactate during resuscitation is similarly associated with a poor prognosis. This evidence is discussed in further detail later.

### Lactate as a biomarker in the diagnosis of sepsis

Severe sepsis is part of the inflammatory cascade that occurs in the setting of infection, from systemic inflammatory response syndrome (SIRS) to sepsis, sepsis with organ hypoperfusion, and finally septic shock. Elevated lactate (most commonly ≥4 mmol/L, though upper limits of normal may vary for a given laboratory) is a marker of sepsis-induced hypoperfusion, even in the absence of frank septic shock.[47] This cutoff was used for entry into pivotal human sepsis trials, including the early goal-directed therapy (EGDT) protocol by Rivers and colleagues,[48] whose entry criteria included suspected infection with at least 2 SIRS criteria and either systolic blood pressure of 90 mm Hg or less or lactate of 4 mmol/L or greater. The same threshold was incorporated into the Surviving Sepsis Campaign guidelines for early identification of sepsis in 2008 with grade 1C evidence[26] and used as an entry criterion for the follow-up early goal-directed therapy ProCESS trial.[49]

### Lactate as a prognostic biomarker in sepsis

Not only does lactate serve as an important biomarker for the diagnosis of sepsis but it is also very clearly associated with increased risk for mortality in patients with sepsis, in both the ICU and emergency department setting.[50,51] Even a moderate elevation of lactate (range 2.1–≤4.0 mmol/L) has been associated with an increased risk of death in normotensive patients who present with sepsis.[52,53]

In addition to the importance of baseline lactate levels, the clearance of lactate during the first 6 hours of sepsis treatment is highly associated with mortality. For example, patients who fail to decrease their lactate level by at least 10% within this timeframe are twice as likely to die as those who reach that threshold.[54] Two randomized controlled trials (RCTs) have evaluated targeting lactate clearance as an end point in early sepsis resuscitation. A trial conducted by the EMShockNet Investigators showed a 17% mortality rate in subjects randomized to lactate clearance-guided resuscitation versus 23% in those randomized to central venous oxygen saturation–guided resuscitation, with the conclusion that this resuscitation goal was noninferior and led to very similar early fluid resuscitation.[55] Another RCT randomized patients to routine EGDT or to lactate measurement every 2 hours for the first 8 hours; although lactate clearance was not appreciably different between the 2 groups, the lactate group did receive more fluids, inotropes, and had a lower hospital mortality after adjustment for severity of illness.[56] Measurement of 6-hour lactate clearance was included in the 2012 Surviving Sepsis guidelines with grade 2C evidence.[47]

## Broader Metabolic Profiling in Sepsis

Although lactate is a highly useful biomarker for sepsis diagnosis and prognosis, it is highly nonspecific and often elevated in patients without sepsis (type B lactic acidosis). Given the myriad metabolic changes induced by sepsis, it makes sense that changes in many other metabolites in addition to lactate would occur.

Metabolomics, the study of chemical products (metabolites) used and produced by cellular metabolism, measures small molecules, including lipids, nucleotides, amino acids, carbohydrates, and even drug metabolites. Metabolomics is a rapidly growing field of study in genomics, in part because it represents the end of the genomic cascade, from single nucleotide polymorphism and methylation changes (many of which are present at birth) through gene expression, protein translation, and finally to metabolic changes. These last genomic markers (gene expression, protein translation, and metabolites) are dynamic and can change in response to environmental perturbations, making them particularly compelling as potential biomarkers in sepsis. The human plasma metabolome includes greater than 4000 metabolites identified to date; however, because the human metabolome is not complete, this is likely an underestimate.[57] Metabolic profiling was previously extremely technically difficult, limiting

exploration of the metabolic changes in sepsis beyond single-metabolite studies in small numbers of individuals. However, recent technological advances in liquid and gas chromatography and mass spectroscopy now allow high-resolution screening of the human metabolome.[58]

A full discussion of technical aspects of metabolic profiling and analysis is beyond the scope of this review, but can be found elsewhere.[59,60] Briefly, metabolic profiling is usually performed in a 2-step fashion: (1) a combination of gas and/or lipid chromatography is used to separate metabolites followed by (2) mass spectroscopy or nuclear magnetic resonance (NMR) mass spectroscopy for quantification. Untargeted metabolic profiling is designed to measure all metabolites in a given sample, whereas targeted profiling is designed to identify a fixed subset of metabolites of interest. Both methods have their strengths. The major advantage of untargeted profiling is the lack of bias and broader ability to discover novel, unanticipated metabolites; but limitations include the substantial time and cost required to definitively characterize newly identified metabolites and the lack of absolute quantification of metabolites. Even in untargeted profiling, resolution of metabolites based on hydrophilicity and size may vary depending on the strategy used, with greatest resolution across a part of the metabolite spectrum. Conversely, targeted metabolomic profiling identifies only a subset of metabolites (often on the order of 100–500); but use of internal calibration standards allows both absolute quantification and high confidence in the individual metabolites attained.

To date, several groups including the authors' own have performed broader metabolic profiling in sepsis to test whether incorporation of multiple metabolites could serve as prognostic indicators in sepsis. Plasma metabolomic changes associated with sepsis mortality published to date are summarized in **Table 2**. The studies vary dramatically in (1) sample size, (2) metabolites measured, and (3) modeling method used to differentiate survivors versus nonsurvivors. Given these varying methodologies in study design, coupled with high correlation among many metabolites, it is perhaps not surprising that the metabolites identified vary greatly across studies. Although settling on one particular metabolic network is, premature at this time, it is worth noting that all studies reveal profound metabolic derangements in sepsis, most (but by no means all) metabolites are upregulated; these changes extend far beyond the anaerobic metabolism/lactate cycle. Identifying the optimal network of metabolites, establishing the importance of these networks across varied populations with sepsis,

**Table 2**
Published metabolomic studies in sepsis

| Reference | No. of Cases/Controls[a] | Control Population | Metabolites Profiled | Analytical Strategy | Final Metabolites |
|---|---|---|---|---|---|
| Mickiewicz et al,[75] 2013 | 10/10 | Pediatric septic shock survivors | 58 | PCA & PLS | 11 Metabolites (not identified) |
| Langley et al,[76] 2013 | 31/119 33/67 25/65 | Surviving subjects with SIRS or sepsis | >300 | Support vector machine | Cis-4-decenoylcarnitine, 2-methylbutyroylcarnitine, butyroylcarnitine, hexanoylcarnitine, and lactate |
| Rogers et al,[77] 2014 | 30/60 115/34 | Surviving subjects with SIRS or sepsis | 167 | Bayesian Network | Sucrose, mannose, β-hydroxyisovalerate, methionine, and arginine |
| Mickiewicz et al,[78] 2014 | 4/4 | ICU survivors with sepsis | 60 | PLS | Network of 20 (not identified) |

Langley and colleagues[76] and Rogers and colleagues[77] analyses use highly overlapping datasets.

*Abbreviations:* PCA, principal components analysis; PLS, partial least squares.

[a] When multiple case/control populations are shown, these represent the total number for testing and replication populations in that work.

ind addressing whether incorporation of these net-works into critical illness severity models improves their performance in prospective cohorts are all needed to determine the clinical utility of metabolo-nics in sepsis.

Metabolomic profiling in sepsis is still in its infancy, and its diagnostic promise is not yet clear. Even such basic issues as type of body fluid to sample are still evolving. Although the studies summarized in **Table 2** have all focused on serum and plasma, Stringer and colleagues[61] recently suggested that whole-blood sampling may be a better target, as it also reflects endothelial cell metabolism and free hemoglobin level. Additional options include studying samples that reflect a particular organ function in sepsis, for example, urine in acute kidney injury or bronchoalveolar lavage fluid in septic patients with acute respira-tory distress syndrome (ARDS).

## NUTRITION IN PATIENTS WITH SEPSIS

As noted throughout this review, patients with severe sepsis and septic shock have profoundly altered metabolism, with a catabolic state leading to breakdown of both protein and lipids coupled with decreased production of new muscle mass. Critically ill patients have been shown to have a profound loss of muscle mass, a mean of 17% loss of femoral mass by day 10, worse among pa-tients with increased severity of illness.[62] Patients who develop critical illness neuropathy are known

to have both increased ICU length of stay and increased ICU mortality.[63]

Given these substantial metabolic changes in sepsis, the potential to reduce these effects through nutritional therapy has been studied extensively. Major topics include timing, route, rate of nutrition, and the nutrient composition to optimize sepsis survival. The authors highlight the strongest evidence for each of these issues later and in **Table 3**. Although many of these studies are not restricted to only patients with sepsis, most of them include critically ill patients who have sepsis as their primary or secondary ICU risk factor. For further reading on this evidence, several excellent reviews of ICU nutri-tion have been written previously.[64,65]

### Timing of Nutrition

Most critically ill patients are unable to take in adequate oral nutrition, particularly early in the course of critical illness. Although several meta-analyses have suggested a mortality benefit to early feeding within the first 48 hours in critically ill patients,[66] methodological concerns about high potential for bias in the small trials included in these meta-analyses limit their usefulness.

Several recent large, high-quality RCTs are highly relevant. The EDEN trial focused on patients with the ARDS; most of these patients had under-lying sepsis (>70% with either sepsis or pneu-monia as their ARDS risk factor). Patients were

**Table 3**
**Highlighted articles in intensive care unit nutrition**

| Trial (Ref) | Treatment Groups | Population (% Sepsis) | Primary Outcome |
|---|---|---|---|
| EDEN[68] | Trophic vs full feeds in first 6 d | ARDS (>70%) | No change in vent time, infections, 60-d mortality, 1-y physical function |
| Early PN[70] | Early PN vs standard care | ICU patients with short-term contraindication to EN (6%) | No difference in mortality, early PN had fewer vent days |
| EPaNIC[69] | Early PN vs delayed to day 8 | ICU patients at nutritional risk (22%) | Late PN: 6% more likely to be discharged alive from ICU & hospital, fewer infections |
| SPN[71] | PN or EN if not meeting caloric need by day 3 | ICU patients not meeting nutritional needs by day 3 (~45%) | No change in ICU stay or 60-d mortality, but ↓ vent days |
| REDOXS[72] | Glutamine or antioxidants | ICU patients with 2 or more organ failures (~30%) | ↑ In-hospital & 6-mo mortality in glutamine group; no effect with antioxidants |
| SIGNET[73] | Glutamine or selenium | ICU needing at least 50% of calories via PN (~60%) | No change in mortality or infection rate in all patients |
| OMEGA[74] | Omega-3 fatty acids | ARDS (75% sepsis or pneumonia) | ↓ Vent-free and ICU days, trend toward ↑ 60-d mortality |

enteral nutrition; PN, parental nutrition.

randomized within 48 hours of mechanical ventilation to either trophic or full enteral feeds for the first 6 days. Despite a marked difference in calories (400 vs 1300), there was no difference in duration of mechanical ventilation, infectious complications, or 60-day mortality in the two groups. Patients followed for up to 1 year after discharge also demonstrated no difference in physical or cognitive function based on nutrition strategy.[67] These data suggest that delay of full nutrition up to 6 days is likely safe in patients without baseline malnutrition (who were excluded from these trials).[68]

### Enteral Versus Parenteral Nutrition

Enteral feeding is the accepted first choice for nutrition in critically ill patients who can tolerate it, given consistent evidence of improved outcomes, including fewer infections and improved gut integrity.[65] However, a large proportion of critically ill patients have relative contraindications to enteral feeding and fail to meet their caloric needs in the early days of ICU care. Thus, several large RCTs have been conducted to address the timing of initiation of parental nutrition (PN) in high-risk ICU patients.

The EPaNIC trial randomized 4640 critically ill subjects at high risk for malnutrition to receive either early PN (glucose $\times$ 48 hours then full-caloric PN) or a late-initiation group that did not receive PN until day 8. The late-initiation strategy was associated with faster recovery (6% increased likelihood of discharge alive from ICU and hospital) and fewer ICU infections.[69] The Early PN Trial randomized 1372 with short-term contraindications to enteral feeding to receive either early PN versus pragmatic standard care (of the latter group, 29% commenced enteral nutrition, 27% parenteral, and 40% unfed). The early PN strategy led to no difference in 60-day mortality but fewer days of mechanical ventilation.[70] Finally, the SPN trial randomized 305 critically ill patients who were reaching less than 60% of nutrition targets by day 3 to receive either PN or enteral nutrition. They found substantially lower rates of infection in the PN group (the primary outcome).[71] Cumulatively, these trials suggest that PN and full nutrition can be delayed for at least 7 days in most critically ill patients with normal nutritional status at presentation and that any advantages to early PN initiation are likely modest.

### Role of Macronutrient and Micronutrient Replacement

Sepsis is characterized by marked systemic inflammation, with increased production of reactive oxygen species and a depletion of antioxidant nutrients associated with increased mortality, as discussed earlier.[27] Not surprisingly, numerous trials of therapeutic administration of macronutrients and antioxidants have been performed in an attempt to improve sepsis mortality. Although many small RCTs and subsequent meta-analyses have shown encouraging trends toward improved sepsis mortality,[39] this has not borne out in larger RCTs to date, which are summarized in **Table 3**.

Low glutamine levels are associated with worse prognosis in critical illness; it has, thus, been the subject of several large RCTs. The REDOXS trial randomized 1223 critically ill patients to receive glutamine, antioxidants (including selenium, zinc, vitamins C, E, and β carotene), both, or placebo. The groups that received glutamine had higher in-hospital and 6-month mortality, whereas antioxidants had no effect.[72] The SIGNET trial randomized 500 subjects to a lower dose of glutamine (approximately one-third the dose in REDOXS) and identified no difference in mortality or new infections in all patients randomized.[73]

The ARDS Network OMEGA trial randomized 272 patients with ARDS (75% with sepsis or pneumonia as their ARDS risk factor) to receive omega-3 fatty acids, which favor production of less active prostaglandins and leukotrienes. The trial was stopped early for futility, with patients receiving supplements having fewer ventilator-free and ICU free days and a trend toward higher 60-day hospital mortality.[74] Although multiple studies have identified deficiencies of specific nutrients/metabolites in septic patients, there are currently no data to support the use of replacement therapy in sepsis.

### SUMMARY

In summary, sepsis is characterized by profound metabolic changes. Some of these metabolic changes contribute to sepsis pathophysiology, and others (eg, high lactate, hyperglycemia, low selenium and zinc) are recognized markers of ICU outcomes. Given these profound metabolic changes, numerous large-scale trials have been designed to optimize nutrition in the ICU, though most have failed to show that nutrition strategies improve outcomes for septic patients, at least early in the ICU course of patients with adequate baseline nutrition.

Finally, technical advances in metabolomic profiling have enabled cheaper, high-resolution testing than was previously available. The option to simultaneously examine multiple metabolic pathways in large populations is now more feasible and will likely allow a more nuanced picture of the metabolic changes that occur in sepsis. As these data emerge in the coming years, developing a more individualized approach to metabolism and nutrition in septic patients may become possible.

## REFERENCES

1. Michie HR. Metabolism of sepsis and multiple organ failure. World J Surg 1996;20(4):460–4.
2. Alberda C, Gramlich L, Jones N, et al. The relationship between nutritional intake and clinical outcomes in critically ill patients: results of an international multicenter observational study. Intensive Care Med 2009;35(10):1728–37.
3. Casaer MP, Van den Berghe G. Nutrition in the acute phase of critical illness. N Engl J Med 2014;370(25): 2450–1.
4. Khardori R, Castillo D. Endocrine and metabolic changes during sepsis: an update. Med Clin North Am 2012;96(6):1095–105.
5. Cooper MS, Stewart PM. Corticosteroid insufficiency in acutely ill patients. N Engl J Med 2003;348(8): 727–34.
6. Catalano RD, Parameswaran V, Ramachandran J, et al. Mechanisms of adrenocortical depression during Escherichia coli shock. Arch Surg 1984;119(2): 145–50.
7. Sprung CL, Annane D, Keh D, et al. Hydrocortisone therapy for patients with septic shock. N Engl J Med 2008;358(2):111–24.
8. Meyer S, Schuetz P, Wieland M, et al. Low triiodothyronine syndrome: a prognostic marker for outcome in sepsis? Endocrine 2011;39(2):167–74.
9. Norbury WB, Jeschke MG, Herndon DN. Metabolism modulators in sepsis: propranolol. Crit Care Med 2007;35(9 Suppl):S616–20.
10. Chu CA, Sindelar DK, Igawa K, et al. The direct effects of catecholamines on hepatic glucose production occur via alpha(1)- and beta(2)-receptors in the dog. Am J Physiol Endocrinol Metab 2000;279(2):E463–73.
11. Lang CH. Sepsis-induced insulin resistance in rats is mediated by a beta-adrenergic mechanism. Am J Physiol 1992;263(4 Pt 1):E703–11.
12. Elenkov IJ, Wilder RL, Chrousos GP, et al. The sympathetic nerve–an integrative interface between two supersystems: the brain and the immune system. Pharmacol Rev 2000;52(4):595–638.
13. Oberbeck R. Therapeutic implications of immune-endocrine interactions in the critically ill patients. Curr Drug Targets Immune Endocr Metabol Disord 2004;4(2):129–39.
14. Blackwell TS, Christman JW. Sepsis and cytokines: current status. Br J Anaesth 1996;77(1):110–7.
15. Rittirsch D, Flierl MA, Ward PA. Harmful molecular mechanisms in sepsis. Nat Rev Immunol 2008; 8(10):776–87.
16. Tracey KJ, Beutler B, Lowry SF, et al. Shock and tissue injury induced by recombinant human cachectin. Science 1986;234(4775):470–4.
17. Molloy RG, Mannick JA, Rodrick ML. Cytokines, sepsis and immunomodulation. Br J Surg 1993; 80(3):289–97.
18. Marshall JC. Why have clinical trials in sepsis failed? Trends Mol Med 2014;20(4):195–203.
19. Englert JA, Fink MP. The multiple organ dysfunction syndrome and late-phase mortality in sepsis. Curr Infect Dis Rep 2005;7(5):335–41.
20. Brealey D, Singer M. Mitochondrial dysfunction in sepsis. Curr Infect Dis Rep 2003;5(5):365–71.
21. VanderMeer TJ, Wang H, Fink MP. Endotoxemia causes ileal mucosal acidosis in the absence of mucosal hypoxia in a normodynamic porcine model of septic shock. Crit Care Med 1995;23(7):1217–26.
22. Boekstegers P, Weidenhofer S, Pilz G, et al. Peripheral oxygen availability within skeletal muscle in sepsis and septic shock: comparison to limited infection and cardiogenic shock. Infection 1991; 19(5):317–23.
23. Sair M, Etherington PJ, Peter Winlove C, et al. Tissue oxygenation and perfusion in patients with systemic sepsis. Crit Care Med 2001;29(7):1343–9.
24. Fink MP. Bench-to-bedside review: cytopathic hypoxia. Crit Care 2002;6(6):491–9.
25. Levy E, Slusser RJ, Ruebner BH. Hepatic changes produced by a single dose of endotoxin in the mouse. Electron microscopy. Am J Pathol 1968; 52(2):477–502.
26. Trager K, DeBacker D, Radermacher P. Metabolic alterations in sepsis and vasoactive drug-related metabolic effects. Curr Opin Crit Care 2003;9(4): 271–8.
27. Brealey D, Brand M, Hargreaves I, et al. Association between mitochondrial dysfunction and severity and outcome of septic shock. Lancet 2002;360(9328): 219–23.
28. Marik PE, Raghavan M. Stress-hyperglycemia, insulin and immunomodulation in sepsis. Intensive Care Med 2004;30(5):748–56.
29. Hirasawa H, Oda S, Nakamura M. Blood glucose control in patients with severe sepsis and septic shock. World J Gastroenterol 2009;15(33):4132–6.
30. Turina M, Fry DE, Polk HC Jr. Acute hyperglycemia and the innate immune system: clinical, cellular, and molecular aspects. Crit Care Med 2005;33(7):1624–33.
31. Taylor JH, Beilman GJ. Hyperglycemia in the intensive care unit: no longer just a marker of illness severity. Surg Infect (Larchmt) 2005;6(2):233–45.
32. Druml W, Heinzel G, Kleinberger G. Amino acid kinetics in patients with sepsis. Am J Clin Nutr 2001;73(5):908–13.
33. Su L, Li H, Xie A, et al. Dynamic changes in amino acid concentration profiles in patients with sepsis. PLoS One 2015;10(4):e0121933.

34. Wendel M, Paul R, Heller AR. Lipoproteins in inflammation and sepsis. II. Clinical aspects. Intensive Care Med 2007;33(1):25–35.

35. Pontes-Arruda A, Martins LF, de Lima SM, et al. Enteral nutrition with eicosapentaenoic acid, gamma-linolenic acid and antioxidants in the early treatment of sepsis: results from a multicenter, prospective, randomized, double-blinded, controlled study: the INTERSEPT study. Crit Care 2011;15(3):R144.

36. Manzanares W, Langlois PL, Hardy G. Update on antioxidant micronutrients in the critically ill. Curr Opin Clin Nutr Metab Care 2013;16(6):719–25.

37. Forceville X, Vitoux D, Gauzit R, et al. Selenium, systemic immune response syndrome, sepsis, and outcome in critically ill patients. Crit Care Med 1998;26(9):1536–44.

38. Angstwurm MW, Engelmann L, Zimmermann T, et al. Selenium in intensive care (SIC): results of a prospective randomized, placebo-controlled, multiple-center study in patients with severe systemic inflammatory response syndrome, sepsis, and septic shock. Crit Care Med 2007;35(1):118–26.

39. Manzanares W, Dhaliwal R, Jiang X, et al. Antioxidant micronutrients in the critically ill: a systematic review and meta-analysis. Crit Care 2012;16(2):R66.

40. Allingstrup M, Afshari A. Selenium supplementation for critically ill adults. Cochrane Database Syst Rev 2015;(7):CD003703.

41. Haase H, Rink L. Functional significance of zinc-related signaling pathways in immune cells. Annu Rev Nutr 2009;29:133–52.

42. Knoell DL, Julian MW, Bao S, et al. Zinc deficiency increases organ damage and mortality in a murine model of polymicrobial sepsis. Crit Care Med 2009;37(4):1380–8.

43. Besecker BY, Exline MC, Hollyfield J, et al. A comparison of zinc metabolism, inflammation, and disease severity in critically ill infected and noninfected adults early after intensive care unit admission. Am J Clin Nutr 2011;93(6):1356–64.

44. Jansen TC, van Bommel J, Bakker J. Blood lactate monitoring in critically ill patients: a systematic health technology assessment. Crit Care Med 2009;37(10):2827–39.

45. Levraut J, Ciebiera JP, Chave S, et al. Mild hyperlactatemia in stable septic patients is due to impaired lactate clearance rather than overproduction. Am J Respir Crit Care Med 1998;157(4 Pt 1):1021–6.

46. Cohen RD, Woods HF. Clinical and biochemical aspects of lactic acidosis. Oxford: Blackwell Scientific Publications; 1976.

47. Dellinger RP, Levy MM, Rhodes A, et al. Surviving sepsis campaign: international guidelines for management of severe sepsis and septic shock: 2012. Crit Care Med 2013;41(2):580–637.

48. Rivers E, Nguyen B, Havstad S, et al. Early goal-directed therapy in the treatment of severe sepsis and septic shock. N Engl J Med 2001;345(19):1368–77.

49. Angus DC, Yealy DM, Kellum JA, et al. Protocol-based care for early septic shock. N Engl J Med 2014;371(4):386.

50. Aduen J, Bernstein WK, Khastgir T, et al. The use and clinical importance of a substrate-specific electrode for rapid determination of blood lactate concentrations. JAMA 1994;272(21):1678–85.

51. Shapiro NI, Howell MD, Talmor D, et al. Serum lactate as a predictor of mortality in emergency department patients with infection. Ann Emerg Med 2005;45(5):524–8.

52. Mikkelsen ME, Miltiades AN, Gaieski DF, et al. Serum lactate is associated with mortality in severe sepsis independent of organ failure and shock. Crit Care Med 2009;37(5):1670–7.

53. Howell MD, Donnino M, Clardy P, et al. Occult hypoperfusion and mortality in patients with suspected infection. Intensive Care Med 2007;33(11):1892–9.

54. Nguyen HB, Rivers EP, Knoblich BP, et al. Early lactate clearance is associated with improved outcome in severe sepsis and septic shock. Crit Care Med 2004;32(8):1637–42.

55. Jones AE, Shapiro NI, Trzeciak S, et al. Lactate clearance vs central venous oxygen saturation as goals of early sepsis therapy: a randomized clinical trial. JAMA 2010;303(8):739–46.

56. Jansen TC, van Bommel J, Schoonderbeek FJ, et al. Early lactate-guided therapy in intensive care unit patients: a multicenter, open-label, randomized controlled trial. Am J Respir Crit Care Med 2010;182(6):752–61.

57. Wishart DS, Jewison T, Guo AC, et al. HMDB 3.0–the human metabolome database in 2013. Nucleic Acids Res 2013;41(Database issue):D801–7.

58. Dettmer K, Aronov PA, Hammock BD. Mass spectrometry-based metabolomics. Mass Spectrom Rev 2007;26(1):51–78.

59. Dunn WB, Ellis DI. Metabolomics: current analytical platforms and methodologies. Trends Analyt Chem 2005;24(4):285–94.

60. Korman A, Oh A, Raskind A, et al. Statistical methods in metabolomics. In: Anisimova M, editor. Evolutionary genomics, 856. New York: Humana Press; 2012. p. 381–413.

61. Stringer KA, Younger JG, McHugh C, et al. Whole blood reveals more metabolic detail of the human metabolome than serum as measured by 1H-NMR spectroscopy: implications for sepsis metabolomics. Shock 2015;44(3):200–8.

62. Puthucheary ZA, Rawal J, McPhail M, et al. Acute skeletal muscle wasting in critical illness. JAMA 2013;310(15):1591–600.

63. Garnacho-Montero J, Madrazo-Osuna J, Garcia-Garmendia JL, et al. Critical illness polyneuropathy: risk factors and clinical consequences. A cohort

study in septic patients. Intensive Care Med 2001; 27(8):1288–96.

64. Casaer MP, van den Berghe G. Nutrition in the acute phase of critical illness. N Engl J Med 2014;370(13): 1227–36.

65. Martindale RG, McClave SA, Vanek VW, et al. Guidelines for the provision and assessment of nutrition support therapy in the adult critically ill patient: Society of Critical Care Medicine and American Society for Parenteral and Enteral Nutrition: executive summary. Crit Care Med 2009;37(5):1757–61.

66. Doig GS, Heighes PT, Simpson F, et al. Early enteral nutrition, provided within 24 h of injury or intensive care unit admission, significantly reduces mortality in critically ill patients: a meta-analysis of randomised controlled trials. Intensive Care Med 2009; 35(12):2018–27.

67. Needham DM, Dinglas VD, Bienvenu OJ, et al. One year outcomes in patients with acute lung injury randomised to initial trophic or full enteral feeding: prospective follow-up of EDEN randomised trial. BMJ 2013;346:f1532.

68. National Heart Lung and Blood Institute Acute Respiratory Distress Syndrome Clinical Trials Network, Rice TW, Wheeler AP, et al. Initial trophic vs full enteral feeding in patients with acute lung injury: the EDEN randomized trial. JAMA 2012; 307(8):795–803.

69. Casaer MP, Mesotten D, Hermans G, et al. Early versus late parenteral nutrition in critically ill adults. N Engl J Med 2011;365(6):506–17.

70. Doig GS, Simpson F, Sweetman EA, et al. Early parenteral nutrition in critically ill patients with short-term relative contraindications to early enteral nutrition: a randomized controlled trial. JAMA 2013; 309(20):2130–8.

71. Heidegger CP, Berger MM, Graf S, et al. Optimisation of energy provision with supplemental parenteral nutrition in critically ill patients: a randomised controlled clinical trial. Lancet 2013;381(9864):385–93.

72. Heyland D, Muscedere J, Wischmeyer PE, et al. A randomized trial of glutamine and antioxidants in critically ill patients. N Engl J Med 2013;368(16): 1489–97

73. Andrews PJ, Avenell A, Noble DW, et al. Randomised trial of glutamine, selenium, or both, to supplement parenteral nutrition for critically ill patients. BMJ 2011;342:d1542.

74. Rice TW, Wheeler AP, Thompson BT, et al. Enteral omega-3 fatty acid, gamma-linolenic acid, and antioxidant supplementation in acute lung injury. JAMA 2011;306(14):1574–81.

75. Mickiewicz B, Vogel HJ, Wong HR, et al. Metabolomics as a novel approach for early diagnosis of pediatric septic shock and its mortality. Am J Respir Crit Care Med 2013;187(9):967–76.

76. Langley RJ, Tsalik EL, Velkinburgh JC, et al. An integrated clinico-metabolomic model improves prediction of death in sepsis. Sci Transl Med 2013;5(195): 195ra95.

77. Rogers AJ, McGeachie M, Baron RM, et al. Metabolomic derangements are associated with mortality in critically ill adult patients. PLoS One 2014;9(1):e87538.

78. Mickiewicz B, Duggan GE, Winston BW, et al. Metabolic profiling of serum samples by 1H nuclear magnetic resonance spectroscopy as a potential diagnostic approach for septic shock. Crit Care Med 2014;42(5):1140–9.

# Neuroanatomy and Physiology of Brain Dysfunction in Sepsis

Aurelien Mazeraud[a,b,c], Quentin Pascal, DVM[a],
Franck Verdonk[a,b], Nicholas Heming, MD, PhD[c],
Fabrice Chrétien, MD, PhD[a,b,d], Tarek Sharshar, MD, PhD[a,c,e],*

## KEYWORDS

- Sepsis-associated encephalopathy • Sepsis • Neuroinflammation • Amygdala • Hippocampus
- Neuroanatomy

## KEY POINTS

- Sepsis-associated encephalopathy induces acute and long-term brain dysfunction.
- Its pathophysiology involves neuroinflammation, microcirculatory alterations, and excitotoxicity.
- Excitotoxicity might occur in specific areas and be involved in the increased mortality, psychological disorders, and cognitive impairment reported in septic patients.

## INTRODUCTION

Sepsis-associated encephalopathy (SAE), a major complication of sepsis, is characterized by impaired consciousness, including delirium and coma. Additionally SAE associates with changes in electroencephalogram (EEG) patterns.[1–3] Neuroimaging is usually unremarkable; white matter hyperintensities or some evidence of ischemic stroke may be seen.[4,5] SAE is associated with increased mortality[6] as well as long-term cognitive impairments,[7–10] including impaired memory, attention and verbal fluency difficulties,[7,8] and psychological disorders including depression,[8] anxiety, and posttraumatic stress disorders.[11–13] The pathophysiology of SAE remains unclear; 3 major processes seem to be involved, including diffuse neuroinflammation, circulatory dysfunction, and excitotoxicity. Whereas neuroinflammation and microcirculatory alterations are diffuse, pathologic examination of the brain of fatal cases of sepsis consistently exhibits increased apoptosis in specific structures (ie, the amygdala, *nucleus tractus solitarii* and *locus ceruleus*). These structures activate in response to stress and are especially sensitive to hypoxia, leading to excitotoxic processes, structural changes, and neurologic dysfunction.[14,15] Theses structural dysfunctions may be responsible for the clinical signs of sepsis-associated brain dysfunction. We review the clinical characteristics of SAE and present an overview of the current knowledge of its pathophysiology.

## CLINICAL PRESENTATION
### Acute Brain Response During Sepsis

The response of the central nervous system to sepsis is triggered by multiple peripheral

This work was supported by DIM Malinf PhD grant and funding by the Société de Réanimation de Langue Française.

[a] Institut Pasteur - Unité Histopathologie Humaine et Modèles Animaux, Département Infection et Épidémiologie, Rue du docteur roux, Paris 75724 Cedex 15, France; [b] Sorbonne Paris Cité, Paris Descartes University, Rue de l'école de médecine, Paris 75006, France; [c] General Intensive Care, Assistance Publique Hopitaux de Paris, Raymond Poincaré Teaching Hosptal, Garches 92380, France; [d] Laboratoire de Neuropathologie, Centre Hospitalier Sainte Anne, 1 rue cabanis, Paris 75014, France; [e] Versailles-Saint Quentin University, Avenue de Paris, Versailles 78000, France

* Corresponding author. Human Histopathology and Animal Models Unit, Infection and Epidemiology Department, Institut Pasteur, Rue du docteur roux, Paris 75724 Cedex 15, France.
*E-mail address:* tarek.sharshar@rpc.aphp.fr

Clin Chest Med 37 (2016) 333–345
http://dx.doi.org/10.1016/j.ccm.2016.01.013
0272-5231/16/$ – see front matter © 2016 Elsevier Inc. All rights reserved.

mediators involving complexly interconnected structures that control both the behavior and cognition, as well as the autonomic and neuroendocrine systems, which in turn drive the immune response.[16–20] This response may broadly be described as either adapted to the severity of sepsis or maladapted/pathologic.[21,22] Such a distinction supposes that the response of the central nervous system may either contribute to the recovery from or a worsening of sepsis. However, such a categorization is not based on well-established clinicobiological criteria. Before disruption of the blood–brain barrier (BBB), 2 distinct pathways are responsible of transmitting inflammatory signals to the brain, namely, the vagal nerve, which senses peripheral inflammatory mediators and transfers the information to the medullary autonomic nuclei,[23,24] and the circumventricular organs, which enables the passage of inflammatory mediators into the cerebral parenchyma.[25,26] The neural first centers to be activated through these neural pathways during sepsis are the *nucleus tractus solitarii* and *locus ceruleus*,[23,24] which are involved in the control of blood pressure, heart rate, and arousal. These neural centers then relay the signal to the other autonomic nuclei as well as the behavioral and neuroendocrine centers. Thus, behavioral changes, coined sickness behavior, are the earliest feature of sepsis.[15] Sickness behavior is characterized by decreased interaction with the environment (social withdrawal), impaired cognitive function (psychomotor retardation, impaired attention), and altered vigilance (anxiety, hypersomnia, fatigue, sleepiness), as well as eating disorders (anorexia, weight loss, thirst). Sickness behavior is partly a physiologic reaction to stress associated with reduced metabolic expenditure. Impaired attention or fluctuating vigilance found in SAE are similar to signs exhibited during hypoactive delirium.[27] Anxiety, which is regulated by the limbic system, may have deleterious effects when too intense. The exact significance and prognostic value of anxiety and behavioral changes in critically ill patients are currently being assessed in a prospective multicenter observational study (ClinicalTrials.gov, NCT02355626).

Sepsis may be associated with acute brain dysfunction, or encephalopathy, characterized by altered consciousness ranging from delirium to coma[6,28] and with focal deficits[5] or even seizures.[29] Delirium induced by sepsis is usually hypoactive, although the hyperactive subtype that is associated with agitation may also be observed.[27] In sedated critically ill patients, abolished brainstem reflexes may be a marker of brainstem dysfunction.[30] Acute brain dysfunction should routinely be identified using validated scales assessing the existence of delirium (ie, Intensive Care Delirium Screening Checklist or Confusion Assessment Method for the ICU),[31] coma (Glasgow Coma Scale), as well as brainstem reflexes in comatose patients (Full Outline of UnResponsiveness [FOUR] score).[32] A full medical history followed by clinical examination and routine blood chemistry are required to reject other causes of acute brain dysfunction including electrolyte disturbance, renal or liver dysfunction, drug side effects (notably antibiotic overdose), and alcohol or drug withdrawal. Cerebrospinal fluid should be obtained whenever meningitis is suspected (in the absence of contraindication) and vitamins $B_1$ and $B_6$ systematically given to alcoholic or malnourished patients.

## Neurophysiologic Tests and Neuroimaging Procedures

SAE may be associated with anomalous EEG patterns. Observed EEG patterns include slow waves, rhythmic delta or theta activity, triphasic waves or burst suppression, periodic epileptiform discharges, electrographic seizures, and absent reactivity.[1,2,5,29] The prevalence of these neurophysiologic patterns depend on the severity of encephalopathy,[1] the severity and the time course (ie, acute vs postacute phase) of sepsis, the type of patients (medical vs surgical), and the prior use of sedation.[1,29] A recent prospective study assessed 110 subjects monitored by standard EEG within 3 days of admission to the intensive care unit (ICU) for sepsis. Predominant theta rhythm was observed in 48%, low voltage in 65%, triphasic waves in 6%, periodic epileptiform discharges in 19%, electrographic seizure in 15%, and absence of reactivity in 25% of cases.[1] Electrographic seizures were associated with delirium at the time of recording, whereas a delta-predominant rhythm was associated with the subsequent occurrence of delirium. Continuous EEG makes the detection of periodic epileptiform discharges and electrographic seizure easier[29]; however, its routine use is not recommended.[2] Of note, none of the previously mentioned pattern is specific for sepsis. Several classifications grading EEG patterns have been described, including the classification of Synek and the classification of Young, which was specifically developed for septic patients.[1] EEG monitoring does not demonstrably impact the management or the outcome of septic associated brain dysfunction and is therefore not recommended in routine care. However, EEG monitoring in septic patients developing an acute brain dysfunction helps to define its severity and prognosis and can help physicians to rule out potentially treatable conditions (such as *status epilepticus*). EEG monitoring may also help to detect focal brain injuries; cerebral imaging is not always safely available in the critically ill.

Few studies undertook to document the result of cerebral imaging in septic patients. Using MRI, we showed that patients with septic shock who developed delirium, coma, seizures, or a focal deficit exhibited evidence of white matter hyperdensities (21%) or ischemic stroke (18%).[5] White matter hyperdensities may be associated with long-term cognitive impairment. Ischemic stroke is associated with coma, focal neurologic signs, and unfavorable outcomes. Although cerebral imaging is a promising field pertaining to the exploration of the pathophysiology of SAE, systematic brain imaging is currently not recommended in routine clinical practice. Cerebral imaging should be requested in case of focal deficit or seizure and in case of delirium or coma of unexplained cause. Although a computed tomography scan is the appropriate tool for documenting intracranial hemorrhage, a MRI is more specific for obtaining evidence of any other type of process.[5,33] Additionally, increased plasma levels of the S100b or neuron-specific enolase proteins have been reported during SAE. Their clinical relevance, however, remains controversial.[4,33–37]

### Short- and Long-term Outcomes

Acute brain dysfunction during sepsis is associated with increased mortality, long-term cognitive impairment, and psychological disorders.[7–9] The mechanisms leading to increased mortality are still not fully elucidated. An ongoing clinical and neurophysiologic study (ClinicalTrials.gov, NCT01796509) is based on the hypothesis that increased mortality relates to brainstem dysfunction, which controls both vital functions and modulates the immune response.[23] Factors during acute brain dysfunction associated with mortality include severity of coma,[6] EEG changes (ie, absence of reactivity, malignant pattern),[1] ischemic stroke,[5] and abolition of the cough reflex in sedated patients.[30]

One-third of critical ill patients present long-term neuropsychological impairment including memory, attention, verbal fluency, and executive function impairment.[8] The main risk factors of long-term cognitive impairment include the duration of delirium in the ICU and the existence of sepsis. Being hospitalized for sepsis increases by 10% the prevalence of cognitive decline after ICU discharge, especially in elderly patients, and the odds of being impaired is multiplied by 3.3.[38,39] Additionally, neurodegenerative diseases increase the risk of infection (notably of pulmonary aspiration). Psychological disorders occurring after acute brain dysfunction include anxiety, depression, and to a lesser extent posttraumatic stress disorders.[13] Psychological disorders have, along with cognitive impairment, a major impact on the functional status and quality of life after an episode of acute illness. Overall, after an episode of sepsis, up to 41% of affected patients are subsequently unable to handle a full-time employment.[40]

## PATHOPHYSIOLOGY OF SEPSIS-ASSOCIATED ENCEPHALOPATHY

Encephalopathy is the consequence of neuronal dysfunction, which may be induced by multiple microenvironmental factors. The neuronal microenvironment is tightly regulated by the BBB as well as astrocytes and microglial cells.[41] The BBB regulates the transport of metabolites and energy substrates to the neurons and the removal of toxic compounds. Astrocytes are involved in maintaining the integrity of the BBB, constituting with endothelial cells and pericytes the neurovascular complex.[42] This neurovascular complex regulates the electrolytic balance and the metabolic support to neurons. Microglial cells are in charge of the immune surveillance of the brain as well as synaptic pruning.

The pathophysiology of SAE is complex, combining intertwined and time-dependent processes affecting brain cells (eg, neurons and glial cells), cell–cell interactions (eg, neuron–glial interactions and interactions among the neurovascular complex), as well as whole structures responsible of cerebral functions (eg, memory, attention, and consciousness). Neuroinflammation, ischemia, and neurotoxicity are the main processes implicated in SAE,[43] which involve respectively, the activation of microglial cells,[44] a dysfunction of neurovascular coupling and of micro/macrocirculation,[45] and cell bioenergetics failure[46–48] (**Fig. 1**). Next, we will summarize the evidence supporting the occurrence of these processes at the tissue level as well as the associated cellular dysfunctions (**Table 1**).

### Neuroinflammation

Activation of microglial cells is a major step in every neuroinflammatory processes. Microglial cells are activated by inflammatory mediators released or passed into the brain through disruption of the BBB or brain areas deprived of the BBB. Whereas microglial cells seem to activate early and are responsible of an early

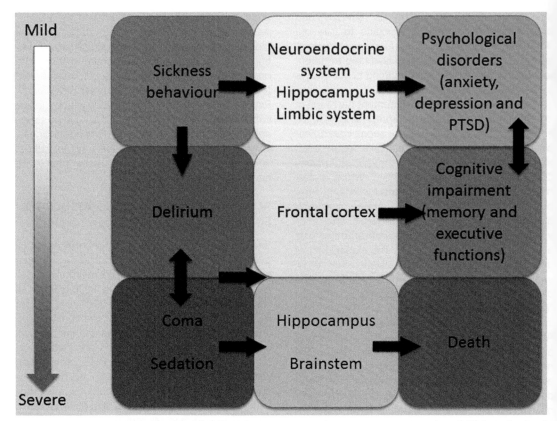

**Fig. 1.** Schematic representation of pathophysiologic processes during sepsis-associated encephalopathy (SAE). PTSD, posttraumatic stress disorder.

neuroinflammatory process, a crosstalk between microglial cells and astrocytic cells might amplify this phenomenon and lead to cellular damage.

*Microglia*

The microglia is the population of mononuclear phagocytes of the brain, involved in immune defense and synaptic stripping. Microglia are antigen presenting cells that, when activated secrete mediators including excitoxic mediators, such as glutamate and interleukins. Microglia activation, which is mediated by lipopolysaccharide and cytokines, is characterized by morphologic changes: cells shift from a hyperramified to an ameboid form. Activated microglia also acquire specific immunologic characteristics ranging from proinflammatory (M1) to antiinflammatory (M2) phenotypes and consequently may have either neuroprotective or neurotoxic properties. Microglia activation increases the cellular metabolic demand, which may result in oxidative stress and mitochondrial dysfunction. Multiple experimental interventions modulating microglia activity show promising results, including antiinflammatory factors[49] minocycline,[50] cholinergic

inhibition,[51] and vagal nerve stimulation.[52] Microglia activation and the parenchymal expression of cytokines and inducible nitric oxide synthase[53,54] are the most consistent neuropathologic features of SAE, both in septic animal[55–57] and patients.[54,58] Microglia immunologic and morphologic changes over the course of SAE have been poorly investigated. We have shown experimentally that tight glucose control dampened microglia activation.[59] The failure of a randomized clinical trial, based on an original and convincing hypothesis that postulated that restoring cholinergic inhibition by rivastigmine administration could decrease microglia activation, indicates that manipulating the microglia is hazardous.[60]

*Astrocytes*

Astrocyes are specialized glial cells assembled in networks providing energy and growth factors to neurons as well as maintaining homeostasis of the neuronal microenvironment. Astrocytes also regulate the synaptic activity through the reuptake of glutamate and the release of neurotransmitters. They interact with capillary endothelial cells, actively participating in the formation and integrity

**Table 1**
Homeostatic cellular function in the brain and pathophysiology during sepsis-associated encephalopathy

| | Cell Type | Homeostatic Function | Cellular Changes | Mechanisms | Consequences |
|---|---|---|---|---|---|
| Glial cells | Astrocytes | Synaptic plasticity,[105] neurovascular coupling,[75] microenvironment homeostasy,[105] BBB formation | Astrogliosis in mouse model[59] but not in patients | Unknown | ↗ BBB permeability, Neuroinflammation, Mediator of tissue damage[105] |
| | Oligodendrocytes | Myelin sheath formation and maintain | Unknown | Unknown | Worse myelination development,[106] potently cognitive impairment |
| | Microglial cells | Innate immune system of the central nervous system[44] Inflammatory cell recruitment | Microgliosis,[54,58,63] modification of their activation state, M1 or M2 phenotype | Vagal nerve stimulation[52,107] IL-1β[49] and TNF-α[57] exposure, Other activating factors | Excitotoxic compound release[106] iNOS expression[54] Neuroinflammation |
| Blood vessels | Endothelial cells | Blood vessel lining in their lumen, Role in coagulation, vasoconstriction and vasodilation, inflammation, | Endothelial activation, Inflammatory mediator leakage and production, Cell recruitement[108] | TNF-α and other cytokine exposure[109] | ↗ BBB permeability, Microthrombi, Infarct, Ischemic lesions[5,58] |
| | Pericytes | Blood vessel stabilization, vasoconstriction, vasodilation[110] | Unknown | — | ↗ BBB permeability, Microthrombi, ischemic lesion, infarct, Supply/demand oxygen inadequation[5] |
| Choroid plexus | Ependymal cell | Cerebrospinal fluid production, and resorption, Information processing | Unknown | — | — |
| | Neurons | Information processing | Dysfunction (long-term potentiation[95]) apoptosis[54,58] | Glutamate excitotoxicity, Metabolic impairment | Cognitive impairment[7,9,64] |

*Abbreviations:* ↗ increased BBB permeability; BBB, blood–brain barrier; IL, interleukin; iNOS, inducible nitric oxide synthase; TNF, tumor necrosis factor.

of the BBB. Neuroinflammation also involves astrocytes because they are able to secrete various mediators.[61] Animal studies have reported astrocyte proliferation, or astrogliosis, during SAE. However, no neuropathologic study has found similar findings in man. This lack of astrocytic activation contrasts with evidence of BBB impairment.[5,62] Most of these studies relied solely on immunostaining of the glial fibrillary acid protein associated with morphologic analysis, tools that are insufficient for detecting molecular changes or to investigate the glial network or neuro–glial interactions. Complementary analysis using specific techniques, such as proteomic and genomic analysis as well as cellular neurophysiologic explorations, are necessary.

### Cellular metabolism
Neuroinflammation increases the metabolic and bioenergetic demand, which may[63,64] result in oxidative stress and mitochondrial dysfunction. Indeed, early mitochondrial dysfunction has been detected in the brain of septic animals, resulting in the production of reactive oxygen or nitrogen species. The production of reactive oxygen or nitrogen species is proapoptotic, affecting both glial cells and neurons. The experimental benefit associated with tight blood glucose control might be a consequence of reduced mitochondrial dysfunction and oxidative stress.

### Ischemic Process

Adequate cerebral perfusion is ensured by the autoregulation of the cerebral blood flow, ensuring the maintenance of cerebral blood flow despite variations of cerebral perfusion pressure.[37] At the microcirculatory level, gliovascular units adjust the cerebral blood flow to the energetic needs of a given area. Ischemic damage including lacunae or large ischemic strokes occurs frequently during SAE.[58] Post mortem studies demonstrate that diffuse lacunar ischemia is present in all fatal cases of septic shock. Ischemic stroke is observed in approximately one-quarter of septic shock patients who develop acute brain dysfunction.[58] Cerebral ischemia during sepsis associates with disseminated intravascular coagulopathy[5] and is responsible of high mortality rates. Animal and human macrocirculatory studies report contradictory findings, because of a discrepancy in monitoring techniques and because of variations regarding the severity and time course of the disease. Interestingly, impaired autoregulation seems to precede the occurrence of delirium in septic patients.[37,65] However, there is no evidence supporting the need to monitor or even to optimize macrocirculatory parameters in septic patients.

### The gliovascular unit
The gliovascular unit is composed of endothelial cells and their basal membrane, of the perivascular endfeet of astrocytes, and of pericytes. Cerebral endothelial cells are connected by tight junctions and possess a high number of mitochondria that provide the energy required for the active transport of metabolites from the circulation to the brain. Astrocytic endfeet and endothelial cells are coupled, via the connexin 43, to ensure an adequate metabolic supply to neurons.[66,67] Astrocytic endfeet also regulate water and ionic homeostasis through the transmembrane channel Aquaporin-4, which is implicated in brain edema formation. Capillary pericytes enable the dilation and constriction of cerebral vessels, regulating the microcirculation.

Sepsis is characterized by a dysfunction of endothelial tight junctions enabling the passage of systemic inflammatory and neurotoxic mediators into the brain.[62,68] Other pathophysiologic phenomena occurring during sepsis include secretion within the brain parenchyma of inflammatory mediators, adhesion and transcytosis of inflammatory cells, activation of the coagulation cascade, and formation of microthrombi, which worsen the impairment of capillary endothelium.[69] Activation of endothelial cells occurs both in neuroinflammatory and in ischemic processes. Impairment of the BBB during sepsis has been well documented experimentally,[68,70,71] and in septic patients.[4,5] Activated complement and tumor necrosis factor-α are major triggers of BBB dysfunction. Aquaporin 4 expression has also been reported to be increased during sepsis; however, its exact role is not understood fully.[57]

### Neurovascular coupling
Neurovascular coupling entails a close temporal relationship between local neuronal activity and cerebral bloodflow.[72] The astrocyte network, through gap junctions enables the propagation of a calcium wave, from the synapse to the perivascular astrocyte,[73] which then induces the synthesis and release of vasoactive substances such as nitric oxide, arachidonic acid, or their byproducts.[73,74] These substances are vasodilatory, inducing leiomyocyte and pericyte relaxation.[41] Impaired neurovascular coupling is found in both acute and chronic disease, such as stroke or hypertension.[75,76] Impaired neurovascular coupling has also been described in sepsis[77] and might be related to the increased release of arachidonic acid and nitric oxide, which are also incriminated in the septic related impairment of autoregulation.

## Neuronal Dysfunction

Clinical signs of SAE are the result of impaired neurotransmission, involving the β-adrenergic system,[78] the γ-amino butyric acid (GABA) receptor system,[79] and the cholinergic system.[64] The imbalance between dopaminergic and cholinergic neurotransmission is incriminated in delirium in the critically ill.[80] However, cholinergic drugs, such as rivastigmine[60] or antidopaminergic drugs, such as haloperidol, do not reduce the incidence or duration of delirium, indicating that restoring this balance pharmacologically is not easy. The use of GABA agonists, such as benzodiazepines, actually increases the risk of brain dysfunction in critically ill patients,[9] whereas this risk is reduced by noradrenergic drugs, such as dexmedetomidine.[81,82] Neurotransmission is impaired by nitric oxide and circulating neurotoxic amino acids, including ammonium, tyrosine, tryptophan, and phenylalanine, all of which are released in excess by the liver and muscles during sepsis.[83–85] The concomitant decrease in branched chain amino acids might potentiate their neurotoxic effect.[83–85] Metabolic disorders, resulting from kidney and liver failure, contribute to neurotransmitter impairment, and facilitate the accumulation of drugs that are administered to septic patients (eg, sedatives, analgesics, and antibiotics).

Glutamate excitoxicity contributes to neuronal apoptosis during sepsis, through metabolic failure leading to intracellular ionic disturbance ultimately leading to apoptosis. Ascorbate is an antioxidant that is able to attenuate excitotoxic insults secondary to glutamate release. The recycling and export of ascorbate by astrocytes are inhibited during sepsis,[55,86] accounting for decreased concentrations of ascorbate in the plasma and cerebrospinal fluid during SAE.[87] When activated, microglia release large amounts of glutamate contributing to the excitotoxic process in SAE. Finally, some specific brain areas that are activated during sepsis (the amygdala, locus coeruleus) suffer from impaired metabolic supply, suggesting that excitotoxicity might be responsible for apoptosis observed in these centers.

## FUNCTIONAL ANATOMY OF THE CENTRAL NERVOUS SYSTEM DURING SEPSIS

Clinical findings are associated with changes in areas of the brain that might be involved in sequelae after sepsis. The relation between clinical findings and anatomic structures are summarized in **Fig. 2**.

### Brainstem

The brainstem has 3 main functions, namely to control (1) arousal via the reticular activating ascending substance (RAAS), (2) brainstem reflexes, (3) vital functions, including the cardiovascular, respiratory, and immune systems. Clinical and neuropathologic observations hint at the possibility of a brainstem dysfunction in sepsis.[30] Impaired alertness is one of the major clinical features of SAE, indicating a dysfunction of the RAAS. The absence of EEG reactivity, which has been shown to be of prognostic value during sepsis, also supports a dysfunction of the RAAS.[1] Additionally, in sedated and non–brain injured critically ill patients (mostly septic), the abolition of the cough reflex and oculocephalogyre response was independently associated with increased ICU mortality and the occurrence of delirium after discontinuation of sedation.[30] Heart rate variability was found to be impaired and associated with a worse outcome during sepsis.[21,88] This phenomenon, which also occurs in experimental sepsis, reflects a decreased sympathetic activity originating from autonomic centers of the brainstem. Interestingly, neuropathologic studies found that medullary autonomic centers, but also the locus coeruleus, which is the noradrenergic nucleus of the RAAS, are liable to neuronal apoptosis during sepsis.[23,54] This corroborates the experimental finding that an lipopolysaccharide challenge induces oxidative stress and apoptosis within the autonomic centers, preceding the occurrence of arterial hypotension. The prevalence of delirium in septic patients may be decreased by the use of dexmedetomidine, an α2 adrenergic receptor agonist possessing antiapoptotic properties.[81] As mentioned, 2 brainstem structures are major pathways in the response to stress. The first is the vagal nerve, which signals autonomic centers of the presence of peripheral inflammation.[24] This signaling involves various mediators, including cytokines. The area postrema, which is deprived of BBB, allows the passage of circulating inflammatory mediators into the brainstem. Excessive inflammatory signaling may even be deleterious. We have reported, in a septic shock patient, a case of multifocal necrotizing leukoencephalopathy, characterized by an overexpression of inflammatory cytokines within the pons.[89] Our hypothesis is that a brainstem dysfunction might account for increased mortality and the occurrence of delirium during sepsis.

### Hypothalamus and Pituitary Gland

It has been clearly established that sepsis is associated with neuroendocrine disorders affecting all axes.[17–19,23,25,67,90] During the acute stage of sepsis, the secretion of hypophyseal hormones is increased and the expression of their peripheral

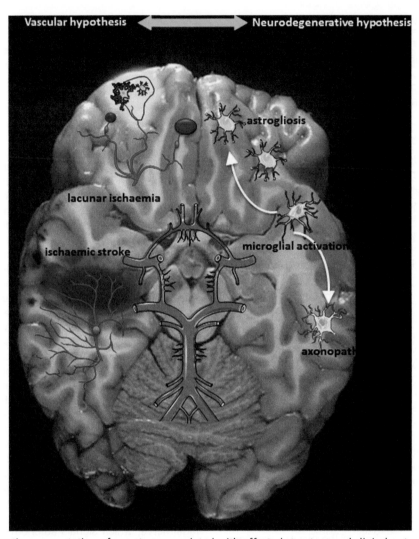

**Fig. 2.** Schematic representation of symptoms correlated with affected structure and clinical outcome.

receptors is downregulated. Prolonged sepsis is characterized by a decrease in pituitary hormone release.[91] Indeed, septic shock may be complicated by relative adrenal insufficiency associated with increased mortality, which responds to substitutive opotherapy.[22,90] Septic shock may also be associated with impaired osmoregulation of vasopressin, resulting from a depolarization of osmoreceptors.[17,18,20] Interestingly, osmoreceptors are located within circumventricular organs and their dysfunction might be induced by inflammatory cytokines.

## Hippocampus, Frontal Cortex, and Amygdala

Memory impairment is indicative of a dysfunction of the hippocampus. The frontal cortex may also be implicated in memory impairment as well as

attention and executive function impairment. Hippocampal atrophy, a major feature of Alzheimer disease, occurs in sepsis survivors and correlates with memory impairment.[92] Experimental studies, using tests such as open field, step avoidance, and water maze tests,[93,94] have demonstrated the existence of protracted hippocampal dysfunction in septic rats or mice. This hippocampal dysfunction correlates with impairment of long-term potentiation,[95] with late-occurring neuronal death, microglial activation, astrogliosis, and increased oxidative stress.[57,95] These phenomena can be partially reversed in tumor necrosis factor receptor[57] or caspase 1 knockout models or by pharmacologic interventions (minocycline,[50] antioxidant peptides,[46] cholinesterase inhibitors[51,60]). Additionally, interleukin-1β–receptor antagonist prevent the intense epsis related neuroinflammatory process,[49] reduce BBB permeability, reactive oxygen species production, and to prevent hippocampus and amygdala-related cognitive impairment. It has to be noted that the hippocampus is highly sensitive to tissue hypoxia, as observed in animal models of hypoxemia,[92,96] and that microcirculatory might be of high importance in the hippocampus. Despite these promising results observed in animal models of sepsis, no pharmacologic treatment in man has been found to have a beneficial effect on memory performance after sepsis.[60]

Anxiety, depression and posttraumatic stress disorder are frequent complications of sepsis, all involving the amygdala and its connections with the medial prefrontal cortex.[16] The amygdala presents early and intense microglial and neuronal apoptosis during sepsis.[23,54] A recent clinical study showed that hydrocortisone prevents posttraumatic stress disorder.[97] Indeed, corticosteroids have been shown to desensitize the amygdala to stressful stimuli and helps resolve the aftermath of stress.[14] This effect might rely either on the direct effect of steroids or on an epigenetic effect of the drug,[98] which are not fully understood but are particularly involved in aversive memory formation.[99]

The frontal cortex is composed of the prefrontal cortex and other sensorimotor areas. One study found ultrastructural anomalies of the sensorimotor cortex occurring in a dog model of endotoxinic shock.[100] Overall, few studies sought to understand prefrontal sequelae after sepsis. Prefrontal cortex–related cognitive function such as memorization and verbal fluency are frequently disabled after sepsis.[7] Lower brain-derived neutrophic factor and neuronal calcium sensor-1 concentration,[101] both implied in the maintenance of dopaminergic neurons, were associated with cognitive impairment and neuronal loss in the prefrontal cortex. Finally, psychological stress in rats potentiated neuroinflammation during SAE mostly through adrenal axis modulation.[102] These data suggest that postseptic cognitive impairment and psychological disorders might be secondary to neuroinflammation, affecting particularly the frontal cortex.[59,62,103] Epidemiologic, neuropathologic and experimental evidence links neuroinflammation with neurodegeneration. Sepsis is a primary or reactivating event, which may promote the occurrence or worsen the course of neurodegenerative diseases.[7,38] No treatment targeting neuroinflammation has exhibited any benefit for preventing or reducing cognitive dysfunction in neurodegenerative diseases. Cerebral ischemia is a major cause of dementia and could therefore be one of the processes linking sepsis to long-term cognitive decline. It would be of interest to assess whether the prevention of ischemic damage during the acute stage of sepsis is beneficial for the cognitive outcome. In addition to these mechanisms, axonal damage might be involved in SAE. Indeed, one may argue that white matter damage observed on MRI may partly be owing to an axonopathy. Interestingly, the first neuroradiologic studies suggested that white matter lesions induced by sepsis were associated with cognitive decline.[4,5,104]

## SUMMARY

Sepsis is the most frequent and severe cause of brain dysfunction in critically ill patients. The pathophysiology of SAE is complex and results of both inflammatory and ischemic processes that affect the frontal cortex, the hippocampus, and the brainstem. The diagnosis of encephalopathy relies essentially on neurologic examination and EEG, upon which cerebral imaging might be indicated. Its main differential diagnosis is a central nervous system infection, which must be ruled out whenever suspected. The treatment of SAE is based on ensuring the resolution of sepsis.

## ACKNOWLEDGMENTS

The authors thank Urska Intihar and Cédric Thepenier for their critical reading.

## REFERENCES

1. Azabou E, Magalhaes E, Braconnier A, et al. Early standard electroencephalogram abnormalities predict mortality in septic intensive care unit patients. PLoS One 2015;10:e0139969.
2. Hosokawa K, Gaspard N, Su F, et al. Clinical neurophysiological assessment of sepsis-associated brain dysfunction: a systematic review. Crit Care 2014;18:674.
3. Punia V, Garcia CG, Hantus S. Incidence of recurrent seizures following hospital discharge in patients with LPDs (PLEDs) and nonconvulsive seizures recorded on continuous EEG in the critical care setting. Epilepsy Behav 2015;49:250–4.
4. Piazza O, Cotena S, De Robertis E, et al. Sepsis associated encephalopathy studied by MRI and cerebral spinal fluid S100B measurement. Neurochem Res 2009;34:1289–92.
5. Polito A, Eischwald F, Maho AL, et al. Pattern of brain injury in the acute setting of human septic shock. Crit Care 2013;17:R204.
6. Ely EW, Shintani A, Truman B, et al. Delirium as a predictor of mortality in mechanically ventilated

patients in the intensive care unit. JAMA 2004;291: 1753–62.

7. Iwashyna TJ, Ely EW, Smith DM, et al. Long-term cognitive impairment and functional disability among survivors of severe sepsis. JAMA 2010; 304:1787–94.

8. Jackson JC, Hart RP, Gordon SM, et al. Six-month neuropsychological outcome of medical intensive care unit patients. Crit Care Med 2003;31:1226–34.

9. Pandharipande PP, Girard TD, Ely EW. Long-term cognitive impairment after critical illness. N Engl J Med 2013;369:1306–16.

10. Guerra C, Linde-Zwirble WT, Wunsch H. Risk factors for dementia after critical illness in elderly Medicare beneficiaries. Crit Care 2012;16:R233.

11. Boer KR, van Ruler O, van Emmerik AA, et al. Factors associated with posttraumatic stress symptoms in a prospective cohort of patients after abdominal sepsis: a nomogram. Intensive Care Med 2008;34:664–74.

12. Schelling G, Briegel J, Roozendaal B, et al. The effect of stress doses of hydrocortisone during septic shock on posttraumatic stress disorder in survivors. Biol Psychiatry 2001;50:978–85.

13. Jensen JF, Thomsen T, Overgaard D, et al. Impact of follow-up consultations for ICU survivors on post-ICU syndrome: a systematic review and meta-analysis. Intensive Care Med 2015;41: 763–75.

14. Henckens MJ, van Wingen GA, Joels M, et al. Time-dependent effects of corticosteroids on human amygdala processing. J Neurosci 2010;30: 12725–32.

15. Dantzer R. Cytokine-induced sickness behavior: where do we stand? Brain Behav Immun 2001; 15:7–24.

16. Muscatell KA, Dedovic K, Slavich GM, et al. Greater amygdala activity and dorsomedial prefrontal-amygdala coupling are associated with enhanced inflammatory responses to stress. Brain Behav Immun 2015;43:46–53.

17. Siami S, Bailly-Salin J, Polito A, et al. Osmoregulation of vasopressin secretion is altered in the post-acute phase of septic shock. Crit Care Med 2010; 38:1962–9.

18. Siami S, Polito A, Porcher R, et al. Thirst perception and osmoregulation of vasopressin secretion are altered during recovery from septic shock. PLoS One 2013;8:e80190.

19. Sonneville R, Guidoux C, Barrett L, et al. Vasopressin synthesis by the magnocellular neurons is different in the supraoptic nucleus and in the paraventricular nucleus in human and experimental septic shock. Brain Pathol 2010;20: 613–22.

20. Stare J, Siami S, Trudel E, et al. Effects of peritoneal sepsis on rat central osmoregulatory neurons

21. mediating thirst and vasopressin release. J Neurosci 2015;35:12188–97.

21. Annane D, Trabold F, Sharshar T, et al. Inappropriate sympathetic activation at onset of septic shock: a spectral analysis approach. Am J Respir Crit Care Med 1999;160:458–65.

22. Annane D, Sébille V, Charpentier C, et al. Effect of treatment with low doses of hydrocortisone and fludrocortisone on mortality in patients with septic shock. JAMA 2002;288:862–71.

23. Carlson DE, Chiu WC, Fiedler SM, et al. Central neural distribution of immunoreactive Fos and CRH in relation to plasma ACTH and corticosterone during sepsis in the rat. Exp Neurol 2007; 205:485–500.

24. Reyes E-P, Abarzúa S, Martin A, et al. LPS-induced c-Fos activation in NTS neurons and plasmatic cortisol increases in septic rats are suppressed by bilateral carotid chemodenervation. Adv Exp Med Biol 2012;758:185–90.

25. Sharshar T, Hopkinson NS, Orlikowski D, et al. Science review: the brain in sepsis–culprit and victim. Crit Care 2005;9:37–44.

26. Fry M, Ferguson AV. The sensory circumventricular organs: brain targets for circulating signals controlling ingestive behavior. Physiol Behav 2007;91: 413–23.

27. Peterson JF, Pun BT, Dittus RS, et al. Delirium and its motoric subtypes: a study of 614 critically ill patients. J Am Geriatr Soc 2006;54:479–84.

28. Mehta S, Cook D, Devlin JW, et al. Prevalence, risk factors, and outcomes of delirium in mechanically ventilated adults. Crit Care Med 2015;43:557–66.

29. Oddo M, Carrera E, Claassen J, et al. Continuous electroencephalography in the medical intensive care unit. Crit Care Med 2009;37:2051–6.

30. Sharshar T, Porcher R, Siami S, et al. Brainstem responses can predict death and delirium in sedated patients in intensive care unit. Crit Care Med 2011; 39:1960–7.

31. Ely EW, Margolin R, Francis J, et al. Evaluation of delirium in critically ill patients: validation of the Confusion Assessment Method for the Intensive Care Unit (CAM-ICU). Crit Care Med 2001;29: 1370–9.

32. Wijdicks EFM, Bamlet WR, Maramattom BV, et al. Validation of a new coma scale: the FOUR score. Ann Neurol 2005;58:585–93.

33. Piazza O, Russo E, Cotena S, et al. Elevated S100B levels do not correlate with the severity of encephalopathy during sepsis. Br J Anaesth 2007;99:518–21.

34. Grandi C, Tomasi CD, Fernandes K, et al. Brain-derived neurotrophic factor and neuron-specific enolase, but not S100β, levels are associated to the occurrence of delirium in intensive care unit patients. J Crit Care 2011;26:133–7.

35. Macedo RC, Tomasi CD, Giombelli VR, et al. Lack of association of S100β and neuron-specific enolase with mortality in critically ill patients. Rev Bras Psiquiatr 2013;35:267–70.

36. Nguyen DN, Spapen H, Su F, et al. Elevated serum levels of S-100?? Protein and neuron-specific enolase are associated with brain injury in patients with severe sepsis and septic shock. Crit Care Med 2006;34:1967–74.

37. Pfister D, Siegemund M, Dell-Kuster S, et al. Cerebral perfusion in sepsis-associated delirium. Crit Care 2008;12:R63.

38. Shah FA, Pike F, Alvarez K, et al. Bidirectional relationship between cognitive function and pneumonia. Am J Respir Crit Care Med 2013;188: 586–92.

39. Shen H-N, Lu C-L, Li C-Y. Dementia increases the risks of acute organ dysfunction, severe sepsis and mortality in hospitalized older patients: a national population-based study. PLoS One 2012;7: e42751.

40. Rothenhäusler H-B, Ehrentraut S, Stoll C, et al. The relationship between cognitive performance and employment and health status in long-term survivors of the acute respiratory distress syndrome: results of an exploratory study. Gen Hosp Psychiatry 2001;23:90–6.

41. Hall CN, Reynell C, Gesslein B, et al. Capillary pericytes regulate cerebral blood flow in health and disease. Nature 2014;508:55–60.

42. Abbott NJ, Rönnbäck L, Hansson E. Astrocyte-endothelial interactions at the blood-brain barrier. Nat Rev Neurosci 2006;7:41–53.

43. Adam N, Kandelman S, Mantz J, et al. Sepsis-induced brain dysfunction. Expert Rev Anti Infect Ther 2013;11:211–21.

44. Hoogland ICM, Houbolt C, van Westerloo, et al. Systemic inflammation and microglial activation: systematic review of animal experiments. J Neuroinflammation 2015;12:114.

45. Taccone FS, Su F, De Deyne C, et al. Sepsis is associated with altered cerebral microcirculation and tissue hypoxia in experimental peritonitis. Crit Care Med 2014;42:e114–22.

46. Galley HF. Bench-to-bedside review: targeting antioxidants to mitochondria in sepsis. Crit Care 2010; 14:230.

47. Brealey D, Brand M, Hargreaves I, et al. Association between mitochondrial dysfunction and severity and outcome of septic shock. Lancet 2002; 360(9328):219–23. Available at: http://discovery.ucl.ac.uk/7447/.

48. Comim CM, Rezin GT, Scaini G, et al. Mitochondrial respiratory chain and creatine kinase activities in rat brain after sepsis induced by cecal ligation and perforation. Mitochondrion 2008;8: 313–8.

49. Mina F, Comim CM, Dominguini D, et al. IL1-β involvement in cognitive impairment after sepsis. Mol Neurobiol 2014;49:1069–76.

50. Adembri C, Selmi V, Vitali L, et al. Minocycline but not tigecycline is neuroprotective and reduces the neuroinflammatory response induced by the superimposition of sepsis upon traumatic brain injury. Crit Care Med 2014;42:e570–82.

51. Comim CM, Pereira JG, Steckert A, et al. Rivastigmine reverses habituation memory impairment observed in sepsis survivor rats. Shock 2009;32: 270–1.

52. Niederbichler AD, Papst S, Claassen L, et al. Burn-induced organ dysfunction: vagus nerve stimulation attenuates organ and serum cytokine levels. Burns 2009;35:783–9.

53. Yokoo H, Chiba S, Tomita K, et al. Neurodegenerative evidence in mice brains with cecal ligation and puncture-induced sepsis: preventive effect of the free radical scavenger edaravone. PLoS One 2012;7:e51539.

54. Sharshar T, Gray F, Lorin de la Grandmaison G, et al. Apoptosis of neurons in cardiovascular autonomic centres triggered by inducible nitric oxide synthase after death from septic shock. Lancet 2003;362:1799–805.

55. Korcok J, Wu F, Tyml K, et al. Sepsis inhibits reduction of dehydroascorbic acid and accumulation of ascorbate in astroglial cultures: intracellular ascorbate depletion increases nitric oxide synthase induction and glutamate uptake inhibition. J Neurochem 2002;81:185–93.

56. Guo H, Wai PY, Mi Z, et al. Osteopontin mediates Stat1 degradation to inhibit iNOS transcription in a cecal ligation and puncture model of sepsis. Surgery 2008;144:182–8.

57. Alexander JJ, Jacob A, Cunningham P, et al. TNF is a key mediator of septic encephalopathy acting through its receptor, TNF receptor-1. Neurochem Int 2008;52:447–56.

58. Sharshar T, Annane D, de la Grandmaison GL, et al. The neuropathology of septic shock. Brain Pathol 2004;14:21–33.

59. Sonneville R, Derese I, Marques MB, et al. Neuropathological correlates of hyperglycemia during prolonged polymicrobial sepsis in mice. Shock 2015;44:245–51.

60. van Eijk MMJ, Roes KC, Honing ML, et al. Effect of rivastigmine as an adjunct to usual care with haloperidol on duration of delirium and mortality in critically ill patients: a multicentre, double-blind, placebo-controlled randomised trial. Lancet 2010; 376:1829–37.

61. Retamal MA, Froger N, Palacios-Prado N, et al. Cx43 hemichannels and gap junction channels in astrocytes are regulated oppositely by proinflammatory cytokines released from activated

microglia. J Neurosci Off J Soc Neurosci 2007;27: 13781–92.

62. Papadopoulos MC, Lamb FJ, Moss RF, et al. Faecal peritonitis causes oedema and neuronal injury in pig cerebral cortex. Clin Sci 1999;96: 461–6.

63. Lemstra AW, Groen in't Woud JC, Hoozemans JJ, et al. Microglia activation in sepsis: a case-control study. J Neuroinflammation 2007;4:4.

64. Semmler A, Frisch C, Debeir T, et al. Long-term cognitive impairment, neuronal loss and reduced cortical cholinergic innervation after recovery from sepsis in a rodent model. Exp Neurol 2007;204: 733–40.

65. Schramm P, Klein KU, Falkenberg L, et al. Impaired cerebrovascular autoregulation in patients with severe sepsis and sepsis-associated delirium. Crit Care 2012;16:R181.

66. Rouach N, Koulakoff A, Abudara V, et al. Astroglial metabolic networks sustain hippocampal synaptic transmission. Science 2008;322:1551–5.

67. Escartin C, Rouach N. Astroglial networking contributes to neurometabolic coupling. Front Neuroenergetics 2013;5:4.

68. Davies DC. Blood-brain barrier breakdown in septic encephalopathy and brain tumours. J Anat 2002;200:639–46.

69. Østergaard L, Granfeldt A, Secher N, et al. Microcirculatory dysfunction and tissue oxygenation in critical illness. Acta Anaesthesiol Scand 2015;59(10):1246–59.

70. Weiss N, Miller F, Cazaubon S, et al. The blood-brain barrier in brain homeostasis and neurological diseases. Biochim Biophys Acta 2009;1788:842–57.

71. Jeppsson B, Freund HR, Gimmon Z, et al. Blood-brain barrier derangement in sepsis: cause of septic encephalopathy? Am J Surg 1981;141:136–42.

72. Sá-Pereira I, Brites D, Brito MA. Neurovascular unit: a focus on pericytes. Mol Neurobiol 2012;45:327–47.

73. Mulligan SJ, MacVicar BA. Calcium transients in astrocyte endfeet cause cerebrovascular constrictions. Nature 2004;431:195–9.

74. Koehler RC, Roman RJ, Harder DR. Astrocytes and the regulation of cerebral blood flow. Trends Neurosci 2009;32:160–9.

75. Petzold GC, Murthy VN. Role of astrocytes in neurovascular coupling. Neuron 2011;71:782–97.

76. Bélanger M, Allaman I, Magistretti PJ. Brain energy metabolism: focus on astrocyte-neuron metabolic cooperation. Cell Metab 2011;14:724–38.

77. Rosengarten B, Krekel D, Kuhnert S, et al. Early neurovascular uncoupling in the brain during community acquired pneumonia. Crit Care 2012; 16:R64.

78. Kadoi Y, Saito S, Kunimoto F, et al. Impairment of the brain beta-adrenergic system during experimental endotoxemia. J Surg Res 1996;61:496–502.

79. Kadoi Y, Saito S. An alteration in the gamma-aminobutyric acid receptor system in experimentally induced septic shock in rats. Crit Care Med 1996;24:298–305.

80. van Gool WA, van de Beek D, Eikelenboom P. Systemic infection and delirium: when cytokines and acetylcholine collide. Lancet 2010;375:773–5.

81. Pandharipande PP, Pun BT, Herr DL, et al. Effect of sedation with dexmedetomidine vs lorazepam on acute brain dysfunction in mechanically ventilated patients: the MENDS randomized controlled trial. JAMA 2007;298:2644–53.

82. Pandharipande PP, Sanders RD, Girard TD, et al. Effect of dexmedetomidine versus lorazepam on outcome in patients with sepsis: an a priori-designed analysis of the MENDS randomized controlled trial. Crit Care 2010;14:R38.

83. Freund PR, Hobbs SF, Rowell LB. Cardiovascular responses to muscle ischemia in man–dependency on muscle mass. J Appl Physiol 1978;45: 762–7.

84. Basler T, Meier-Hellmann A, Bredle D, et al. Amino acid imbalance early in septic encephalopathy. Intensive Care Med 2002;28:293–8.

85. Berg RM, Taudorf S, Bailey DM, et al. Cerebral net exchange of large neutral amino acids after lipopolysaccharide infusion in healthy humans. Crit Care 2010;14:R16.

86. Wilson JX, Dragan M. Sepsis inhibits recycling and glutamate-stimulated export of ascorbate by astrocytes. Free Radic Biol Med 2005;39:990–8.

87. Voigt K, Kontush A, Stuerenburg HJ, et al. Decreased plasma and cerebrospinal fluid ascorbate levels in patients with septic encephalopathy. Free Radic Res 2002;36:735–9.

88. Korach M, Sharshar T, Jarrin I, et al. Cardiac variability in critically ill adults: influence of sepsis. Crit Care Med 2001;29:1380–5.

89. Sharshar T, Gray F, Poron F, et al. Multifocal necrotizing leukoencephalopathy in septic shock. Crit Care Med 2002;30:2371–5.

90. Aboab J, Polito A, Orlikowski D, et al. Hydrocortisone effects on cardiovascular variability in septic shock: a spectral analysis approach. Crit Care Med 2008;36:1481–6.

91. Schroeder S, Wichers M, Klingmüller D, et al. The hypothalamic-pituitary-adrenal axis of patients with severe sepsis: altered response to corticotropin-releasing hormone. Crit Care Med 2001;29:310–6.

92. Di Paola M, Caltagirone C, Fadda L, et al. Hippocampal atrophy is the critical brain change in patients with hypoxic amnesia. Hippocampus 2008; 18:719–28.

93. Liu L, Xie K, Chen H, et al. Inhalation of hydrogen gas attenuates brain injury in mice with cecal ligation and puncture via inhibiting neuroinflammation,

oxidative stress and neuronal apoptosis. Brain Res 2014;1589:78–92.

94. Gao R, Tang YH, Tong JH, et al. Systemic lipopoly-saccharide administration-induced cognitive impairments are reversed by erythropoietin treatment in mice. Inflammation 2015;38:1949–58.

95. Imamura Y, Wang H, Matsumoto N, et al. Interleukin-1β causes long-term potentiation deficiency in a mouse model of septic encephalopathy. Neuroscience 2011;187:63 0.

96. Müller M, Somjen GG. Intrinsic optical signals in rat hippocampal slices during hypoxia-induced spreading depression-like depolarization. J Neurophysiol 1999;82:1818–31.

97. Schelling G, Stoll C, Kapfhammer HP, et al. The effect of stress doses of hydrocortisone during septic shock on posttraumatic stress disorder and health-related quality of life in survivors. Crit Care Med 1999;27:2678–83.

98. Hunter RG. Epigenetic effects of stress and corticosteroids in the brain. Front Cell. Neurosci 2012;6:18.

99. Steckert AV, Comim CM, Igna DM, et al. Effects of sodium butyrate on aversive memory in rats submitted to sepsis. Neurosci Lett 2015;595:134–8.

100. Polyanin KI, Bardakhch'yan EA. Ultrastructure of components of the functional element of the senso-motor cortex in endotoxin shock. Neurosci Behav Physiol 1984;14:54–9.

101. Comim CM, Silva NC, Mina F, et al. Evaluation of NCS-1, DARPP-32, and neurotrophins in hippocampus and prefrontal cortex in rats submitted to sepsis. Synapse 2014;68:474–9.

102. de Pablos RM, Villarán RF, Argüelles S, et al. Stress increases vulnerability to inflammation in the rat prefrontal cortex. J Neurosci 2006;26:5709–19.

103. Ari I, Kafa IM, Kurt MA. Perimicrovascular edema in the frontal cortex in a rat model of intraperitoneal sepsis. Exp Neurol 2006;198:242–9.

104. Stubbs DJ, Yamamoto AK, Menon DK. Imaging in sepsis-associated encephalopathy–insights and opportunities. Nat Rev Neurol 2013;9:551–61.

105. Sofroniew MV, Vinters HV. Astrocytes: biology and pathology. Acta Neuropathol 2010;119:7–35.

106. Cardoso FL, Herz J, Fernandes A, et al. Systemic inflammation in early neonatal mice induces transient and lasting neurodegenerative effects. J Neuroinflammation 2015;12:82.

107. Cai B, Chen F, Ji Y, et al. Alpha7 cholinergic-agonist prevents systemic inflammation and improves survival during resuscitation. J Cell Mol Med 2009;13:3774–85.

108. Reis PA, Estato V, da Silva TI, et al. Statins decrease neuroinflammation and prevent cognitive impairment after cerebral malaria. PLoS Pathog 2012;8:e1003099.

109. Dunne JL, Ballantyne CM, Beaudet AL, et al. Control of leukocyte rolling velocity in TNF-α-induced inflammation by LFA-1 and Mac-1. Blood 2002;99:336–41.

110. Correale J, Villa A. Cellular elements of the blood-brain barrier. Neurochem Res 2009;34:2067–77.

# Beyond the Golden Hours
## Caring for Septic Patients After the Initial Resuscitation

Jean P. Gelinas, MD, Keith R. Walley, MD*

## KEYWORDS

- Sepsis • Resuscitation • Delirium • Mechanical ventilation • Immune function

## KEY POINTS

- Recognition and management of agitation, delirium, and pain are essential.
- Low tidal volumes and low mean airway pressures during mechanical ventilation should be used.
- The adverse consequences of volume overload can be avoided by careful assessment of volemia.
- Following the initial septic inflammatory response, immune function is profoundly altered, which increases susceptibility to an array of persistent viral infections.

## INTRODUCTION

Critically ill patients consume approximately 20% of hospital resources, which amounts to 1% of the gross domestic product of the United States.[1] Sepsis and septic shock are among the leading causes of intensive-care-unit (ICU) admission worldwide resulting in about 2 million ICU admissions per year for sepsis.[2] Encouragingly, mortality and morbidity are decreasing. A retrospective observational study of 100,000 Australian and New Zealand patients with severe sepsis showed that mortality rates between 2000 and 2012 decreased from 35% to a little more than 18%. Patients with severe sepsis were actually discharged in greater numbers when compared with other groups. Younger patients with severe sepsis without significant comorbidities had mortality rates less than 5%.[3] Some fraction of this improvement in survival might be explained by administrative coding modifications or by exclusion of patients for whom ICU admission is potentially futile.[4–7] However, over the last few decades it has become generally recognized that early antibiotics and timely resuscitation, optimally driven by a resuscitation algorithm or protocol, have made a real difference.[3,8,9]

In addition, several fundamental improvements in the practice of critical care have contributed. Here the authors review care in the period after the initial resuscitation to identify features that may also have contributed to improvement in sepsis and septic shock outcomes. In particular, the authors highlight post–acute phase management of agitation and delirium, mechanical ventilation, hemodynamic management, blood transfusion, nutrition, and briefly touch on immune function. The authors make the case that decreasing invasiveness when possible will have synergistic benefits for our patients.

The septic shock literature has a surprisingly low ratio of positive result[10–13] versus negative result[14–21] randomized clinical trials when improved survival is the end point. The relative paucity of clearly positive trials and management guidelines that sometimes make conflicting recommendations[22,23] can make it challenging for clinicians. This point is particularly true for the management of patients after the first several hours of resuscitation. Here the authors attempt

Disclosure Statement: The authors have nothing to disclose.
Centre for Heart Lung Innovation, St. Paul's Hospital, University of British Columbia, 1081 Burrard Street, Vancouver, British Columbia V6Z 1Y6, Canada
* Corresponding author.
E-mail address: Keith.Walley@hli.ubc.ca

Clin Chest Med 37 (2016) 347–365
http://dx.doi.org/10.1016/j.ccm.2016.01.006
0272-5231/16/$ – see front matter © 2016 Elsevier Inc. All rights reserved.

to strike a reasonable balance in the face of significant uncertainty.

## AGITATION AND DELIRIUM

Patients frequently come to the ICU already suffering from pain and acute cognitive dysfunction.[24] Cognitive dysfunction is associated with increased overall mortality, and this increased mortality is frequently because of respiratory complications.[25] Although there is little disagreement as to the management end points of analgesia, sedation, and treatment of delirium (calm, comfortable, and cooperative patients treated so as to maximize short- and long-term psychological and overall outcomes[23,26–28]), there is considerable variability in opinion as to how pain, agitation, and delirium (PAD) interact and how they should be managed.

### Importance of Agitation and Delirium

Patients with agitation and delirium cannot participate fully in weaning and rehabilitation and are at increased risk of accidental self-injury.

Agitation and delirium are also frequent and costly causes of intubation.[29,30] ICU procedures and the medications used to treat pain and agitation can themselves increase delirium and cause respiratory, musculoskeletal, cardiovascular, or digestive complications. PAD and its management interact with just about every aspect of clinical care[28,31–40] (Fig. 1). Cognitive impairment following critical illness has long-term adverse consequences.[41,42] Even mild sepsis is an independent risk factor for developing subsequent dementia.[43,44] The length of the delirious episode correlates with long-term functional outcome and mortality.[32,35,45,46] Delirium can be seen as a phenotype of acute brain failure, and its prevention is sometimes consider a marker of quality of care.[47] Our understanding of modalities to prevent and treat cognitive dysfunction is incomplete.[28,47–52]

### Treatment of Pain, Agitation, and Delirium

The Society of Critical Care Medicine's (SCCM) 2013 published guidelines[22] encourage caregivers to adopt a structured, holistic multidisciplinary

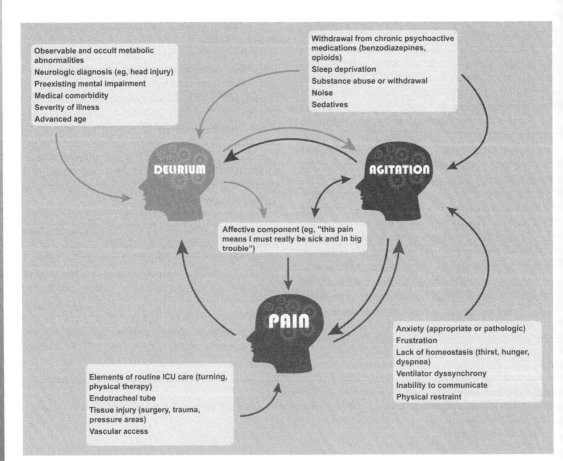

**Fig. 1.** Contributors to PAD and their interactions are illustrated.

approach to the prevention, evaluation, and treatment of PAD in critically ill patients. Using relatively simple ICU PAD care bundles (**Table 1**), the SCCM's guidelines incorporate early mobilization, exercise, daily spontaneous breathing trials (SBTs), and sedation minimization as strategies for the prevention of PAD.[22] Introduction of these bundles is associated with improved outcomes.[53] Early mobilization,[54–56] avoidance of certain medications like anticholinergics[47] and longer-acting benzodiazepines,[57] adaptation of the ICU environment to maximize natural nocturnal sleep,[24] nighttime use of ear plugs,[58] and using patients' usual eyeglasses and hearing aids can improve appropriate sensory awareness and reduce morbidity.[47]

### Early mobilization and exercise

Septic patients are often malnourished and deconditioned at presentation.[59] Additionally, the inflammatory and immune responses to infection and critical illness further reduce muscle mass[60] and increase risk of critical illness neuromyopathy. Respiratory and limb muscles tend to become weak together.[61] Nutrition[62] and exercise[55] are interlinked. A randomized trial of 104 mechanically ventilated ICU patients showed that patients who received routine physical exercise and mobilization had significantly less delirium, earlier extubation, and were significantly more likely to have an independent functional status at discharge.[55] Needham and colleagues[63] found that decreasing sedation and increasing rehabilitation treatments and early mobilization in patients ventilated for 4 or more days resulted in a decreased incidence of delirium and a decreased length of ICU stay. Keys to implementation were education, modification of order sets so that the default favors decreased sedation and increased mobilization, changing sedation practice from use of continuous intravenous infusions of benzodiazepines and narcotics to as-needed bolus doses, and changing staffing to include physiotherapy and occupational therapy.

### Spontaneous breathing trials and decreased sedation

Daily interruption of sedation decreases time to extubation[64] and subsequently has been incorporated into guidelines[65,66] along with protocolized sedation management.[67] However, daily sedation interruption[68,69] has not consistently been adopted by care providers,[70–73] in part because of variable trials results.[74] Use of long half-life benzodiazepines may account for some of the discrepancy between trials. Use of no sedation (and narcotic analgesics as needed) compared with propofol and/or midazolam (and narcotic

analgesia as needed) demonstrated that the group receiving no sedation had earlier extubation and discharge from the ICU but higher rates of delirium and more frequent need of haloperidol.[75] Combining daily wakening with SBTs demonstrated benefit and highlights the multifactorial nature of critical care.[11]

## Specific Medications for Sedation, Agitation, and Delirium

There is ample literature comparing various medications for management of sedation, agitation, and delirium in the hospital and ICU.[76] As indicated earlier, agitation and delirium are best dealt with initially by nonpharmacologic means, recognizing that pharmacologic treatment of anxiety and delirium are often necessary and essential.

### Dexmedetomidine

Dexmedetomidine may permit earlier extubation and cause less delirium when compared with midazolam[77] or lorazepam.[78] Both dexmedetomidine and propofol can contribute to hypotension,[79] and dexmedetomidine may cause bradycardia and first-degree atrioventricular block. Although dexmedetomidine does not produce as deep a sedative effect,[79] it may leave patients calm and interactive with a higher Richmond Agitation-Sedation Scale score than comparable benzodiazepine sedation. A meta-analysis of 20 studies done in 2612 ICU patients found that the use of dexmedetomidine was associated with a lower risk of neurocognitive dysfunction when compared with other treatment modalities.[80]

### Propofol

Propofol is a useful, titratable sedative in the critical care setting. Given its ubiquitous use, it is important to recognize the propofol-related infusion syndrome (PRIS), which is an uncommon but potentially fatal syndrome described in children[81,82] and adults receiving prolonged propofol infusions in the ICU. Its most extreme manifestations include cardiac failure, rhabdomyolysis, metabolic acidosis, renal failure, and death.[83] The use of vasopressors is associated with propofol toxicity.[84–87] In a large prospective study, 11 of 1017 patients (1.1%) developed PRIS, often within 24 hours of initiation of propofol infusion. A high index of suspicion should be maintained in all patients receiving propofol, particularly when combined with vasopressor support.

### Haloperidol and other delirium medication

Evidence to support the use of medication to prevent delirium is weak, and choice of medications used to treat delirium is far from settled.[22,47,88,89]

**Table 1**
**The Society of Critical Care Medicine's current care bundles for intensive-care-unit pain, agitation, and delirium are shown**

| A | Pain | Agitation | Delirium |
|---|------|-----------|----------|
| Assess | Assess pain ≥4× per shift & as needed<br>Preferred pain assessment tools:<br>• Patients able to self-report → NRS (0–10)<br>• Unable to self-report → BPS (3–12) or CPOT (0–8)<br>Patients are in significant pain if NRS ≥4, BPS >5, CPOT ≥3 | Assess agitation ≥4× per shift & as needed<br>Preferred sedation assessment tools:<br>• RASS (−5 to +4) or SAS (1–7)<br>• Neuromuscular blockade → suggest using brain function monitoring<br>Depth of agitation, sedation defined as:<br>• Agitated if RASS = +1 to +4 or SAS = 5–7<br>• Awake and calm if RASS = 0 or SAS = 4<br>• Lightly sedated if RASS = −1 to −2 or SAS = 3<br>• Deeply sedated if RASS = −3 to −5 or SAS = 1–2 | Assess delirium every shift & as needed<br>Preferred delirium assessment tools:<br>• CAM-ICU (+ or −)<br>• ICDSC (0–8)<br>Delirium present if:<br>• CAM-ICU is positive<br>• ICDSC ≥4 |
| Treat | Treat pain within 30 min then reassess:<br>• Nonpharmacologic treatment: relaxation therapy<br>• Pharmacologic treatment<br>○ Non-neuropathic pain → IV opioids +/− nonopioid analgesics<br>○ Neuropathic pain → gabapentin or carbamazepine + IV opioids<br>○ Post abdominal aortic aneurysm, rib fractures → thoracic epidurals | Targeted sedation or DSI (goal: patients purposely follow commands without agitation): RASS = −2–0, SAS = 3–4<br>• If undersedated (RASS >0, SAS >4) assess/treat pain → treat with sedatives as needed (non-benzodiazepines preferred unless ETOH or benzodiazepine withdrawal is suspected)<br>awake and calm if RASS = 0 or SAS = 4<br>• If oversedated (RASS <−2, SAS <3), hold sedatives until a target, then restart at 50% of the previous dose | • Treat pain as needed<br>• Reorient patients, familiarize surroundings, use patients' eyeglasses, hearing aids as needed<br>• Pharmacologic treatment<br>○ Avoid benzodiazepine unless ETOH or benzodiazepine withdrawal is suspected<br>○ Avoid rivastigmine<br>○ Avoid antipsychotics if ↑ risk of torsades de pointes |
| Prevent | • Administer preprocedural analgesia and/or nonpharmacologic interventions (eg, relaxation therapy)<br>• Treat pain first, then sedate | • Consider daily SBT, early mobility, and exercise when patients are at goal sedation level, unless contraindicated<br>• EEG monitoring if<br>○ At risk for seizures<br>○ Burst suppression therapy is indicated for ↑ ICP | • Identify delirium risk factors: dementia, HTN, ETOH abuse, high severity of illness, coma, benzodiazepine administration<br>• Avoid benzodiazepine use in those at ↑ risk for delirium<br>• Mobilize and exercise patients early<br>• Promote sleep (control light noise, cluster patient care activities, decrease nocturnal stimuli)<br>• Restart baseline psychiatric medications, if indicated |

| B | Pain | Agitation | Delirium |
|---|------|-----------|----------|
| Assess | • Percentage of time patients are monitored for pain ≥4× per shift<br>• Demonstrate local compliance and implementation integrity over time in the use of ICU pain scoring systems | • Percentage of time sedation assessments are performed ≥4× per shift<br>• Demonstrate local compliance and implementation integrity overtime in the use of ICU sedation scoring systems | • Percentage of time delirium assessments are performed every shift<br>• Demonstrate local compliance and implementation integrity over time in the use of ICU delirium assessment tools |
| Treat | • Percentage of time ICU patients are in significant pain (ie, NRS ≥4, BPS ≥6, or CPOT ≥3)<br>• Percentage of time treatment is initiated within 30 s of detecting significant pain | • Percentage of time patients are either optimally sedated or successfully achieve target sedation during DSI trials (ie, RASS = −2–0, SAS = 3–4)<br>• Percentage of time ICU patients are *undersedated* (RASS >0, SAS >4)<br>• Percentage of time ICU patients are *oversedated* (RASS <−2, SAS <3) or fail to undergo DSI trials | • Percentage of time delirium is present in ICU patients (CAM-ICU is positive or ICDSC ≥4)<br>• Percentage of time benzodiazepines are administered to patients with documented delirium (not due to ETOH or benzodiazepine withdrawal) |
| Prevent | • Percentage of time patients receive preprocedural analgesia therapy and/or nonpharmacologic interventions<br>• Percentage of compliance with institutional-specific ICU pain management protocols | • Percentage of failed attempts at SBTs due to either over or under sedation<br>• Percentage of patients undergoing EEG monitoring if<br>  ○ At risk for seizures<br>  ○ Burst suppression therapy is indicated for ↑ ICP<br>• Percentage of compliance with institutional-specific ICU sedation/agitation management protocols | • Percentage of patients receiving daily physical therapy and early mobility<br>• Percentage of compliance with ICU sleep-promotion strategies<br>• Percentage of compliance with institutional-specific ICU delirium prevention and treatment protocols |

*Abbreviations:* AAA, abdominal aortic aneurysm; BPS, behavioural pain scale; CAM-ICU, confusion assessment method for the ICU; CPOT, Critical Care Pain Observation Tool; DSI, daily sedation interruption; EEG, electroencephalogram; ETOH, ethanol; HTN, hypertension; ICDSC, intensive care delirium screening checklist; ICP, intracranial pressure; IV, intravenous; NRS, numeric rating scale; RASS, Richmond Agitation-Sedation Scale; SAS, sedation-agitation scale; SBT, spontaneous breathing trial.

*From* Barr J, Fraser GL, Puntillo K, et al. Clinical practice guidelines for the management of pain, agitation, and delirium in adult patients in the intensive care unit. Crit Care Med 2013;41(1):292–3; with permission.

Haloperidol and other antipsychotics are also associated with prolonged QTc intervals, which can idiosyncratically lead to torsade de pointes.[90–94] Monitoring for QTc prolongation and checking magnesium and potassium levels, when appropriate, could potentially be useful to minimize complications arising from haloperidol and antipsychotic drug use.[94]

### Ramelteon and melatonin receptor agonists

Melatonin receptor agonists might be useful in diminishing sleep disturbances and delirium in the ICU.[95,96] Administration of prophylactic melatonin receptor agonists have been shown to decrease delirium in elderly patients admitted to the medical ward[97] but not in patients with hip fractures.[98] Ramelteon is the first melatonin receptor agonist to be approved for the treatment of insomnia and is more potent than previous melatonin receptor agonists.[99] A recent small multicentric trial evaluating the use of ramelteon in 67 elderly Japanese patients admitted to the ICU or the ward showed a significant decrease in delirium in patients treated with prophylactic ramelteon versus placebo (3% vs 32%).[100]

## MECHANICAL VENTILATION

In this section the authors focus on ventilation from the perspective of patients with sepsis or septic shock while keeping in mind multisystem interactions. The authors also examine less invasive ventilation strategies as they pertain to septic patients.

### Small Tidal Volumes, Low Plateau Pressures

The Surviving Sepsis guidelines recommend that septic patients who have acute respiratory distress syndrome (ARDS) be treated with smaller tidal volumes and plateau pressures while, if necessary, tolerating permissive hypercapnia.[101–103] An extensive review of mostly perioperative trials[104] similarly recommends that high tidal volumes and high plateau pressures be avoided. In a meta-analysis of 6 trials (n = 1297 patients) low tidal volume targeted at 6 mL/kg lean body mass reduced mortality (relative risk 0.74).[105] Much of the beneficial effect may be related to the concomitant maintenance of plateau pressures less than approximately 30 cm $H_2O$.[105] Obesity confounds standard airway pressure measurements. Positive end-expiratory pressure (PEEP) and plateau measurements from the endotracheal tube may reach high levels, whereas lung inflation (eg, on a chest radiograph) may be low.[106] Measurement of esophageal pressure, as a surrogate of pleural pressure, allows the calculation of transpulmonary pressure and can reveal that an obese chest wall results in artifactually elevated airway pressure measurements without lung hyperinflation. In this case, transpulmonary pressures (airway pressure minus esophageal pressure) can then be used to guide application of positive airway pressure.

### Earliest Possible Extubation

Daily SBTs[107,108] are an established and accepted part of critical care practice. A 2008 study by Girard and colleagues[11] conducted in the medical ICUs of 4 tertiary care hospitals found an impressive one life saved for every 7 patients treated when comparing protocol-guided spontaneous awakening combined with SBTs versus trials without changes to sedation. Prolonged intubation and mechanical ventilation, beyond what is absolutely essential, results in increased risk of ventilator-associated pneumonia, agitation and self-harm (eg, self-extubation without deflation of the endotracheal tube cuff), increased use of harmful sedative and antipsychotic drugs, increased delirium, and so forth.

### Noninvasive Positive Pressure Ventilation

#### Selection of patients for noninvasive positive pressure

Identifying patients who are most likely to benefit[109–114] or not likely to benefit[115–118] from noninvasive positive pressure ventilation (NPPV) is an ongoing process.[119] The highest level of evidence supporting the use of noninvasive mechanical ventilation is available for patients with chronic obstructive pulmonary disease (COPD) exacerbations, facilitation of weaning/extubation in patients with COPD, cardiogenic pulmonary edema, and for use in certain selected immunosuppressed patients.[120–123] A detailed analysis of this topic is beyond the scope of this article, and readers are referred to 2 excellent general NPPV reviews[121,124] and to some more specific or focused Cochrane reviews.[125–127]

From the perspective of patients experiencing respiratory failure in the context of sepsis and septic shock, the evidence to support routine use of NPPV is less well established. A small study of patients with severe community-acquired pneumonia showed NPPV to be safe and effective while significantly decreasing the need for endotracheal intubation compared with patients who did not receive any NPPV. There was even a slight decrease in mortality rates at 2 months. Patients who had baseline COPD benefitted more from NPPV.[128] A large multicenter trial evaluating NPPV in a non-COPD patient population with hypoxic respiratory failure found that patients with sepsis or septic shock, pneumonia, and ARDS vere significantly more likely to fail NPPV and need intubation than other enrolled patients.[129]

### Current guidelines for noninvasive positive pressure ventilation in sepsis

The Surviving Sepsis Campaign's guidelines suggest that NPPV be used in a minority of patients with sepsis-induced ARDS in whom the benefits of NPPV are thought to outweigh the risks[23] (Fig. 2). One of the studies cited by the Surviving Sepsis Campaign's guidelines evaluates the outcome of 54 patients with progressive hypoxic respiratory failure treated with bilevel positive airway pressure (BIPAP) or continuous positive airway pressure (CPAP) and found that 38 of these patients (21 BIPAP and 17 CPAP) went on to require intubation. Although sepsis alone was not a predictor of failure, all patients with shock (of whatever origin) failed noninvasive support. Higher Acute Physiology and Chronic Health Evaluation and Sepsis-related Organ Failure Assessment (SOFA) scores and lower $PaO_2$/fraction of inspired oxygen were also associated with failure of CPAP and BIPAP.[130] Thus, the role for NPPV is limited in sepsis and not recommended for patients with septic shock.

### HEMODYNAMIC MANAGEMENT: FLUIDS AND VASOPRESSORS

Early goal-directed therapy[12] fundamentally changed the standard of care in resuscitation of patients with septic shock, so much so that careful studies of differences between current standard of care and original EGDT (Early Goal-Directed

Therapy) algorithms (PROCESS and ARISE) were very similar, both in practices of care and in excellent outcomes.[14,15] All standard and experimental early goal-directed protocols that have recently been tested[14,15,17] highlight and then address 3 key clinical questions: First, is volume resuscitation adequate? Second, has a minimum mean arterial pressure been achieved? Third, is oxygen delivery to vital organs sufficient? Although resuscitation protocols have typically been limited to the first 6 hours of care, these 3 key clinical questions should continue to be addressed after the initial resuscitation.

### Fluid Choice

In sepsis, there is no clear evidence that one type of fluid is best. Instead, the important issue is whether fluid resuscitation is adequate (or excessive). The SAFE study randomized nearly 7000 critically ill patients (1218 with sepsis) to receive either 4% albumin or sodium chloride 0.9% as a resuscitation fluid. No significant differences in mortality or new organ failure were observed.[131] Subsequent post hoc analysis of the data suggested that the subgroup of patients with severe sepsis might have had a slightly better outcome if given albumin instead of saline.[132] This idea was tested prospectively by the ALBIOS investigators who found no difference in survival outcomes in 1818 patients with severe sepsis randomized to receiving 20% albumin and crystalloids (with an end goal of keeping albumin levels >30 g per liter) versus crystalloids alone.[133] Thus, any difference in patient outcomes between

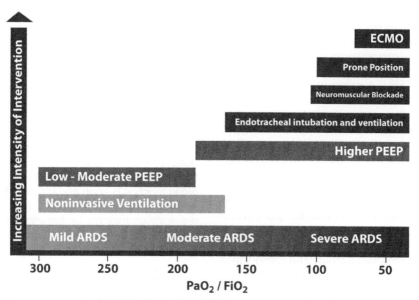

**Fig. 2.** Ventilator management of ARDS is illustrated. ECMO, extracorporeal membrane oxygenation; $Fio_2$, fraction of inspired oxygen.

crystalloids and albumin is so small as to be undetectable and clinically insignificant. In contrast, use of starches in resuscitation results in adverse clinical outcomes. In patients with severe sepsis, the use of starch solutions increased renal failure resulted in more renal replacement therapy, lower platelet counts, more transfusion requirements, and a trend toward increased 90-day mortality.[134] Subsequent trials confirmed that the use of starch solutions increased the incidence of renal failure and death.[135,136] A subsequent multicenter open-labeled ICU trial in 2857 primarily septic patients evaluating the use of various colloids (1414 patients treated with gelatins, dextrans, hydroxyethyl starches, 4% or 20% of albumin) versus crystalloids (1443 patients) showed no difference in the prospective primary outcome of 28-day survival.[137]

Although crystalloids are widely used and recommended as the mainstay of fluid therapy in sepsis,[23] little is known about which particular crystalloid is better. Isotonic saline solutions can cause hyperchloremic metabolic acidosis and have been linked with increased kidney injury and possibly increased mortality when given in large doses to ICU patients.[138,139] Accordingly, there is increasing use of balanced salt solutions (eg, lactated Ringer, Hartmann solution, Plasmalyte) although they themselves have their own metabolic issues.[140] No robust randomized controlled trials have been conducted demonstrating significant differences in clinical outcomes between different crystalloid solutions.

### How Much Volume Resuscitation?

Recent early goal-directed therapy trials did not show any advantage to any particular fluid therapy or dosing. By conventional standards doses of fluid administered in these trials might be considered modest.[14,15,17] A multicenter randomized trial of 1000 mostly septic patients with ARDS evaluated conservative versus liberal fluid administration. The type of fluid (saline, Ringer, Plasmalyte, or albumin but no synthetic colloids) was left to the discretion of the treating physician, and furosemide administration was an important part of the protocol. The 60-day mortality was similar in the conservative versus the liberal groups (25.5% vs 28.4%). The conservative group had a very significantly smaller 7-day cumulative fluid balance ($-136 \pm 491$ mL vs $6992 \pm 502$ mL) compared with the liberal group. The conservative group had better oxygenation and spent significantly less time being ventilated and not in the ICU. Patients in the conservative fluid management group did not require more dialysis and did not have more episodes of shock, but they did have more minor metabolic abnormalities consistent with receiving less fluid and more furosemide.[141] More recently, post hoc analysis of the Vasopressin and Septic Shock Trial demonstrated that those patients who received volume resuscitation beyond the Surviving Sepsis Campaign guidelines had greatly increased mortality.[142] Although not definitive, these large studies highlight the problem of excessive fluid administration.

### Intravascular Volume Assessment

Fluid administration to restore intravascular volume and, consequently, adequate oxygen delivery has traditionally been seen as a major end point to optimal fluid administration.[143] At the same time, excessive administration of fluids past the first 6 hours of resuscitation might simply produce edema and increase complications.[141,143–145]

Determining which patients could potentially benefit from increased fluid administration is often difficult. Generally, multiple measurements should be considered ranging from clinical examination to sophisticated imaging. Clinical examination should assess tissue turgor, venous pressures, and end-organ function. Catheter-enabled venous pressure measurement is helpful when central venous pressures (CVPs) are very low (likely fluid responsive) or very high (not likely to be fluid responsive) but are often not informative for the wide range of intermediate CVP values (4–16 mm Hg). Arterial pressure measurement can be helpful. Variation in arterial pulse pressure with respiration suggests fluid responsiveness. In a related manner, changes in the amplitude of the pulse oximeter trace with respiration suggest possible fluid responsiveness. Similarly, echocardiographically measured changes in inferior vena caval diameter, and other central vein diameter,[146–151] with respiration suggests fluid responsiveness as does a positive response to a passive leg raising test.[146–152] Generally the assessment of adequacy of volume resuscitation should not be based on any one of these measures alone but rather on a consistent pattern involving multiple measures. Even more importantly, evidence suggesting volume responsiveness does not mean that additional volume should always be infused. If organ function is good and potential for significant adverse consequences exist, then further volume resuscitation may not be beneficial. Indeed, often a more useful perspective is to use these measures as evidence to stop further volume resuscitation.

## BLOOD TRANSFUSION

Recently the PROCESS and ARISE trials found no benefit of targeting an elevated hematocrit using blood transfusions during resuscitation of severe sepsis and septic shock.[14,15] The original Transfusion Requirements in Critical Care trial[153] and a recent validation[154] do not find benefit of transfusion more than a threshold of 7 g/dL in patients without myocardial ischemia, active bleeding, or severe hypoxemia.[23]

## Transfusion Threshold

Recently Holst and colleagues[154] evaluated transfusion thresholds of 7 g/dL or less versus 9 g/dL or less using prestorage leukocyte-depleted red cells in 1224 adult patients in septic shock. Patients were excluded for active coronary artery disease and severe bleeding but not for hemodynamic instability. Patients in the higher transfusion threshold group received 2 times as many units of blood. Mortality was no different (43% and 45%) in the low- and high-threshold groups. Ischemic events, other clinical outcomes, and mortality in prespecified subgroups (older patients, sicker patients, and those with cardiovascular disease) were no different between groups.[154] Another restrictive versus liberal transfusion trial of leukocyte-depleted blood studied 648 pediatric ICU patients and found no outcome differences.[155] About 50% of the randomized patients had systemic inflammatory response syndrome, 21% had sepsis, and 5% were in septic shock. With respect to the issue of coronary artery disease, a meta-analysis of 9 nonrandomized observational and 1 small randomized study found that blood transfusions increase mortality in anemic patients suffering from acute coronary disease.[156] In contrast, a small multicentric study of 110 patients evaluating restrictive versus liberal transfusion strategies in patients with active coronary disease did find that patients in the restrictive-treatment group had twice the composite end point of mortality, myocardial infarction, and unscheduled revacularization.[157] A 2012 Cochrane review of 19 randomized trials evaluating liberal versus restrictive transfusion strategies (only 3 of these were done in ICU patients[153,155,158]) found that, in patients without acute coronary artery disease and in the absence of active bleeding, hemoglobin levels of 7 to 8 g/dL are safe and effective at decreasing blood administration.[159]

## Leukodepletion of Blood Products/Age of Blood

Complications directly attributed to leukocytes in allogeneic blood transfusion include nonhemolytic febrile transfusion reactions, transmission of bacterial (*Yersinia enterocolitica*) and viral infections (cytomegalovirus [CMV], human herpes virus [HHV] 8, human T-lymphotropic virus I/II, and possibly other viruses), cytokine-mediated effects, HLA-alloimmunization and platelet transfusion refractoriness, transfusion-related immunomodulation, and graft-versus-host disease.[160–162] Decreases in surgical infection and even mortality have been attributed to leukoreduction, but the exact mechanisms whereby leukoreduction improves surgical outcomes are complex and unclear.[162–165] Transfusion-associated acute lung injury has also been associated with donor leukocytes.[160,161]

A recent randomized controlled trial examined the outcome of 1211 critically ill patients given blood 6.1 ± 4.9 days old versus 22.0 ± 8.4 days old. Mortality (37.0% and 35.3%) and all the secondary outcomes examined showed no differences.[18] Other large recent multicentric studies comparing the use of new versus old blood in cardiac surgery[166] and in premature very low birth weight infants[167] did not find any benefit to administering fresh blood.

## NUTRITION

Malnutrition has serious economic[168] and medical consequences, which include higher short-and long-term mortality.[169–171] Many patients with sepsis start off being malnourished,[59] and nutritional support during hospitalization is often inadequate.[172] Simply feeding patients without taking into consideration mobilization and exercise is suboptimal. An excellent recent review by Casaer and Van den Berghe[173] dissects the now large volume of clinical trials evaluating different types of feeding strategies in critically ill patients.

## Enteral Nutrition

Earlier and more aggressive nutritional administration may seem sensible, but the data do not clearly support it. A large trial of 1000 patients with ARDS compared trophic-feeding (400 kcal/d) with full-feeding (1300 kcal/d) and found no difference in any of the outcome measures studied except that those with more feeding vomited more, received more prokinetics and insulin, and had higher blood glucose values. Albumin and protein levels were similar in both groups.[174] This big trial is important because it is consistent with another large study showing no benefit[175] and because it contradicts previous smaller trials supporting hypocaloric nutrition[176–178] or higher caloric intake.[179–182] Mobilization and exercise generally have not been taken into consideration.

A multicentric trial comparing permissive underfeeding (40%–60% of caloric requirements) versus standard enteral feeding (70%–100% of caloric requirements) while maintaining equal protein dosage (1.2–1.5 g per kilogram of body weight per day) in 894 critically ill mostly ventilated patients (96.7%) was recently published. Roughly 30% of patients were admitted with severe sepsis. The study protocol provided suggestions on the selection of enteral formulas, but the decision was left to the clinical team. Study centers used their own insulin protocols, with a target blood glucose level of 4.4 to 10.0 mmol/L (80–180 mg/dL) in both groups. The 90-day mortality (primary end point) was 27.2% (permissive-underfeeding group) versus 28.9% (standard-feeding group). ICU mortality, in-hospital mortality, and 28-day mortality or 180-day mortality were all similar. Serial SOFA scores, nitrogen balance, body weight, multiple markers of nutrition status, the number of days free from mechanical ventilation, and the number of ICU-free days did not differ significantly between the two. In addition, there were no significant between-group differences with respect to hypoglycemia, hypokalemia, hypomagnesemia, hypophosphatemia, transfusion of packed red cells, ICU-acquired infections, diarrhea, or feeding intolerance. Post hoc analysis showed that incident renal-replacement therapy was required less frequently in the permissive-underfeeding group than in the standard-feeding group (7.1% vs 11.4%). Patients in the permissive-underfeeding group had lower blood glucose levels and reduced insulin requirements but no evidence of decreased protein catabolism.[183]

### Gastric Residuals

Using gastric residuals to guide use of tube feeding does not prevent complications or improve outcomes but does decrease the amount of feedings administered.[184,185] One study compared no gastric measurements at all versus using 250 mL of residue as a cutoff,[185] whereas the other compared gastric residuals of 200 mL and 500 mL as determinants of feeding. Erythromycin has been shown to be a better prokinetic than metoclopramide, but both treatments wane in efficacy with time; refractory patients to either treatments tend to respond when both are administered together.[186]

### Parenteral Nutritional Support

A large study of more than 4600 critically ill patients evaluated the use of early parenteral nutrition with progressive enteral feeding versus late parenteral feeding with progressive tube feeding and found that patients who received parenteral nutrition early had more infections and spent more time on a ventilator and in the ICU. Six-minute walk tests done just before discharge were similar. Post hoc subgroup analyses showed surgical patients fare particularly worse with early parenteral nutrition. All the patients in this trial had aggressive glucose control.[187] Other studies have also failed to show a benefit of early parenteral nutrition.[173]

In 2014, the CALORIES Trial reported the randomization of 2400 critically ill but previously not malnourished patients into a group receiving parenteral nutrition and a comparator group receiving enteral nutrition. Feeding was started at day 3 in both groups. Mortality at 30 days (33% vs 34%) was similar, and most of the secondary outcomes except for vomiting and hypoglycemia were also similar. Tight glycemic control was not used.[188]

## VIRAL REACTIVATION

Over the past few years numerous studies, based on downregulating the host proinflammatory response (anti–tumor necrosis factor, interleukin 1 receptor antagonist, and so forth), have repeatedly failed to alter outcomes. Because of these multiple clinical trial failures many have questioned preconceived notions and concepts regarding sepsis and sepsis-related multiple organ dysfunction syndrome (MODS).[189–195]

Hotchkiss and colleagues[196] recently postulated that patients suffering from sepsis not only exhibited many of the signs of immunosuppression but that this immune state could also be implicated in many subsequent disease processes, including ongoing unresolved infections, infection with relatively nonvirulent pathogens, and reactivation of certain viruses like CMV and herpes simplex virus (HSV). Hotchkiss and Moldawer[197] noted that many of the mechanisms operating in sepsis are also present in oncology. They speculated that monitoring of septic and oncological immune function could potentially be evaluated by looking at viral reactivation. Stimulation of the immune system as done with various cancers like melanoma, renal carcinoma and non–small cell lung cancer could prove to be beneficial in patients with immune depression secondary to sepsis.[197] In a trial comparing viral reactivation in critically ill septic patients, critically ill nonseptic patients, and healthy patients, critically ill septic patients had frequent quantitative-polymerase-chain-reaction confirmation of reactivation of CMV, Epstein-Barr (EBV), HSV, HHV-6, and TTV (transfusion tansmitted virus) as well as Polyomaviruses BK and JC in urine compared with matched nonseptic ICU controls and healthy individuals. Viremia seemed to be a risk factor for opportunistic infections, and it also progressed with time. Viremia with CMV, EBV, HSV, and HHV-6 was associated with higher SOFA scores; patients with CMV viral reactivation had significantly higher 90-day mortality. The mechanisms by which viruses are able to reactivate are not clear, but immunosuppression may be an important contributor. Conceivably high viral loads are a contributing factor to patients developing MODS, but this study cannot differentiate whether viremia is a cause of MODS and death or simply a marker of severity of illness.[198]

Interestingly and maybe simply coincidentally, the previously mentioned viral reactivation study found viral reactivation to approximately start when MODS often develops. As the investigators point out, it is impossible to know whether reactivated viruses represent an epiphenomenon or contribute to MODS and mortality. Using information learned from patients intentionally immunosuppressed for various organ transplants, we know that biopsies of various presumably affected organs frequently confirmed causality of viral infection to specific organ dysfunction.[199,200] Critically ill patients traditionally thought to not be immunocompromised have often been shown to have CMV colitis on colonic biopsy. This finding in itself is a paradigm shift in our understanding of disease patterns in the ICU.[201] Septic patients dying in the ICU have also been

---

**Box 1**
**Recommendations for clinical practice**

*Agitation and delirium*

Recognition is key, often enabled by the use of protocolized care bundles (see **Table 1**).

Minimize use of sedatives, particularly benzodiazepines.

Adapt ICU environment to maximize natural nocturnal sleep.

Increase mobilization and exercise.

Use the patients' eyeglasses and hearing aids.

*Mechanical ventilation*

For controlled mechanical ventilation use tidal volumes of 6 mL/kg lean body mass.

Maintain inspiratory plateau pressures less than 30 cm $H_2O$.

Measurement of esophageal pressure should be considered in obese patients to calculate transpulmonary pressure when setting PEEP levels.

Use daily SBTs.

NPPV should be considered for specific indications.

*Fluid resuscitation*

Starch-based colloid solutions should not be used.

Balanced salt solutions (eg, lactated Ringer, Hartmann solution, Plasmalyte) reduce the incidence of hyperchloremic metabolic acidosis and may improve renal function.

Early aggressive fluid resuscitation is usefully driven by resuscitation protocols.

Assessment of volemia soon after initial fluid resuscitation is essential to avoid unnecessary additional fluid resuscitation and volume overload.

Volemia may be assessed using a combination of clinical examination (organ function, such as urine output, jugular venous pressure), static pressure measurement (CVP, pulmonary capillary wedge pressure), dynamic measurements (blood pressure response to passive leg raising, pulse pressure variation, inferior vena caval diameter variation using goal-directed echocardiography, and so forth), and direct flow measurements (thermodilution cardiac output and other devices).

*Blood transfusion*

Given the evidence, the authors favor transfusing leukocyte-depleted red blood cells of any reasonable age to septic patients with a hemoglobin less than 7.

*Nutrition*

There is no clear evidence that early institution of nutrition is beneficial.

shown to have biochemical, flow cytometric, and immunohistochemical findings consistent with immunosuppression on autopsy findings performed rapidly after death.[202]

Again none of the aforementioned observations prove causality, but the authors think these observations are important and that this could be a promising area for future research.

## SUMMARY

Following initial resuscitation of sepsis and septic shock, outcomes improve with attention to several key features. These features include recognition of PAD and treatment with reduced use of sedatives coupled with increased patient engagement, mobilization, and exercise (**Box 1**). Use of low tidal volumes and low mean airway pressures during mechanical ventilation are helpful. A key hemodynamic principle following early aggressive volume resuscitation is subsequent careful assessment to avoid unnecessary additional volume administration and the adverse consequences of frank volume overload. Substantial evidence now supports a lower hemoglobin transfusion threshold of 7 g/dL. Nutrition is important, but a rush to initiate enteral or parenteral feeds is not clearly supported by the current evidence. Following the initial septic inflammatory response, immune function is profoundly altered, which increases susceptibility to an array of persistent viral infections.

## REFERENCES

1. Milbrandt EB, Kersten A, Rahim MT, et al. Growth of intensive care unit resource use and its estimated cost in Medicare. Crit Care Med 2008;36(9): 2504–10.
2. Daniels R. Surviving the first hours in sepsis: getting the basics right (an intensivist's perspective). J Antimicrob Chemother 2011;66(Suppl 2):ii11–23.
3. Kaukonen K-M, Bailey M, Suzuki S, et al. Mortality related to severe sepsis and septic shock among critically ill patients in Australia and New Zealand, 2000-2012. JAMA 2014;311(13):1308–9.
4. Lindenauer PK, Lagu T, Shieh M-S, et al. Association of diagnostic coding with trends in hospitalizations and mortality of patients with pneumonia, 2003-2009. JAMA 2012;307(13):1405–13.
5. Hall WB, Willis LE, Medvedev S, et al. The implications of long-term acute care hospital transfer practices for measures of in-hospital mortality and length of stay. Am J Respir Crit Care Med 2012; 185(1):53–7.
6. Lagu T, Rothberg MB, Shieh M-S, et al. Hospitalizations, costs, and outcomes of severe sepsis in the United States 2003 to 2007. Crit Care Med 2012; 40(3):754–61.
7. Khandelwal N, Kross EK, Engelberg RA, et al. Estimating the effect of palliative care interventions and advance care planning on ICU utilization: a systematic review. Crit Care Med 2015;43(5): 1102–11.
8. Stevenson EK, Rubenstein AR, Radin GT, et al. Two decades of mortality trends among patients with severe sepsis: a comparative meta-analysis* Crit Care Med 2014;42(3):625–31.
9. Levy MM, Rhodes A, Phillips GS, et al. Surviving sepsis campaign. Crit Care Med 2015;43(1):3–12.
10. Ventilation with lower tidal volumes as compared with traditional tidal volumes for acute lung injury and the acute respiratory distress syndrome. The Acute Respiratory Distress Syndrome Network. N Engl J Med 2000;342(18):1301–8.
11. Girard TD, Kress JP, Fuchs BD, et al. Efficacy and safety of a paired sedation and ventilator weaning protocol for mechanically ventilated patients in intensive care (Awakening and Breathing Controlled trial): a randomised controlled trial. Lancet 2008;371(9607):126–34.
12. Rivers E, Nguyen B, Havstad S, et al. Early goal-directed therapy in the treatment of severe sepsis and septic shock. N Engl J Med 2001;345(19): 1368–77.
13. Bernard GR, Vincent JL, Laterre PF, et al. Efficacy and safety of recombinant human activated protein C for severe sepsis. N Engl J Med 2001;344(10): 699–709.
14. The ProCESS Investigators. A randomized trial of protocol-based care for early septic shock. N Engl J Med 2014;370(18):1683–93.
15. ARISE Investigators, ANZICS Clinical Trials Group, Peake SL, et al. Goal-directed resuscitation for patients with early septic shock. N Engl J Med 2014; 371(16):1496–506.
16. Asfar P, Meziani F, Hamel J-F, et al. High versus low blood-pressure target in patients with septic shock. N Engl J Med 2014;370(17):1583–93.
17. Mouncey PR, Osborn TM, Power GS, et al. Trial of early, goal-directed resuscitation for septic shock. N Engl J Med 2015;372(14):1301–11.
18. Lacroix J, Hébert PC, Fergusson DA, et al. Age of transfused blood in critically ill adults. N Engl J Med 2015;372(15):1410–8.
19. Russell JA, Walley KR, Singer J, et al. Vasopressin versus norepinephrine infusion in patients with septic shock. N Engl J Med 2008;358(9):877–87.
20. Abraham E, Laterre P-F, Garg R, et al. Drotrecogin alfa (activated) for adults with severe sepsis and a low risk of death. N Engl J Med 2005;353(13): 1332–41.
21. Nadel S, Goldstein B, Williams MD, et al. Drotrecogin alfa (activated) in children with severe sepsis: a

multicentre phase III randomised controlled trial. Lancet 2007;369(9564):836–43.

22. Barr J, Fraser GL, Puntillo K, et al. Clinical practice guidelines for the management of pain, agitation, and delirium in adult patients in the intensive care unit. Crit Care Med 2013;263–306.

23. Dellinger RP, Levy MM, Rhodes A, et al. Surviving Sepsis Campaign: international guidelines for management of severe sepsis and septic shock: 2012. Crit Care Med 2013;41(2):580–637.

24. Brummel NE, Girard TD. Preventing delirium in the intensive care unit. Crit Care Clin 2013;29(1): 51–65.

25. Marik PE, Kaplan D. Aspiration pneumonia and dysphagia in the elderly. Chest 2003;124(1): 328–36.

26. Jacobi J, Fraser GL, Coursin DB, et al. Clinical practice guidelines for the sustained use of sedatives and analgesics in the critically ill adult. Crit Care Med 2002;30(1):119–41.

27. Barr J, Kishman CP, Jaeschke R. The methodological approach used to develop the 2013 pain, agitation, and delirium clinical practice guidelines for adult ICU patients. Crit Care Med 2013;41(9 Suppl 1):S1–15.

28. Reade MC, Finfer S. Sedation and delirium in the intensive care unit. N Engl J Med 2014;370(5): 444–54.

29. Kuchinski J, Tinkoff G, Rhodes M, et al. Emergency intubation for paralysis of the uncooperative trauma patient. J Emerg Med 1991;9(1–2):9–12.

30. Morrison RS, Siu AL. Survival in end-stage dementia following acute illness. JAMA 2000; 284(1):47–52.

31. Ely EW, Gautam S, Margolin R, et al. The impact of delirium in the intensive care unit on hospital length of stay. Intensive Care Med 2001;27(12):1892–900.

32. Ely EW, Shintani A, Truman B, et al. Delirium as a predictor of mortality in mechanically ventilated patients in the intensive care unit. JAMA 2004; 291(14):1753–62.

33. Muakkassa FF, Marley RA, Workman MC, et al. Hospital outcomes and disposition of trauma patients who are intubated because of combativeness. J Trauma 2010;68(6):1305–9.

34. Girard TD, Jackson JC, Pandharipande PP, et al. Delirium as a predictor of long-term cognitive impairment in survivors of critical illness. Crit Care Med 2010;38(7):1513–20.

35. Lin S-M, Liu C-Y, Wang C-H, et al. The impact of delirium on the survival of mechanically ventilated patients. Crit Care Med 2004;32(11):2254–9.

36. Myhren H, Ekeberg O, Tøien K, et al. Posttraumatic stress, anxiety and depression symptoms in patients during the first year post intensive care unit discharge. Crit Care 2010; 14(1):R14.

37. Stein-Parbury J, McKinley S. Patients' experiences of being in an intensive care unit: a select literature review. Am J Crit Care 2000;9(1):20–7.

38. Hall JB, Schweickert W, Kress JP. Role of analgesics, sedatives, neuromuscular blockers, and delirium. Crit Care Med 2009;37(Suppl 10): S416–21.

39. Jones C, Griffiths RD, Humphris G, et al. Memory, delusions, and the development of acute posttraumatic stress disorder-related symptoms after intensive care. Crit Care Med 2001;29(3): 573–80.

40. Vincent J-L, Norrenberg M. Intensive care unit-acquired weakness: framing the topic. Crit Care Med 2009;37(Suppl 10):S296–8.

41. Iwashyna TJ, Ely EW, Smith DM, et al. Long-term cognitive impairment and functional disability among survivors of severe sepsis. JAMA 2010; 304(16):1787–94.

42. Ehlenbach WJ, Hough CL, Crane PK, et al. Association between acute care and critical illness hospitalization and cognitive function in older adults. JAMA 2010;303(8):763–70.

43. Tate JA, Snitz BE, Alvarez KA, et al. Infection hospitalization increases risk of dementia in the elderly. Crit Care Med 2014;42(5):1037–46.

44. Shah FA, Pike F, Alvarez K, et al. Bidirectional relationship between cognitive function and pneumonia. Am J Respir Crit Care Med 2013;188(5): 586–92.

45. Pisani MA, Kong SYJ, Kasl SV, et al. Days of delirium are associated with 1-year mortality in an older intensive care unit population. Am J Respir Crit Care Med 2009;180(11):1092–7.

46. Pandharipande PP, Girard TD, Jackson JC, et al. Long-term cognitive impairment after critical illness. N Engl J Med 2013;369(14):1306–16.

47. Inouye SK, Westendorp RGJ, Saczynski JS. Delirium in elderly people. Lancet 2014;383(9920): 911–22.

48. Milbrandt EB, Angus DC. Bench-to-bedside review: critical illness-associated cognitive dysfunction–mechanisms, markers, and emerging therapeutics. Crit Care 2006;10(6):238.

49. Campbell NL, Khan BA, Farber M, et al. Improving delirium care in the intensive care unit: the design of a pragmatic study. Trials 2011;12(1):139.

50. Skrobik Y, Chanques G. The pain, agitation, and delirium practice guidelines for adult critically ill patients: a post-publication perspective. Ann Intensive Care 2013;3(1):9.

51. Gunther ML, Morandi A, Krauskopf E, et al. The association between brain volumes, delirium duration, and cognitive outcomes in intensive care unit survivors: the VISIONS cohort magnetic resonance imaging study*. Crit Care Med 2012;40(7): 2022–32.

52. Morandi A, Rogers BP, Gunther ML, et al. The relationship between delirium duration, white matter integrity, and cognitive impairment in intensive care unit survivors as determined by diffusion tensor imaging: the VISIONS prospective cohort magnetic resonance imaging study*. Crit Care Med 2012;40(7):2182–9.

53. Levy MM, Dellinger RP, Townsend SR, et al. The Surviving Sepsis Campaign: results of an international guideline-based performance improvement program targeting severe sepsis. Crit Care Med 2010;38(2):367–74.

54. Bailey P, Thomsen GE, Spuhler VJ, et al. Early activity is feasible and safe in respiratory failure patients. Crit Care Med 2007;35(1):139–45.

55. Schweickert WD, Pohlman MC, Pohlman AS, et al. Early physical and occupational therapy in mechanically ventilated, critically ill patients: a randomised controlled trial. Lancet 2009;373(9678):1874–82.

56. Needham DM. Mobilizing patients in the intensive care unit: improving neuromuscular weakness and physical function. JAMA 2008; 300(14):1685–90.

57. Pandharipande P, Shintani A, Peterson J, et al. Lorazepam is an independent risk factor for transitioning to delirium in intensive care unit patients. Anesthesiology 2006;104(1):21–6.

58. Van Rompaey B, Elseviers MM, Van Drom W, et al. The effect of earplugs during the night on the onset of delirium and sleep perception: a randomized controlled trial in intensive care patients. Crit Care 2012;16(3):R73.

59. Singh H, Watt K, Veitch R, et al. Malnutrition is prevalent in hospitalized medical patients: are house staff identifying the malnourished patient? Nutrition 2006;22(4):350–4.

60. Reid CL, Campbell IT, Little RA. Muscle wasting and energy balance in critical illness. Clin Nutr 2004;23(2):273–80.

61. De Jonghe B, Bastuji-Garin S, Durand M-C, et al. Respiratory weakness is associated with limb weakness and delayed weaning in critical illness. Crit Care Med 2007;35(9):2007–15.

62. Weijs PJM. Fundamental determinants of protein requirements in the ICU. Curr Opin Clin Nutr Metab Care 2014;17(2):183–9.

63. Needham DM, Korupolu R, Zanni JM, et al. Early physical medicine and rehabilitation for patients with acute respiratory failure: a quality improvement project. Arch Phys Med Rehabil 2010;91(4): 536–42.

64. Kress JP, Pohlman AS, O'Connor MF, et al. Daily interruption of sedative infusions in critically ill patients undergoing mechanical ventilation. N Engl J Med 2000;342(20):1471–7.

65. Dellinger RP, Carlet JM, Masur H, et al. Surviving Sepsis Campaign guidelines for management of severe sepsis and septic shock. Crit Care Med 2004;32(3):858–73.

66. Morandi A, Brummel NE, Ely EW. Sedation delirium and mechanical ventilation: the "ABCDE" approach. Curr Opin Crit Care 2011;17(1):43–9.

67. Mehta S, Burry L, Cook D, et al. Daily sedation interruption in mechanically ventilated critically ill patients cared for with a sedation protocol: a randomized controlled trial. JAMA 2012;308(19): 1985–92.

68. Tanios MA, de Wit M, Epstein SK, et al. Perceived barriers to the use of sedation protocols and daily sedation interruption: a multidisciplinary survey. J Crit Care 2009;24(1):66–73.

69. Roberts RJ, de Wit M, Epstein SK, et al. Predictors for daily interruption of sedation therapy by nurses: a prospective, multicenter study. J Crit Care 2010; 25(4):660.e1–7.

70. Mehta S, Burry L, Fischer S, et al. Canadian survey of the use of sedatives, analgesics, and neuromuscular blocking agents in critically ill patients. Crit Care Med 2006;34(2):374–80.

71. Patel RP, Gambrell M, Speroff T, et al. Delirium and sedation in the intensive care unit: survey of behaviors and attitudes of 1384 healthcare professionals. Crit Care Med 2009;37(3):825–32.

72. Martin J, Franck M, Sigel S, et al. Changes in sedation management in German intensive care units between 2002 and 2006: a national follow-up survey. Crit Care 2007;11(6):R124.

73. Devlin JW, Tanios MA, Epstein SK. Intensive care unit sedation: waking up clinicians to the gap between research and practice. Crit Care Med 2006;34(2):556–7.

74. Augustes R, Ho KM. Meta-analysis of randomised controlled trials on daily sedation interruption for critically ill adult patients. Anaesth Intensive Care 2011;39(3):401–9.

75. Strøm T, Martinussen T, Toft P. A protocol of no sedation for critically ill patients receiving mechanical ventilation: a randomised trial. Lancet 2010; 375(9713):475–80.

76. Roberts DJ, Haroon B, Hall RI. Sedation for critically ill or injured adults in the intensive care unit: a shifting paradigm. Drugs 2012;72(14):1881–916.

77. Riker RR, Shehabi Y, Bokesch PM, et al. Dexmedetomidine vs midazolam for sedation of critically ill patients: a randomized trial. JAMA 2009;301(5): 489–99.

78. Pandharipande PP, Pun BT, Herr DL, et al. Effect of sedation with dexmedetomidine vs lorazepam on acute brain dysfunction in mechanically ventilated patients: the MENDS randomized controlled trial. JAMA 2007;298(22):2644–53.

79. Jakob SM, Ruokonen E, Grounds RM, et al. Dexmedetomidine vs midazolam or propofol for sedation during prolonged mechanical

ventilation: two randomized controlled trials. JAMA 2012;307(11):1151–60.

80. Li B, Wang H, Wu H, et al. Neurocognitive dysfunction risk alleviation with the use of dexmedetomidine in perioperative conditions or as ICU sedation: a meta-analysis. Medicine (Baltimore) 2015;94(14):e597.

81. Parke TJ, Stevens JE, Rice AS, et al. Metabolic acidosis and fatal myocardial failure after propofol infusion in children. five case reports. BMJ 1992; 305(6854):613–6.

82. Bray RJ. Propofol infusion syndrome in children. Paediatr Anaesth 1998;8(6):491–9.

83. Vasile B, Rasulo F, Candiani A, et al. The pathophysiology of propofol infusion syndrome: a simple name for a complex syndrome. Intensive Care Med 2003;29(9):1417–25.

84. Schroeppel TJ, Fabian TC, Clement LP, et al. Propofol infusion syndrome: a lethal condition in critically injured patients eliminated by a simple screening protocol. Injury 2014;45(1): 245–9.

85. Kam PCA, Cardone D. Propofol infusion syndrome. Anaesthesia 2007;62(7):690–701.

86. Ahlen K, Buckley CJ, Goodale DB, et al. The "propofol infusion syndrome": the facts, their interpretation and implications for patient care. Eur J Anaesthesiol 2006;23(12):990–8.

87. Wong JM. Propofol infusion syndrome. Am J Ther 2010;17(5):487–91.

88. Hirota T, Kishi T. Prophylactic antipsychotic use for postoperative delirium: a systematic review and meta-analysis. J Clin Psychiatry 2013;74(12): e1136–44.

89. Joffe AM, Coursin DB, Coursin DR. Why all the confusion about confusion? Crit Care Med 2010; 38(2):695–6.

90. Hatta K, Takahashi T, Nakamura H, et al. The association between intravenous haloperidol and prolonged QT interval. J Clin Psychopharmacol 2001;21(3):257–61.

91. Hassaballa HA, Balk RA. Torsade de pointes associated with the administration of intravenous haloperidol: a review of the literature and practical guidelines for use. Expert Opin Drug Saf 2003; 2(6):543–7.

92. Sharma ND, Rosman HS, Padhi ID, et al. Torsades de pointes associated with intravenous haloperidol in critically ill patients. Am J Cardiol 1998;81(2): 238–40.

93. U.S. Food and Drug Administration. Haloperidol labeling updated. React Wkly 2007;1170(1):2.

94. Muzyk AJ, Rivelli SK, Jiang W, et al. A computerized physician order entry set designed to improve safety of intravenous haloperidol utilization: a retrospective study in agitated hospitalized patients. Drug Saf 2012;35(9):725–31.

95. Bourne RS, Mills GH. Melatonin: possible implications for the postoperative and critically ill patient. Intensive Care Med 2006;32(3):371–9.

96. Bellapart J, Boots R. Potential use of melatonin in sleep and delirium in the critically ill. Br J Anaesth 2012;108(4):572–80.

97. Al-Aama T, Brymer C, Gutmanis I, et al. Melatonin decreases delirium in elderly patients: a randomized, placebo-controlled trial. Int J Geriatr Psychiatry 2011;26(7):687–94.

98. de Jonghe A, van Munster BC, Goslings JC, et al. Effect of melatonin on incidence of delirium among patients with hip fracture: a multicentre, double-blind randomized controlled trial. CMAJ 2014; 186(14):E547–56.

99. Simpson D, Curran MP. Ramelteon: a review of its use in insomnia. Drugs 2008;68(13):1901–19.

100. Perkisas SMT, Vandewoude MFJ. Ramelteon for prevention of delirium in hospitalized older patients. JAMA 2015;313(17):1745–6.

101. Gajic O, Dara SI, Mendez JL, et al. Ventilator-associated lung injury in patients without acute lung injury at the onset of mechanical ventilation. Crit Care Med 2004;32(9):1817–24.

102. Yilmaz M, Keegan MT, Iscimen R, et al. Toward the prevention of acute lung injury: protocol-guided limitation of large tidal volume ventilation and inappropriate transfusion. Crit Care Med 2007; 35(7):1660–6 [quiz: 1667].

103. Determann RM, Royakkers A, Wolthuis EK, et al. Ventilation with lower tidal volumes as compared with conventional tidal volumes for patients without acute lung injury: a preventive randomized controlled trial. Crit Care 2010;14(1):R1.

104. Schultz MJ. Lung-protective mechanical ventilation with lower tidal volumes in patients not suffering from acute lung injury: a review of clinical studies. Med Sci Monit 2008;14(2):RA22–6.

105. Petrucci N, De Feo C. Lung protective ventilation strategy for the acute respiratory distress syndrome. Cochrane Database Syst Rev 2013;(2):CD003844.

106. Aldenkortt M, Lysakowski C, Elia N, et al. Ventilation strategies in obese patients undergoing surgery: a quantitative systematic review and meta-analysis. Br J Anaesth 2012;109(4):493–502.

107. Esteban A, Frutos F, Tobin MJ, et al. A comparison of four methods of weaning patients from mechanical ventilation. Spanish Lung Failure Collaborative Group. N Engl J Med 1995;332(6):345–50.

108. Ely EW, Baker AM, Dunagan DP, et al. Effect on the duration of mechanical ventilation of identifying patients capable of breathing spontaneously. N Engl J Med 1996;335(25):1864–9.

109. Brochard L, Mancebo J, Wysocki M, et al. Noninvasive ventilation for acute exacerbations of chronic obstructive pulmonary disease. N Engl J Med 1995;333(13):817–22.

110. Meduri GU. Noninvasive positive-pressure ventilation in patients with acute respiratory failure. Clin Chest Med 1996;17(3):513–53.

111. Keenan SP, Kernerman PD, Cook DJ, et al. Effect of noninvasive positive pressure ventilation on mortality in patients admitted with acute respiratory failure: a meta-analysis. Crit Care Med 1997;25(10):1685–92.

112. Antonelli M, Conti G, Rocco M, et al. A comparison of noninvasive positive-pressure ventilation and conventional mechanical ventilation in patients with acute respiratory failure. N Engl J Med 1998; 339(7):429–35.

113. Plant PK, Owen JL, Elliott MW. Early use of non-invasive ventilation for acute exacerbations of chronic obstructive pulmonary disease on general respiratory wards: a multicentre randomised controlled trial. Lancet 2000;355(9219):1931–5.

114. Levy M, Tanios MA, Nelson D, et al. Outcomes of patients with do-not-intubate orders treated with noninvasive ventilation. Crit Care Med 2004; 32(10):2002–7.

115. Wysocki M, Tric L, Wolff MA, et al. Noninvasive pressure support ventilation in patients with acute respiratory failure. A randomized comparison with conventional therapy. Chest 1995;107(3):761–8.

116. Barbé F, Togores B, Rubí M, et al. Noninvasive ventilatory support does not facilitate recovery from acute respiratory failure in chronic obstructive pulmonary disease. Eur Respir J 1996;9(6):1240–5.

117. Esteban A, Frutos-Vivar F, Ferguson ND, et al. Noninvasive positive-pressure ventilation for respiratory failure after extubation. N Engl J Med 2004; 350(24):2452–60.

118. Keenan SP, Sinuff T, Cook DJ, et al. Does noninvasive positive pressure ventilation improve outcome in acute hypoxemic respiratory failure? A systematic review. Crit Care Med 2004;32(12):2516–23.

119. Lemiale V, Resche-Rigon M, Azoulay E, Study Group for Respiratory Intensive Care in Malignancies Groupe de Recherche en Réanimation Respiratoire du patient d'Onco-Hématologie. Early non-invasive ventilation for acute respiratory failure in immunocompromised patients (IVNIctus): study protocol for a multicenter randomized controlled trial. Trials 2014;15(1):372.

120. Winck JC, Azevedo LF, Costa-Pereira A, et al. Efficacy and safety of non-invasive ventilation in the treatment of acute cardiogenic pulmonary edema–a systematic review and meta-analysis. Crit Care 2006;10(2):R69.

121. Nava S, Hill N. Non-invasive ventilation in acute respiratory failure. Lancet 2009;374(9685):250–9.

122. Hilbert G, Gruson D, Vargas F, et al. Noninvasive ventilation in immunosuppressed patients with pulmonary infiltrates, fever, and acute respiratory failure. N Engl J Med 2001;344(7):481–7.

123. Antonelli M, Conti G, Bufi M, et al. Noninvasive ventilation for treatment of acute respiratory failure in patients undergoing solid organ transplantation: a randomized trial. JAMA 2000;283(2):235–41.

124. Ambrosino N, Vagheggini G. Noninvasive positive pressure ventilation in the acute care setting: where are we? Eur Respir J 2008;31(4):874–86.

125. Burns KEA, Meade MO, Premji A, et al. Noninvasive positive-pressure ventilation as a weaning strategy for intubated adults with respiratory failure. Cochrane Database Syst Rev 2013;(12):CD004127.

126. Lim WJ, Mohammed Akram R, Carson KV, et al. Non-invasive positive pressure ventilation for treatment of respiratory failure due to severe acute exacerbations of asthma. Cochrane Database Syst Rev 2012;(12):CD004360.

127. Lightowler JV, Wedzicha JA, Elliott MW, et al. Non-invasive positive pressure ventilation to treat respiratory failure resulting from exacerbations of chronic obstructive pulmonary disease: Cochrane systematic review and meta-analysis. BMJ 2003; 326(7382):185.

128. Confalonieri M, Potena A, Carbone G, et al. Acute respiratory failure in patients with severe community-acquired pneumonia. A prospective randomized evaluation of noninvasive ventilation. Am J Respir Crit Care Med 1999;160(5 Pt 1):1585–91.

129. Antonelli M, Conti G, Moro ML, et al. Predictors of failure of noninvasive positive pressure ventilation in patients with acute hypoxemic respiratory failure: a multi-center study. Intensive Care Med 2001; 27(11):1718–28.

130. Rana S, Jenad H, Gay PC, et al. Failure of non-invasive ventilation in patients with acute lung injury: observational cohort study. Crit Care 2006; 10(3):R79.

131. Finfer S, Bellomo R, Boyce N, et al. A comparison of albumin and saline for fluid resuscitation in the intensive care unit. N Engl J Med 2004;350(22):2247–56.

132. SAFE Study Investigators, Finfer S, McEvoy S, et al. Impact of albumin compared to saline on organ function and mortality of patients with severe sepsis. Intensive Care Med 2011;37(1):86–96.

133. Caironi P, Tognoni G, Masson S, et al. Albumin replacement in patients with severe sepsis or septic shock. N Engl J Med 2014;370(15):1412–21.

134. Brunkhorst FM, Engel C, Bloos F, et al. Intensive insulin therapy and pentastarch resuscitation in severe sepsis. N Engl J Med 2008;358(2):125–39.

135. Perner A, Haase N, Guttormsen AB, et al. Hydroxyethyl starch 130/0.42 versus Ringer's acetate in severe sepsis. N Engl J Med 2012;367(2):124–34.

36. Myburgh JA, Finfer S, Bellomo R, et al. Hydroxyethyl starch or saline for fluid resuscitation in intensive care. N Engl J Med 2012;367(20):1901–11.

37. Annane D, Siami S, Jaber S, et al. Effects of fluid resuscitation with colloids vs crystalloids on mortality in critically ill patients presenting with hypovolemic shock: the CRISTAL randomized trial. JAMA 2013;310(17):1809–17.

38. Yunos NM, Bellomo R, Hegarty C, et al. Association between a chloride-liberal vs chloride-restrictive intravenous fluid administration strategy and kidney injury in critically ill adults. JAMA 2012; 308(15):1566–72.

39. Raghunathan K, Shaw A, Nathanson B, et al. Association between the choice of IV crystalloid and in-hospital mortality among critically ill adults with sepsis*. Crit Care Med 2014;42(7): 1585–91.

40. Guidet B, Soni N, Rocca Della G, et al. A balanced view of balanced solutions. Crit Care 2010;14(5):325.

41. National Heart, Lung, and Blood Institute, Acute Respiratory Distress Syndrome (ARDS) Clinical Trials Network, Wiedemann HP, et al. Comparison of two fluid-management strategies in acute lung injury. N Engl J Med 2006;354(24): 2564–75.

42. Boyd JH, Forbes J, Nakada T-A, et al. Fluid resuscitation in septic shock: a positive fluid balance and elevated central venous pressure are associated with increased mortality. Crit Care Med 2011;39(2):259–65.

143. Finfer SR, Vincent J-L, De Backer D. Circulatory shock. N Engl J Med 2013;369(18):1726–34.

144. Myburgh JA. Fluid resuscitation in acute medicine: what is the current situation? J Intern Med 2015; 277(1):58–68.

145. Myburgh JA, Mythen MG. Resuscitation fluids. N Engl J Med 2013;369(13):1243–51.

146. Via G, Price S, Storti E. Echocardiography in the sepsis syndromes. Crit Ultrasound J 2011;3(2): 71–85.

147. Via G, Hussain A, Wells M, et al. International evidence-based recommendations for focused cardiac ultrasound. J Am Soc Echocardiogr 2014; 27(7):683.e1–33.

148. Vieillard-Baron A, Prin S, Chergui K, et al. Hemodynamic instability in sepsis: bedside assessment by Doppler echocardiography. Am J Respir Crit Care Med 2003;168(11):1270–6.

149. Arntfield RT, Millington SJ. Point of care cardiac ultrasound applications in the emergency department and intensive care unit–a review. Curr Cardiol Rev 2012;8(2):98–108.

150. Jones AE, Tayal VS, Sullivan DM, et al. Randomized, controlled trial of immediate versus delayed goal-directed ultrasound to identify the cause of nontraumatic hypotension in emergency department patients. Crit Care Med 2004;32(8):1703–8.

151. Marcelino PA, Marum SM, Fernandes APM, et al. Routine transthoracic echocardiography in a general intensive care unit: an 18 month survey in 704 patients. Eur J Intern Med 2009;20(3):e37–42.

152. Cavallaro F, Sandroni C, Marano C, et al. Diagnostic accuracy of passive leg raising for prediction of fluid responsiveness in adults: systematic review and meta-analysis of clinical studies. Intensive Care Med 2010;36(9):1475–83.

153. Hébert PC, Wells G, Blajchman MA, et al. A multicenter, randomized, controlled clinical trial of transfusion requirements in critical care. Transfusion requirements in critical care investigators, Canadian Critical Care Trials Group. N Engl J Med 1999;340(6):409–17.

154. Holst LB, Haase N, Wetterslev J, et al. Lower versus higher hemoglobin threshold for transfusion in septic shock. N Engl J Med 2014; 371(15):1381–91.

155. Lacroix J, Hébert PC, Hutchison JS, et al. Transfusion strategies for patients in pediatric intensive care units. N Engl J Med 2007;356(16):1609–19.

156. Chatterjee S, Wetterslev J, Sharma A, et al. Association of blood transfusion with increased mortality in myocardial infarction: a meta-analysis and diversity-adjusted study sequential analysis. JAMA Intern Med 2013;173(2):132–9.

157. Carson JL, Brooks MM, Abbott JD, et al. Liberal versus restrictive transfusion thresholds for patients with symptomatic coronary artery disease. Am Heart J 2013;165(6):964–71.e1.

158. Hébert PC, Wells G, Marshall J, et al. Transfusion requirements in critical care. A pilot study. Canadian Critical Care Trials Group. JAMA 1995; 273(18):1439–44.

159. Carson JL, Carless PA, Hébert PC. Transfusion thresholds and other strategies for guiding allogeneic red blood cell transfusion. Cochrane Database Syst Rev 2012;(4):CD002042.

160. Gelinas JP, Stoddart LV, Snyder EL. Thrombocytopenia and critical care medicine. J Intensive Care Med 2001;16(1):1–21.

161. Bassuni WY, Blajchman MA, Al-Moshary MA. Why implement universal leukoreduction? Hematol Oncol Stem Cell Ther 2008;1(2):106–23.

162. Vamvakas EC, Blajchman MA. Transfusion-related immunomodulation (TRIM): an update. Blood Rev 2007;21(6):327–48.

163. Vamvakas EC. White-blood-cell-containing allogeneic blood transfusion and postoperative infection or mortality: an updated meta-analysis. Vox Sang 2007;92(3):224–32.

164. Vamvakas EC. Why have meta-analyses of randomized controlled trials of the association between non-white-blood-cell-reduced allogeneic

blood transfusion and postoperative infection produced discordant results? Vox Sang 2007; 93(3):196–207.

165. Bilgin YM, van de Watering LMG, Eijsman L, et al. Double-blind, randomized controlled trial on the effect of leukocyte-depleted erythrocyte transfusions in cardiac valve surgery. Circulation 2004; 109(22):2755–60.

166. Steiner ME, Ness PM, Assmann SF, et al. Effects of red-cell storage duration on patients undergoing cardiac surgery. N Engl J Med 2015;372(15): 1419–29.

167. Fergusson DA, Hébert P, Hogan DL, et al. Effect of fresh red blood cell transfusions on clinical outcomes in premature, very low-birth-weight infants: the ARIPI randomized trial. JAMA 2012; 308(14):1443–51.

168. Reilly JJ, Hull SF, Albert N, et al. Economic impact of malnutrition: a model system for hospitalized patients. JPEN J Parenter Enteral Nutr 1988;12(4): 371–6.

169. Alberda C, Gramlich L, Jones N, et al. The relationship between nutritional intake and clinical outcomes in critically ill patients: results of an international multicenter observational study. Intensive Care Med 2009;35(10):1728–37.

170. Norman K, Pichard C, Lochs H, et al. Prognostic impact of disease-related malnutrition. Clin Nutr 2008;27(1):5–15.

171. Cederholm T, Jägrén C, Hellström K. Outcome of protein-energy malnutrition in elderly medical patients. Am J Med 1995;98(1):67–74.

172. Cahill NE, Dhaliwal R, Day AG, et al. Nutrition therapy in the critical care setting: what is "best achievable" practice? An international multicenter observational study. Crit Care Med 2010;38(2):395–401.

173. Casaer MP, Van den Berghe G. Nutrition in the acute phase of critical illness. N Engl J Med 2014;370(13):1227–36.

174. National Heart, Lung, and Blood Institute Acute Respiratory Distress Syndrome (ARDS) Clinical Trials Network, Rice TW, Wheeler AP, et al. Initial trophic vs full enteral feeding in patients with acute lung injury: the EDEN randomized trial. JAMA 2012;307(8):795–803.

175. Doig GS, Simpson F, Finfer S, et al. Effect of evidence-based feeding guidelines on mortality of critically ill adults: a cluster randomized controlled trial. JAMA 2008;300(23):2731–41.

176. Ibrahim EH, Mehringer L, Prentice D, et al. Early versus late enteral feeding of mechanically ventilated patients: results of a clinical trial. JPEN J Parenter Enteral Nutr 2002;26(3):174–81.

177. Krishnan JA, Parce PB, Martinez A, et al. Caloric intake in medical ICU patients: consistency of care with guidelines and relationship to clinical outcomes. Chest 2003;124(1):297–305.

178. Arabi YM, Haddad SH, Tamim HM, et al. Near-target caloric intake in critically ill medical-surgical patients is associated with adverse outcomes. JPEN J Parenter Enteral Nutr 2010; 34(3):280–8.

179. Heyland DK, Dhaliwal R, Day A, et al. Validation of the Canadian clinical practice guidelines for nutrition support in mechanically ventilated, critically ill adult patients: results of a prospective observational study. Crit Care Med 2004;32(11):2260–6.

180. Barr J, Hecht M, Flavin KE, et al. Outcomes in critically ill patients before and after the implementation of an evidence-based nutritional management protocol. Chest 2004;125(4):1446–57.

181. Rubinson L, Diette GB, Song X, et al. Low caloric intake is associated with nosocomial bloodstream infections in patients in the medical intensive care unit. Crit Care Med 2004;32(2):350–7.

182. Martin CM, Doig GS, Heyland DK, et al, Southwestern Ontario Critical Care Research Network. Multicentre, cluster-randomized clinical trial of algorithms for critical-care enteral and parenteral therapy (ACCEPT). CMAJ 2004;170(2):197–204.

183. Arabi YM, Aldawood AS, Haddad SH, et al. Permissive underfeeding or standard enteral feeding in critically Ill adults. N Engl J Med 2015;372(25): 2398–408.

184. Montejo JC, Miñambres E, Bordejé L, et al. Gastric residual volume during enteral nutrition in ICU patients: the REGANE study. Intensive Care Med 2010;36(8):1386–93.

185. Reignier J, Mercier E, Le Gouge A, et al. Effect of not monitoring residual gastric volume on risk of ventilator-associated pneumonia in adults receiving mechanical ventilation and early enteral feeding: a randomized controlled trial. JAMA 2013;309(3):249–56.

186. Nguyen NQ, Chapman MJ, Fraser RJ, et al. Erythromycin is more effective than metoclopramide in the treatment of feed intolerance in critical illness. Crit Care Med 2007;35(2):483–9.

187. Casaer MP, Mesotten D, Hermans G, et al. Early versus late parenteral nutrition in critically ill adults. N Engl J Med 2011;365(6):506–17.

188. Harvey SE, Parrott F, Harrison DA, et al. Trial of the route of early nutritional support in critically ill adults. N Engl J Med 2014;371(18):1673–84.

189. Cohen J, Opal S, Calandra T. Sepsis studies need new direction. Lancet Infect Dis 2012; 12(7):503–5.

190. Wenzel RP, Edmond MB. Septic shock — evaluating another failed treatment. N Engl J Med 2012;366:1–3.

191. Williams SCP. After Xigris, researchers look to new targets to combat sepsis. Nat Med 2012; 18(7):1001.

192. Dolgin E. Trial failure prompts soul-searching for critical-care specialists. Nat Med 2012;18(7):1000.

93. Angus DC. The search for effective therapy for sepsis: back to the drawing board? JAMA 2011; 306(23):2614–5.

94. Vincent J-L. The rise and fall of drotrecogin alfa (activated). Lancet Infect Dis 2012;12(9): 649–51.

95. Holder AL, Huang DT. A dream deferred: the rise and fall of recombinant activated protein C. Crit Care 2013;17(2):309.

96. Hotchkiss RS, Monneret G, Payen D. Immunosup pression in sepsis: a novel understanding of the disorder and a new therapeutic approach. Lancet Infect Dis 2013;13(3):260–8.

97. Hotchkiss RS, Moldawer LL. Parallels between cancer and infectious disease. N Engl J Med 2014;371(4):380–3.

198. Walton AH, Muenzer JT, Rasche D, et al. Reactivation of multiple viruses in patients with sepsis. PLoS One 2014;9(2):e98819.

199. Wada K, Kubota N, Ito Y, et al. Simultaneous quantification of Epstein-Barr virus, cytomegalovirus, and human herpesvirus 6 DNA in samples from transplant recipients by multiplex real-time PCR assay. J Clin Microbiol 2007;45(5):1426–32.

200. Gärtner B, Preiksaitis JK. EBV viral load detection in clinical virology. J Clin Virol 2010;48(2):82–90.

201. Siciliano RF, Castelli JB, Randi BA, et al. Cytomegalovirus colitis in immunocompetent critically ill patients. Int J Infect Dis 2014;20:71–3.

202. Boomer JS, To K, Chang KC, et al. Immunosuppression in patients who die of sepsis and multiple organ failure. JAMA 2011;306(23):2594–605.

# Short-term Gains with Long-term Consequences
## The Evolving Story of Sepsis Survivorship

CrossMark

Jason H. Maley, MD[a], Mark E. Mikkelsen, MD, MSCE[a,b,c,*]

## KEYWORDS

- Sepsis • Cognitive impairment • Physical impairment • Infection • Hospital readmission
- Critical care

## KEY POINTS

- Sepsis survivors frequently experience declines in cognitive and physical function.
- Sepsis survivors experience increased cardiovascular risk and are at increased risk for subsequent infections.
- Health care resource use is high among sepsis survivors given the frequency of postacute services at hospital discharge and hospital readmission.
- Health-related quality of life is decreased, and long-term mortality is increased after sepsis.

Sepsis is an acute, life-threatening condition characterized by the human systemic inflammatory response to infection.[1] Sepsis is common, afflicting millions of patients each year in the United States and countless more internationally.[2–4] The incidence of sepsis seems to be increasing,[3] owing in part to an aging population, age-related impaired immunity, and an increasing burden of comorbid conditions.

Although the proportion of in-hospital deaths attributed to sepsis remains extremely high,[5,6] advances in care and heightened awareness of sepsis have led to substantial declines in in-hospital mortality over the last 20 years.[7–13] A stark example of this phenomenon is the trend in mortality in severe sepsis and septic shock trials. In the original early goal-directed therapy trial conducted by Rivers and colleagues[8] between 1997 and 2000, the in-hospital mortality in the control arm receiving usual care at the time was 46.5%. In contrast, the in-hospital mortality in the early goal-directed therapy arm was 30.5%. In 3 multicenter trials published in 2014 and 2015, in-hospital mortality had improved to approximately 20% and 90-day mortality ranged from 19% to 29%.[11–13] In parallel, temporal trends of severe sepsis and septic shock mortality outside of the trial context have revealed similar improvement.[4,7,9,10]

At the intersection of an increasing incidence of sepsis and declining short-term mortality is a growing population of sepsis survivors that has been heralded as a "hidden public health disaster."[14] Over the last decade, an expanding body of literature has emerged to describe the

Funding: The study was supported in part by National Institutes of Health (NINR [National Institute of Nursing Research] R01NR016014), National Heart, Lung, and Blood Institute (NIH NHLBI) Loan Repayment Program, Bethesda, MD (M.E. Mikkelsen).
Disclosures: The authors have no financial or other potential conflicts of interest exist related to the work.
[a] Department of Medicine, Perelman School of Medicine at the University of Pennsylvania, Philadelphia, PA, USA; [b] Division of Pulmonary, Allergy, and Critical Care, Department of Medicine, Perelman School of Medicine at the University of Pennsylvania, Philadelphia, PA, USA; [c] Center for Clinical Epidemiology and Biostatistics, Perelman School of Medicine at the University of Pennsylvania, Philadelphia, PA, USA
* Corresponding author. Division of Pulmonary, Allergy, and Critical Care, Perelman School of Medicine, University of Pennsylvania, Gates 05.042, 3400 Spruce Street, Philadelphia, PA 19104.
E-mail address: mark.mikkelsen@uphs.upenn.edu

Clin Chest Med 37 (2016) 367–380
http://dx.doi.org/10.1016/j.ccm.2016.01.017
0272-5231/16/$ – see front matter © 2016 Elsevier Inc. All rights reserved.

Box 1
**Long-term consequences of sepsis**

Neuropsychological impairment

Physical impairment

Sepsis-induced inflammation and cardiovascular risk

Sepsis-induced immunosuppression

Health care resource use

Long-term health-related quality of life

Long-term mortality

long-term impact of sepsis among survivors. These studies have revealed that long-term cognitive and functional impairment, sustained inflammation and immune dysfunction, increased health care resource use, decreased health-related quality of life, and increased mortality plague many sepsis survivors. The evidence challenges the notion that sepsis is an acute, transient illness, instead revealing that sepsis is an acute illness with lingering consequences that impact one's long-term health. This article provides a state-of-the-art review of the emerging literature of the long-term consequences of sepsis (**Box 1**).

## LONG-TERM NEUROPSYCHOLOGICAL AND PHYSICAL IMPAIRMENTS

Survivors of critical illness frequently experience cognitive and functional impairments that persist after discharge and impact health-related quality of life. In survivors of critical illness, this is known as the post–intensive care syndrome (PICS) and is defined as new or worsening cognition, mental health, and/or physical health that arises after critical illness and endures.[15,16] Severe sepsis and septic shock are common risk factors for these

impairments, although admission to an intensive care unit (ICU) is not a prerequisite for the development of impairments among sepsis survivors.

### Cognitive Impairment

Cognitive impairment seems to be a profound and persistent development in sepsis survivors. In a landmark study, Iwashyna and colleagues[17] examined the impact of severe sepsis on cognitive and physical functions. Using the Health and Retirement Study, a national representative sample of elderly subjects in the United States, serial cognitive and functional assessments were leveraged to compare function after severe sepsis hospitalizations to nonsepsis hospitalizations. The cohort enrolled 1194 elderly patients (mean age, 76.9 years) who experienced 1520 hospitalizations. The rate of moderate to severe cognitive impairment increased from 6.1% before severe sepsis to 16.7% afterward, an absolute increase of 10.6%. After adjustment, for which patients served as their own controls, the odds of moderate to severe cognitive impairment developing after severe sepsis remained 3-fold higher compared with nonsepsis hospitalizations. Approximately 2 years after the initial postsepsis assessment, a nearly identical proportion of severe sepsis survivors were found to have moderately to severely impaired cognition, suggesting that these new impairments persisted (**Fig. 1**). Because only 43% of the severe sepsis episodes included an ICU stay, cognitive impairment after severe sepsis seems to extend to those cared for outside of the ICU as well.

In the largest prospective study of cognitive impairment in ICU survivors, the Bringing to Light the Risk Factors and Incidence of Neuropsychological Dysfunction in ICU Survivors (BRAIN-ICU) investigators assessed patients for cognitive function at 3 and 12 months after hospitalization.[18]

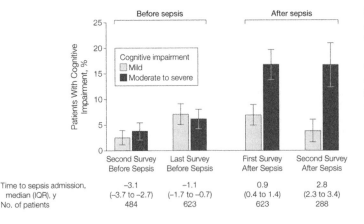

Fig. 1. Cognitive trajectory among elderly severe sepsis survivors. IQR, interquartile range. (*From* Iwashyna TJ, Ely EW, Smith DM, et al. Long-term cognitive impairment and functional disability among survivors of severe sepsis. JAMA 2010;304:1790; with permission.)

Sepsis was the most common diagnosis in this population, present in 30% of the cohort at the time of enrollment. At 3 months, 40% of the patients studied had global cognition scores similar to scores for patients with moderate traumatic brain injury and 26% had scores similar to patients with mild Alzheimer's disease. Cognitive impairment was seen in both younger and older patients, and persisted in large part at 12 months. Consistent with these studies, in a representative study of Medicare beneficiaries, Guerra and colleagues[19] demonstrated that infection and/or severe sepsis were independent risk factors for incident dementia after critical illness.

The neuropathology of sepsis-induced cognitive impairment is being elucidated and seems to be a complex interplay between ischemia, inflammation, oxidative stress, microglial activation, and disruption of the blood–brain barrier.[20] Risk factors for the development of postsepsis cognitive impairment include presepsis factors and physiologic changes that occur during sepsis. Examples of factors present presepsis that modify the risk of cognitive impairment postsepsis include premorbid health conditions (eg, cerebrovascular disease), level of education, and preexisting psychiatric or cognitive impairment.

Incident impairment seems to be independent of age,[18] although cognitive trajectories may decline more rapidly in those with preexisting cognitive impairment and decreased "cognitive reserve."[21] In the acute care setting, decreased cognitive reserve may manifest as delirium.[18,21–23] Because the duration of delirium is independently associated with long-term cognitive impairment after medical and surgical critical illness,[18,21–23] the observation that statin use in the ICU seemed to mitigate delirium development among sepsis patients warrants additional study.[24] Physiologic variables implicated as risk factors for cognitive impairment after critical illness, and common in sepsis include:

- Hypoxemia
- Hypotension
- Glucose dysregulation
- Acute kidney injury requiring renal replacement therapy
- Disordered sleep[19,20,25,26]

## Psychological Morbidity

Psychological impairment among sepsis survivors seems to be common and manifests as:

- Anxiety
- Depression
- Posttraumatic stress disorder (PTSD)[27–30]

After a general critical illness, the point prevalence for depression, anxiety, and PTSD is estimated at 28%, 24%, and 22%, respectively.[27–30] In the BRAIN-ICU study, where sepsis was the most common diagnosis at admission, 37% of survivors of critical illness reported symptoms of mild depression or worse at 3 months and 33% at 12 months.[18] Notably, the symptoms were primarily owing to somatic complaints rather than cognitive–affective symptoms.[18] These findings support the notion that physical impairment may be intimately connected to depressive symptoms that persist in survivors.

In an investigation that examined survivors of critical illness transitioned to acute rehabilitation after discharge, 68% of who were sepsis survivors, 10% were found to have symptoms of PTSD at 3 months and 16% at 6 months.[30] At 3 months, fear of death in the ICU, a diagnosis of sepsis, and the number of traumatic memories from the ICU were associated with symptoms of PTSD; at 6 months, PTSD at 3 months and a lack of social support were associated with symptoms of PTSD.

In the lone longitudinal study to examine patients before and after an episode of sepsis, Davydow and colleagues[31] found a point prevalence of depressive symptoms of 28% after severe sepsis. In the absence of presepsis assessments, it would be reasonable to conclude that sepsis was associated with increased symptoms of depression. However, because the prevalence of depressive symptoms was likewise 28% at 1.2 years before sepsis, the prior conclusion was demonstrated to be erroneous. In the process, it suggested that preexisting depression is common in survivors of sepsis. In concert with evidence that preexisting depression is associated with postsepsis cognitive impairment,[32] these studies reveal that an understanding of depression and its impact on long-term outcomes after sepsis is critical to designing interventions and follow-up at the time of hospital discharge.

In parallel to the patient experience, it is increasingly recognized that family members of ICU survivors experience lasting psychological effects, known as Post-Intensive Care Syndrome–Family (PICS-F).[15,16] Spouses of patients with severe sepsis experience increased depressive symptoms, and female spouses seem to be the most at risk for this complication.[33]

## Physical Impairment and Functional Disability

Sepsis is an established risk factor for the development of critical illness polyneuromyopathy.[27]

In many patients, these physical impairments manifest in a high rate of new functional limitations after severe sepsis—limitations that persisted for at least 5 years after hospitalization in 1 prospective cohort.[17] In this cohort, the deleterious effects of sepsis on physical function seemed to be most pronounced in survivors with no limitations (1.57 new activity of daily living or instrumental activity of daily living limitations) or mild to moderate limitations before sepsis (1.50 new limitations; **Fig. 2**). Together, at the first postsepsis assessment, hospitalization for severe sepsis heralded a cognitive and/or physical decline in 59% of cases. Based on an analysis of Medicare data, it was estimated that 106,311 of 637,867 severe sepsis survivors would incur moderate-to-severe cognitive impairment and 476,862 would incur functional disability after severe sepsis.[34]

Similar to cognitive impairment, the literature on risk factors and mechanisms of functional impairment is limited. Studies of critical illness polyneuromyopathy relate weakness to inflammation and ischemic injury at the level of muscle fibers and motor neurons, developments that may be exacerbated by prolonged immobility.[35,36] After discharge, physical function seems to be modified by neuropsychological function in a bidirectional manner.[35,36] For example, among survivors of acute respiratory distress syndrome (ARDS), many of whom had sepsis as the precipitant of ARDS, depression was associated with incident physical impairment.[37]

## Qualitative Experience of Sepsis Survivors

In general, the qualitative experience of survivors and their caregivers' is consistent with the quantitative research.[38] In a study using semistructured interviews to understand the recovery experience of survivors and their caregivers from the United States and United Kingdom, 5 themes emerged:

- [Lack of] awareness and knowledge of severe sepsis
- Experience of the hospitalization
- Enduring impact of sepsis on survivors
- Impact of sepsis on caregivers
- [Lack of] support after severe sepsis

After discharge, survivors detailed impairments that made self-care challenging, resulted in a loss of independence, and had a profound emotional impact driven by fear of a recurrence of sepsis and sense of burden to caregivers.

A qualitative study of ARDS survivors, 30% of whom had sepsis, used semistructured interviews to examine similar themes of survivor quality of

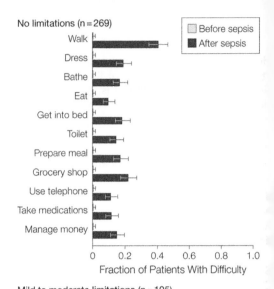

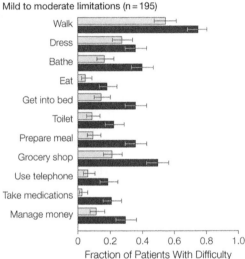

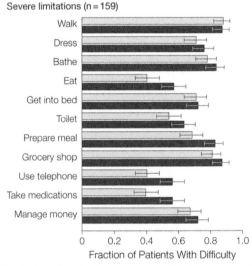

**Fig. 2.** Functional trajectory among elderly severe sepsis survivors according to baseline functioning. (*From* Iwashyna TJ, Ely EW, Smith DM, et al. Long-term cognitive impairment and functional disability among survivors of severe sepsis. JAMA 2010;304:1792; with permission.)

...fe.[39] The 5 key themes that emerged from this study were:

- Pervasive memories of critical care
- Day-to-day impact of new disability
- Critical illness defining sense of self
- Relationship strain and change
- [In]ability to cope with disability.

Again, the loss of independence, fear of cognitive impairment, and impact of lasting disability were prominent features of patient responses, with interviews illuminating the burden of functional impairment.

## SEPSIS-INDUCED INFLAMMATION AND CARDIOVASCULAR RISK

After the acute, hyperinflammatory response to infection subsides, it is postulated that persistent innate immune-mediated inflammation induces long-term organ dysfunction.[40] In support of this hypothesis, increased inflammatory and hemostasis markers after pneumonia predicted all-cause and cardiovascular deaths.[41,42]

Cardiovascular morbidity, in particular, is common during sepsis and manifests through arrhythmia, hypotension and shock, and sepsis-induced cardiomyopathy.[1,43–46] Atrial fibrillation is common during an index sepsis hospitalization, especially in older patients. In a nationally representative study of 60,209 Medicare beneficiaries, Walkey and colleagues[47] found that atrial fibrillation occurred in 25% of sepsis hospitalizations. Nearly three-quarters of the patients had a history of atrial fibrillation, with the remainder experiencing new-onset atrial fibrillation.[47] Factors associated with new-onset atrial fibrillation included older age, white race, illness severity (eg, ICU admission, mechanical ventilation), right heart catheterization, presence of endocarditis, and coronary artery bypass graft surgery. Because many typical cardiovascular comorbidities, such as heart failure, myocardial infarction, hypertension, and valvular disease, were not associated significantly with new-onset atrial fibrillation, it was presumed that mechanisms related to sepsis were the precipitating factors.

In a separate investigation, compared with hospitalized patients without sepsis, new-onset atrial fibrillation was found to be nearly 10-fold higher in severe sepsis patients (5.9% vs 0.6%).[48] Further, severe sepsis patients with new-onset atrial fibrillation were at increased risk of in-hospital stroke (2.6% vs 0.6%) and in-hospital mortality (56% vs 39%).

Beyond the acute care hospitalization, severe sepsis survivors incur increased cardiovascular risk.[49] However, the increased risk seems to be largely owing to prehospitalization factors and seems to reflect a more generalized risk associated with acute hospitalization. Nevertheless, in patients with new-onset, sepsis-associated atrial fibrillation, the 5-year risk of recurrent atrial fibrillation was found to be 55%.[50] Moreover, patients with new-onset atrial fibrillation during sepsis were more likely to be hospitalized over this interval for heart failure (11.2% vs 8.2%) or ischemic stroke (5.3% vs 4.7%) and were more likely to die (74.8% vs 72.1%).[50] Because patients with new-onset atrial fibrillation during sepsis are at increased risk of long-term cardiovascular events, they may benefit from postdischarge surveillance and prevention strategies.

## SEPSIS-INDUCED IMMUNOSUPPRESSION

The host response to an infectious pathogen induces a complex balance between proinflammatory and antiinflammatory processes.[40,51,52] After the exuberant proinflammatory period wanes, a period of immunosuppression may ensue. In this later stage of sepsis, defective immune status may result, in part, from sepsis-induced immune cell apoptosis. Apoptosis impacts the innate and adaptive immune system, and coupled with dysregulation within the cell lines of both systems and T-cell exhaustion, may leave the immune system vulnerable.[40,51,52]

Clinically, sepsis-induced immunosuppression seems to manifest as new, recurrent, or unresolved infections. During an index sepsis hospitalization, 1 investigation of cultures obtained at autopsy consistently revealed unresolved foci of infection.[53] In a separate study that compared 560 critically ill sepsis patients with 161 critically ill patients without sepsis and 164 healthy controls, postsepsis latent viral reactivation was common and reactivation was associated with increased 90-day mortality.[54] Sepsis-induced immunosuppression seems to explain the results of the emerging hospital readmission literature, which has revealed that sepsis survivors are frequently rehospitalized with new, recurrent, or unresolved infections (see Health care resource use in sepsis survivors).

## HEALTH CARE RESOURCE USE IN SEPSIS SURVIVORS

Health care use in sepsis survivors is common, costly, and frequently endures for at least 1 year after discharge. The increased health care use after sepsis includes increased postacute care use at the time of discharge and hospital-based acute care in the weeks and months after discharge. The cost of postsepsis care seems to rival the cost of the initial acute care sepsis hospitalization, confirming that sepsis is a major driver of United States health care. Based on the observed 30- and 180-day readmission rates observed after sepsis, it is estimated that the national burden for these readmissions exceeds $3 and $9 billion, respectively.[55]

### Post–Acute Care Use

At the time of discharge, nearly 3 out of 5 sepsis survivors receive post–acute care services.[6,56] Services include home health services, acute inpatient rehabilitation, and skilled nursing facility or long-term acute care hospital placement.[6,56]

Post–acute care service use seems to be highest after severe sepsis[6] and to be driven by the increased use of skilled care facility placement.[56] For example, in the study by Jones and colleagues,[6] sepsis survivors were 2 times more likely to be discharged to a skilled nursing facility and nearly ten times more likely to be discharged to a long-term acute care hospital. A report from the Agency for Healthcare Research and Quality revealed that discharge to a skilled care facility was nearly 2 times more likely in patients with multiple sepsis admissions.[57] Together, these data suggest that loss of independence is a product of the severity of an acute sepsis event and the cumulative burden over serial events. Potentially related, despite functional impairment after sepsis, the use of acute inpatient rehabilitation was rare and only modestly higher in sepsis survivors (4.3% after nonsepsis hospitalizations vs 3.6% after sepsis hospitalizations and 8.65% after severe sepsis hospitalizations).[6] Whether sepsis survivors are disadvantaged from timely access to inpatient rehabilitation, as a result of healthcare policy that mandates a minimum proportion of rehabilitation recipients fulfill one or more medical conditions (eg, stroke, knee or hip joint replacement), requires further examination.

### Hospital-Based Acute Care Use

Improving care transitions and reducing hospital readmissions are a national priority to control health care costs and improve the quality of care delivered. To incentivize these objectives, the US Patient Protection and Affordable Care Act implemented the hospital readmission reduction program.[58–60] After discharge, sepsis survivors frequently require hospital-based acute care. Hospital-based acute care, in these cases, includes both emergency department (ED) treat-and-release encounters and hospital readmissions. Based on these findings, sepsis has emerged as an important condition to measure and track at the national level.

### Emergency Department Visits

As detailed in 2 studies, the rate of ED treat-and-release visits is modest, at 3.8% to 4.5%.[6,61] Compared with nonsepsis hospitalizations, the rate of ED treat-and-release encounters is actually less after sepsis hospitalizations.[6] In part, this paradoxic finding is related to the extremely high conversion rate to hospital readmission upon ED presentation based on the frequent burden of coexisting conditions, recent events, and presentation (eg, severe sepsis) at the time of readmission.

### Hospital Readmissions

A growing body of literature has revealed that hospital readmission is common after sepsis. Using data from academic medical centers,[6,61] community medical centers,[62] and national data,[55,56,63] the 30-day all-cause hospital readmission rate after sepsis is remarkable in its consistency, ranging from 18% to 26% (**Tables 1** and **2**). By 90, 180, and 365 days, 30% to 42%,[6,61,62,64] 48%,[55] and 63%[64] of sepsis survivors had been readmitted, respectively. Among elderly severe sepsis survivors, only 1 out of 5 survivors were alive and had not been readmitted in the year after discharge.[64]

#### Risk factors

A number of patient-level risk factors for increased readmission risk have been identified and include sociodemographics, insurance status, income status, comorbid conditions, prior hospitalizations, and illness severity (see **Table 2**). In general, factors identified in the nonsepsis readmission literature have also been observed to be risk factors after sepsis.[65]

Among these potential factors, comorbid conditions and prior use were found to be the dominant contributors to post–acute care use and hospital readmissions.[62] Consistent with prior use as a dominant risk factor, a disproportionate number of readmissions are concentrated in a subgroup of high users, because one-quarter of survivors accounted for 77% of rehospitalizations over 6 months in 1 national study.[55]

In general, despite its association with mortality in the acute care hospitalization setting,[67] source of infection has not been identified as a tool to risk stratify at-risk patients, although 1 study did find that gastrointestinal-related sepsis cases may confer an increased risk.[63] Although illness severity has been associated with increased

**Table 1**
Rate, timing, and cause of 30-day hospital readmissions among sepsis survivors

| Study | Population | Rate (%) | Timing (d) | Cause |
|---|---|---|---|---|
| Elixhauser et al,[65] 2013 | Septicemia (n = 696,122) | 21.0 | — | — |
| Liu et al,[62] 2014 | Sepsis (n = 5479) | 17.9 | 11 | Infection (28%–43%) |
| Prescott et al,[64,66] 2014, 2015 | Elderly severe sepsis survivors (n = 1083) | 26.5 | — | Ambulatory care sensitive conditions (42%)[a] |
| Ortego et al,[61] 2015 | Septic shock (n = 269) | 23.4 | 7 (3–15) | Related to comorbid condition/planned (22%) Infection (46%) Cardiovascular/ thromboembolic (18%) Acute kidney injury (6%) Complications of devices (3%) Other (5%) |
| Jones et al,[6] 2015 | Sepsis (n = 1268) | 27.0 | 13 (6–21) | — |
| Jones et al,[6] 2015 | Severe sepsis (n = 2352) | 26.2 | 11 (5–18) | — |
| Goodwin et al,[55] 2015 | Severe sepsis (n = 43,452) | 25.6 | — | — |
| Donnelly et al,[63] 2015[b] | Severe sepsis (n = 216,328) | 19.9 | — | Infection (66.9%) Severe sepsis (40.3%) |
| Chang et al,[56] 2015 | Sepsis (n = 240,198) | 20.4 | — | Infection (59.3%) Septicemia (29.2%) |

Abbreviation: —, not reported.
[a] Ambulatory care sensitivity conditions suggest effective outpatient care exists that could reduce need for hospitalization. Percentage represents expanded ambulatory care sensitive condition diagnoses and includes sepsis, soft tissue infection, acute renal failure and aspiration pneumonitis.[66]
[b] Unplanned 30-day readmission rate.

readmission risk (eg, prolonged duration of stay, procedures during the hospitalization), factors such as acute respiratory failure, use of mechanical ventilation, shock, acute renal failure, and acute neurologic dysfunction have not been identified as risk factors.[6,55]

## Readmission causes

In accord with the evidence supporting sepsis-induced immunosuppression, multiple studies have demonstrated that the majority of unplanned readmissions are owing to infection (see Table 1).[56,61–63,68] Additional causes of unplanned readmissions include cardiovascular and thromboembolic events and acute kidney injury.

## Outcomes associated with hospital readmissions after sepsis

Readmissions among sepsis survivors, compared with readmissions after nonsepsis hospitalizations, are more likely to include an ICU admission, less likely to result in discharge to home, and more likely to result in death or a transition to hospice[6,55,61] (Table 3). In general, the duration of stay for the hospital readmissions was substantial.

## Hospital-level variation in hospital readmissions after sepsis

Across hospitals, there exists substantial variability in the rate of risk-standardized hospital readmissions. Among 209 University HealthSystem Consortium hospitals, the 30-day risk standardized readmission rates ranged from 14.1% to 31.1%.[63] In a separate study, conducted among 325 California hospitals included in the Healthcare Cost and Utilization Project State Inpatient Database, risk-standardized readmission rates ranged from 11.0% to 39.8%. As shown in Table 4, hospital-level risk factors associated with higher risk-standardized readmission rates included greater institutional volume, teaching status, trauma services, geographic location, and lower ICU use rates.[6,55–63]

Given the magnitude of the variability observed, additional study is warranted to understand the differences in sociodemographics, case mix, and discharge practices that could explain the observed differences. Highlighting the need to examine discharge practices, in the only study to examine care transition practice, Ortego and colleagues[61] found that follow-up appointments had

**Table 2**
**Patient-level risk factors associated with hospital readmission after sepsis**

| Risk Factor | References |
|---|---|
| Age (younger) | 6,55,56 |
| Gender | 55,56,63 |
| Race | 56,63 |
| Insurance status (Medicare, Medicaid) | 55,63 |
| Lower income | 56 |
| Urban residence | 56 |
| Comorbid conditions (oncology) | 6,56,61–63 |
| Number of hospitalizations preceding the index sepsis admission | 6,61 |
| Source of sepsis (gastrointestinal infections) | 63 |
| Index hospital duration of stay | 6,55,61–63 |
| Illness severity | 6,62 |
| Procedures | 6 |
| ICU admission (as risk factor) | 62 |
| ICU admission (as protective factor) | 63 |
| Discharge disposition | 55 |
| Low hemoglobin at discharge | 6 |
| High red cell distribution width at discharge | 6 |

Abbreviation: ICU, intensive care unit.

**Table 4**
**Hospital-level risk factors associated with higher risk-standardized readmission rates after sepsis**

| Risk Factor | References |
|---|---|
| Greater institutional volume | 55,63 |
| Teaching status | 63 |
| Trauma services | 63 |
| Geographic location (Northeast) | 63 |
| Lower intensive care unit rates | 63 |

not been made in 41% of septic shock survivors readmitted within 30 days of discharge, and an additional 27% were readmitted before their scheduled appointment.

## Long-term Health-related Quality of Life and Mortality

In a systematic review of 30 publications published between 1994 and 2009, Winters and colleagues[69] examined the long-term health-related quality of life and mortality among sepsis survivors. Compared with controls, sepsis survivors were found to incur an increased mortality risk after discharge.[69] The increased mortality risk was found to be consistent across the illness severity spectrum. Health-related quality of life was lower

**Table 3**
**Readmission outcomes after index sepsis acute care hospitalizations**

| Study | Readmission Duration of Stay (d) (median, interquartile range) | Readmission, ICU Use (%) | Readmission Outcome |
|---|---|---|---|
| Ortego et al,[61] 2015 | 5 (2–14) | 33 | 16% died or transitioned to hospice |
| Jones et al,[6] 2015 | — | 29[a] | 6.6% died, compared with 2.6% after nonsepsis index hospitalization 6.6% transitioned to hospice, compared with 3.5% after nonsepsis index hospitalization |
| Goodwin et al,[55] 2015 | — | — | 4% died |
| Donnelly et al,[63] 2015 | 5 (3–8) | 24 | 6.2% died |
| Chang et al,[56] 2015 | 7 (4–13) | — | 6.5% died, compared with 1.4% in readmissions after acute myocardial infarction and 1.7% in readmissions after congestive heart failure |

Abbreviations: —, not reported; ICU, intensive care unit.
[a] Compared with 17% ICU use in readmissions after nonsepsis hospitalizations.

than population norms before sepsis, and incident sepsis was associated with a consistent decline in health-related quality of life.[69]

Postsepsis mortality seems to be modified by age[62] and to be independent of comorbidities.[70] As an example, within an integrated community health care system, the 1-year postsepsis survival rate was 71% overall, with a high of 94% among survivors less than 45 years of age and a low of 54% among survivors 85 years of age or older.[62] Likewise, in a study that examined Medicare beneficiaries, the 90-day and 1-year mortality rates were 27.5% and 44.2% after severe sepsis, compared with 15.5% and 31.4% for a matched, nonsepsis cohort.[64] Among severe sepsis survivors who died in the year after hospital discharge, 48% died at home, 34% in the hospital, and 18% in a skilled care facility; a minority (34%) were under hospice care at the time of their death.[64]

The impact of sepsis on long-term outcomes extends for years.[69,71] In sepsis survivors from 26 Scottish ICUs, mortality was 58% at 3.5 years, 61% at 5 years, and health-related quality of life, driven in large part by lower physical scores, was lower than population controls.[71] Despite the measured quality of life and "unpleasant" memories of the acute event, 80% of survivors shared that they were satisfied with their quality of life and all reported that they would undergo similar treatment if their critical illness recurred.[71] These latter findings typify the psychological construct of adaptation and the modifiable trait of psychological resilience.

## IMPROVING LONG-TERM OUTCOMES AFTER SEPSIS

Clinicians and investigators are now tasked with identifying interventions, both within the hospital and after discharge, which will accelerate recovery and improve long-term outcomes after sepsis. Based on survivors' qualitative experiences,[38] opportunities to improve outcomes fall under 5 primary aims[72] (**Fig. 3**):

- Increase awareness of the diagnosis of sepsis
- Educate patients and caregivers
- Mitigate risks of physical and neuropsychological impairment
- Prioritize early and sustained rehabilitation
- Coordinate longitudinal care

The cornerstone of the strategy to improve long-term outcomes begins with increasing awareness of the diagnosis of sepsis. In concert, it is essential that patients, caregivers, and outpatient providers be educated on the long-term consequences of

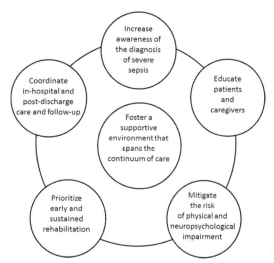

**Fig. 3.** Conceptual framework of strategies to improve long-term outcomes for sepsis survivors. (*From* Maley JH, Mikkelsen ME. Sepsis survivorship: how can we promote a culture of resilience? Crit Care Med 2015;43(2):480; with permission.)

sepsis survivorship. To empower patients and their caregivers, information sharing about the long-term consequences of sepsis should begin during the in-patient hospitalization and continue through recovery as survivors needs evolve.

Mitigating the risk of impairment begins with implementation of practices in the ICU to minimize delirium and preserve physical function. To accomplish these aims, we recommend the use of the ABCDEF bundle,[73,74] a systematic means of ensuring that nurses, physicians, and ICU staff assess for and manage pain, perform both spontaneous awakening and breathing trials, pay attention to the choice of sedation and analgesia, provide delirium monitoring and management, and ensure early mobility and family engagement. The care components included in this bundle have been demonstrated to reduce the duration of delirium and incidence of ventilator-associated events, increase ventilator-free days, and improve functional outcomes at discharge with increased likelihood of return to functional independence.[75–79]

Because sedation is intimately linked to many factors within this bundle, providers must pay close attention to medication choice, duration, and level of sedation. Two randomized controlled trials compared the use of dexmedetomidine, midazolam, and propofol in mechanically ventilated patients, the majority of whom had sepsis. The authors found that patients receiving dexmedetomidine experienced a reduced duration of mechanical ventilation compared with midazolam (median of 123 vs 164 hours; *P* = .03) and improved ability to communicate pain compared with midazolam and propofol.[80]

Experimental animal models have also demonstrated that dexmedetomidine may have protective effects against ischemic brain injury.[81,82] Additionally, the use of lorazepam has been demonstrated to be an independent risk factor for development of delirium in a cohort of mechanically ventilated patients.[83] Our recommended approach, in line with established guidelines,[84] includes analgosedation with an analgesic-first approach that may be combined, if needed, with a propofol- or dexmedetomidine-based sedative regimen.[85]

Early and sustained rehabilitation is essential to recovery from sepsis. Physical rehabilitation in particular may not only improve physical function, but also seems to decrease the duration of delirium[77] and has the potential to improve long-term neuropsychological function,[86] decrease hospital readmission,[87] and improve long-term survival.[88] Additionally, specialized cognitive rehabilitation may play a role in reducing the incidence of lasting cognitive deficits in survivors. A small, randomized trial of ICU survivors with cognitive or physical impairment at discharge examined the efficacy of home-based cognitive and physical rehabilitation. The study, wherein ARDS owing to sepsis was the most common ICU admission diagnosis, demonstrated that patients receiving specialized rehabilitation experienced improved executive function at 3 months of follow-up compared with control subjects.[89]

The use of an ICU diary, a descriptive book detailing a patient's ICU stay, seems to mitigate impairments in mental health and provide much-needed education to patients.[90] The ICU diary is a notebook within which doctors, nurses, family members, and patient visitors can record narrative information and pictures documenting the patient's hospital course, along with messages from visitors. In follow-up after discharge, patients review the diary with a health care provider as a strategy to fill gaps in their memory regarding the hospitalization and to reconcile clouded or inaccurate memories with an accurate depiction of their hospitalization. The ICU diary has been shown to reduce PTSD symptoms in survivors and family members in multiple small prospective studies. However, the use of an ICU diary requires careful coordination of in-hospital and postdischarge care; therefore, its use in the United States has been limited to date.

Care coordination after hospitalization for sepsis remains an enduring challenge for survivors and providers given the frequency of post–acute care use after discharge,[6] the complex needs of sepsis survivors, and the recent realization that timely follow-up is necessary given the frequency of infection-related hospital readmissions in the early postdischarge period. Primary care physicians have traditionally been responsible for follow-up care after an acute care hospitalization. In recent years, follow-up clinics specializing in critical illness survivorship have been established on a limited and primarily investigational basis to address symptoms related to PICS. These clinics provide extensive care coordination between physical and occupational therapists, psychologists and psychiatrists, physical medicine and rehabilitation physicians, pulmonary physicians, and neurologists. Given the impairments and mortality that survivors experience, integration of palliative care into postdischarge practice should be considered as these practices mature. Although the theoretical benefits of ICU follow-up clinics exist, their effectiveness has not been established.[91]

As a result, extensive research is still needed to define the optimal structure of these clinics to maximize patient-centered outcomes. In the interim, it is essential that survivors be prioritized to receive early postdischarge follow-up, and that providers and patients partner during these visits with the shared vision to optimize recovery.[92]

## SUMMARY

Sepsis survivorship is a rapidly growing field that will be a defining aspect of critical care in the coming decades. Extensive literature now demonstrates that the long-term consequences of sepsis include significant and lasting impairment of cognition, physical function, and mental health. These impairments, combined with residual inflammation and immunosuppression, impact long-term health-related quality of life and survival. However, with improved focus on high-quality care across the continuum, and an emphasis on longitudinal coordination of care and rehabilitation after discharge, providers may help patients to convert our short-term success into long-term gains.

## ACKNOWLEDGMENTS

The authors acknowledge prior and present collaborations with Theodore J. Iwashyna, MD, PhD, that informed the present work and for his support to use figures from his prior work herein.

## REFERENCES

1. Angus DC, van der Poll T. Severe sepsis and septic shock. N Engl J Med 2013;369(9):840–51.

2. Angus DC, Linde-Zwirble WT, Lidicker J, et al. Epidemiology of severe sepsis in the United States: analysis of incidence, outcome, and associated costs of care. Crit Care Med 2001;29: 1303–10.

3. Gaieski DF, Edwards JM, Kallan MJ, et al. Benchmarking the incidence and mortality of severe sepsis in the United States. Crit Care Med 2013; 41:1167–74.

4. Kaukonen KM, Bailey M, Suzuki S, et al. Mortality related to severe sepsis and septic shock among critically ill patients in Australia and New Zealand, 2000-2012. JAMA 2014;311(13):1308–16.

5. Liu V, Escobar GJ, Greene JD, et al. Hospital deaths in patients with sepsis from 2 independent cohorts. JAMA 2014;312:90–1.

6. Jones TK, Fuchs BD, Small DS, et al. Post-acute care use and hospital readmission after sepsis. Ann Am Thorac Soc 2015;12(6):904–13.

7. Stevenson EK, Rubenstein AR, Radin GT, et al. Two decades of mortality trends among patients with severe sepsis: a comparative meta-analysis. Crit Care Med 2014;42(3):625–31.

8. Rivers E, Nguyen B, Havstad S, et al. Early goal-directed therapy in the treatment of severe sepsis and septic shock. N Engl J Med 2001; 345:1368–77.

9. Dellinger RP, Levy MM, Rhodes A, et al. Surviving sepsis campaign: international guidelines for management of severe sepsis and septic shock, 2012. Intensive Care Med 2013;39(2):165–228.

10. Levy MM, Rhodes A, Phillips GS, et al. Surviving sepsis campaign: association between performance metrics and outcomes in a 7.5-year study. Crit Care Med 2015;43(1):3–12.

11. The ProCESS Investigators. A randomized trial of protocol-based care for early septic shock. N Engl J Med 2014;370:1683–93.

12. The ARISE Investigators, the ANZICS Clinical Trials Group, Peake SL, et al. Goal-directed resuscitation for patients with early septic shock. N Engl J Med 2014;371:1496–506.

13. Mouncey PR, Osborn TM, Power GS, et al. Trial of early, goal-directed resuscitation for septic shock. N Engl J Med 2015;372:1301–11.

14. Angus DC. The lingering consequences of sepsis: a hidden public health disaster? JAMA 2010;304: 1833–4.

15. Needham DM, Davidson J, Cohen H, et al. Improving long-term outcomes after discharge from intensive care unit: report from a stakeholders' conference. Crit Care Med 2012;40(2):502–9.

16. Elliott D, Davidson JE, Harvey MA, et al. Exploring the scope of post-intensive care syndrome therapy and care: engagement of non-critical care providers and survivors in a second stakeholder meeting. Crit Care Med 2014;42(12):2518–26.

17. Iwashyna TJ, Ely EW, Smith DM, et al. Long-term cognitive impairment and functional disability among survivors of severe sepsis. JAMA 2010;304: 1787–94.

18. Pandharipande PP, Girard TD, Jackson JC, et al. Long-term cognitive impairment after critical illness. N Engl J Med 2013;369(14):1306–16.

19. Guerra C, Linde-Zwirble WT, Wunsch H. Risk factors for dementia after critical illness in elderly Medicare beneficiaries. Crit Care 2012;16(6):R233.

20. Annane D, Sharshar T. Cognitive decline after sepsis. Lancet Respir Med 2015;3(1):61–9.

21. Gross AL, Jones RN, Habtemariam DA, et al. Delirium and long-term cognitive trajectory among persons with dementia. Arch Intern Med 2012; 172(17):1324–31.

22. Saczynski JS, Marcantonio ER, Quach L, et al. Cognitive trajectories after postoperative delirium. N Engl J Med 2012;367:30.

23. Girard TD, Jackson JC, Bernard GR, et al. Delirium as a predictor of long-term cognitive impairment in survivors of critical illness. Crit Care Med 2010; 38(7):1513.

24. Morandi A, Hughes CG, Thompson JL, et al. Statins and delirium during critical illness: a multicenter, prospective cohort study. Crit Care Med 2014; 42(8):1899–909.

25. Mikkelsen ME, Christie JD, Lanken PN, et al. The adult respiratory distress syndrome cognitive outcomes study: long-term neuropsychological function in survivors of acute lung injury. Am J Respir Crit Care Med 2012;185(12):1307–15.

26. Wilcox ME, Brummel NE, Archer K, et al. Cognitive dysfunction in ICU patients: risk factors, predictors, and rehabilitation interventions. Crit Care Med 2013; 41(9 Suppl 1):S81–98.

27. Desai SV, Law TJ, Needham DM. Long-term complications of critical care. Crit Care Med 2011;39: 371–9.

28. Davydow DS, Gifford JM, Desai SV, et al. Depression in general intensive care unit survivors. A systematic review. Intensive Care Med 2009;35: 796–809.

29. Davydow DS, Gifford JM, Desai SV, et al. Posttraumatic stress disorder in general intensive care unit survivors: a systematic review. Gen Hosp Psychiatry 2008;30:421–34.

30. Wintermann GB, Brunkhorst FM, Petrowski K, et al. Stress disorders following prolonged critical illness in survivors of severe sepsis. Crit Care Med 2015; 43(6):1213–22.

31. Davydow DS, Hough CL, Langa KM, et al. Symptoms of depression in survivors of severe sepsis: a prospective cohort study of older Americans. Am J Geriatr Psychiatry 2013;21(9):887–97.

32. Davydow DS, Hough CL, Langa KM. Presepsis depressive symptoms are associated with incident

cognitive impairment in survivors of severe sepsis: a prospective cohort study of older Americans. J Am Geriatr Soc 2012;60(12):2290–6.

33. Davydow DS, Hough CL, Langa KM, et al. Depressive symptoms in spouses of older patients with severe sepsis. Crit Care Med 2012;40(8):2335–41.

34. Iwashyna TJ, Cooke CR, Wunsch H, et al. Population burden of long-term survivorship after severe sepsis among older Americans. J Am Geriatr Soc 2012; 60(6):1070–7.

35. Batt J, dos Santos CC, Cameron JI, et al. Intensive care unit-acquired weakness: clinical phenotypes and molecular mechanisms. Am J Respir Crit Care Med 2013;187(3):238–46.

36. Dos Santos CC, Batt J. ICU-acquired weakness: mechanisms of disability. Curr Opin Crit Care 2012;18(5):509–17.

37. Bienvenu OJ, Colantuoni E, Mendez-Tellez PA, et al. Depressive symptoms and impaired physical function after acute lung injury: a 2-year longitudinal study. Crit Care Med 2012;185(5):517–24.

38. Gallop KH, Kerr CE, Nixon A, et al. A qualitative investigation of patients' and caregivers' experiences of severe sepsis. Crit Care Med 2015;43(2): 296–307.

39. Cox CE, Docherty SL, Brandon DH, et al. Surviving critical illness: acute respiratory distress syndrome as experienced by patients and their caregivers. Crit Care Med 2009;37(10):2702–8.

40. Hotchkiss RS. Sepsis-induced immunosuppression: from cellular dysfunctions to immunotherapy. Nat Rev Immunol 2013;13:862–74.

41. Yende S, D'Angelo G, Kellum JA, et al, GenIMS Investigators. Inflammatory markers at hospital discharge predict subsequent mortality after pneumonia and sepsis. Am J Respir Crit Care Med 2008;177:1242–7.

42. Yende S, D'Angelo G, Mayr F, et al, GenIMS Investigators. Elevated hemostasis markers after pneumonia increases one-year risk of allcause and cardiovascular deaths. PLoS One 2011;6:e22847.

43. Bone RC, Balk RA, Cerra FB, et al. Definitions for sepsis and organ failure and guidelines for the use of innovative therapies in sepsis. The ACCP/SCCM Consensus Conference Committee. American College of Chest Physicians/Society of Critical Care Medicine. Chest 1992;101:1644–55.

44. Calandra T, Cohen J, International Sepsis Forum Definition of Infection in the ICU consensus Conference. The international sepsis forum consensus conference on definitions of infection in the intensive care unit. Crit Care Med 2005;33(7):1538–48.

45. Yende S, Angus DC. Long-term outcomes from sepsis. Curr Infect Dis Rep 2007;9:382–6.

46. Romero-Bermejo FJ, Ruiz-Bailen M, Gil-Cebrian J, et al. Sepsis-induced cardiomyopathy. Curr Cardiol Rev 2011;7(3):163–83.

47. Walkey AJ, Greiner MA, Heckbert SR, et al. Atrial fibrillation among Medicare beneficiaries hospitalized with sepsis: incidence and risk factors. Am Heart J 2013;165(6):949–55.

48. Walkey AJ, Wiener RS, Ghobrial JM, et al. Incident stroke and mortality associated with new-onset atrial fibrillation in patients hospitalized with severe sepsis. JAMA 2011;306(20):2248–54.

49. Yende S, Linde-Zwirble W, Mayr F, et al. Risk of cardiovascular events in survivors of severe sepsis. Am J Respir Crit Care Med 2014;189:1065–74.

50. Walkey AJ, Hammill BG, Curtis LH, et al. Long-term outcomes following development of new-onset atrial fibrillation during sepsis. Chest 2014;146(5):1187–95.

51. Ward PA. Immunosuppression in sepsis. JAMA 2011;306:2618–9.

52. Simon PM, Delude RL, Lee M, et al, GenIMS Investigators. Duration and magnitude of hypotension and monocyte deactivation in patients with community-acquired pneumonia. Shock 2011;36: 553–9.

53. Torgersen C, Moser P, Luckner G, et al. Macroscopic postmortem findings in 235 surgical intensive care patients with sepsis. Anesth Analg 2009;108:1841–7.

54. Walton AH, Muenzer JT, Rasche D, et al. Reactivation of multiple viruses in patients with sepsis. PLoS One 2014;9(6):e98819.

55. Goodwin AJ, Rice DA, Simpson KN, et al. Frequency, cost, and risk factors of readmissions among severe sepsis survivors. Crit Care Med 2015;43:738–46.

56. Chang DW, Tseng CH, Shapiro MF. Rehospitalizations following sepsis: common and costly. Crit Care Med 2015;43(10):2085–93.

57. Sutton J, Friedman B. Trends in septicemia hospitalizations and readmissions in selected HCUP states, 2005 and 2010. HCUP statistical brief #161. Rockville (MD): Agency for Healthcare Research and Quality; 2013. Available at: www.hcup-us.ahrq. gov/reports/statbriefs/sb161.pdf.

58. Centers for Medicare & Medicaid Services: Readmissions reduction program. Available at: www.cms. gov/Medicare/Medicare-Fee-for-Service-Payment/ AcuteInpatientPPS/Readmissions-Reduction-Program. html. Accessed August 9, 2015.

59. Jencks SF, Williams MV, Coleman EA. Rehospitalizations among patients in the Medicare fee-for-service program. N Engl J Med 2009;360:1418–28.

60. Mechanic R. Post-acute care—the next frontier for controlling Medicare spending. N Engl J Med 2014;370:692–4.

61. Ortego A, Gaieski DF, Fuchs BD, et al. Hospital-based acute care use in survivors of septic shock. Crit Care Med 2015;43:729–37.

62. Liu V, Lei X, Prescott HC, et al. Hospital readmission and healthcare utilization following sepsis in community settings. J Hosp Med 2014;9:502–7.

63. Donnelly JP, Hohmann SF, Wang HE. Unplanned re-admissions after hospitalization for severe sepsis at academic medical center-affiliated hospitals. Crit Care Med 2015;43(9):1916–27.

64. Prescott HC, Langa KM, Liu V, et al. Increased one-year health care utilization in survivors of severe sepsis. Am J Respir Crit Care Med 2014;190(1):62–9.

65. Elixhauser A, Steiner C. Readmissions to U.S. hospital by diagnosis, 2010. HCUP statistical brief #161. Rockville (MD): Agency for Healthcare Research and Quality; 2013. Available at: www.hcup-us.ahrq.gov/reports/statbriefs/sb153.pdf.

66. Prescott HC, Langa KM, Iwashyna TJ. Readmission diagnoses after hospitalization for severe sepsis and other acute medical conditions. JAMA 2015; 313(10):1055–7.

67. Leligdowicz A, Dodek PM, Norena M, et al. Association between source of infection and hospital mortality in patients who have septic shock. Am J Respir Crit Care Med 2014;189(10):1204–13.

68. Wang T, Derhovanessian A, De Cruz S, et al. Subsequent infections in survivors of sepsis: epidemiology and outcomes. J Intensive Care Med 2014; 29:87–95.

69. Winters BD, Eberlein M, Leung J, et al. Long-term mortality and quality of life in sepsis: a systematic review. Crit Care Med 2010;38:1276–83.

70. Wang HE, Szychowski JM, Griffin R, et al. Long-term mortality after community-acquired sepsis: a longitudinal population-based cohort study. BMJ Open 2014;4:e004283.

71. Cuthbertson BH, Elders A, Hall S, et al. Mortality and quality of life in the five years after severe sepsis. Crit Care 2013;17(2):R70.

72. Maley JH, Mikkelsen ME. Sepsis survivorship: how can we promote a culture of resilience? Crit Care Med 2015;43(2):479–81.

73. Pandharipande P, Banerjee A, McGrane S, et al. Liberation and animation for ventilated ICU patients: the ABCDE bundle for the back-end of critical care. Crit Care 2010;14(3):157.

74. Morandi A, Brummel NE, Ely EW. Sedation, delirium and mechanical ventilation: the 'ABCDE' approach. Curr Opin Crit Care 2011;17(1):43–9.

75. Girard TD, Kress JP, Fuchs BD, et al. Efficacy and safety of a paired sedation and ventilator weaning protocol for mechanically ventilated patients in intensive care (awakening and breathing controlled trial): a randomised controlled trial. Lancet 2008; 371(9607):126–34.

76. Ely EW, Inouye SK, Bernard GR, et al. Delirium in mechanically ventilated patients: validity and reliability of the confusion assessment method for the intensive care unit (CAM-ICU). JAMA 2001;286: 2703–10.

77. Schweickert WD, Pohlman MC, Pohlman AS, et al. Early physical and occupational therapy in mechanically ventilated, critically ill patients: a randomized, controlled trial. Lancet 2009;373:1874–82.

78. Balas MC, Vasilevskis EE, Olsen KM, et al. Effectiveness and safety of the awakening and breathing coordination, delirium monitoring/management, and early exercise/mobility bundle. Crit Care Med 2014;42(5):1024–36.

79. Klompas M, Anderson D, Trick W, et al. The preventability of ventilator-associated events. The CDC Prevention Epicenters Wake Up and Breathe Collaborative. Am J Respir Crit Care Med 2015; 191(3):292–301.

80. Jakob SM, Ruokonen E, Grounds RM, et al. Dexmedetomidine vs midazolam or propofol for sedation during prolonged mechanical ventilation: two randomized controlled trials. JAMA 2012; 307(11):1151–60.

81. Dahmani S, Rouelle D, Gressens P, et al. Effects of dexmedetomidine on hippocampal focal adhesion kinase tyrosine phosphorylation in physiologic and ischemic conditions. Anesthesiology 2005;103(5): 969–77.

82. Sonneville R, Verdonk F, Rauturier C, et al. Understanding brain dysfunction in sepsis. Ann Intensive Care 2013;3(1):15.

83. Pandharipande P, Shintani A, Peterson J, et al. Lorazepam is an independent risk factor for transitioning to delirium in intensive care unit patients. Anesthesiology 2006;104(1):21–6.

84. Barr J, Fraser GL, Puntillo K, et al. Clinical practice guidelines for the management of pain, agitation, and delirium in adult patients in the Intensive Care Unit. Crit Care Med 2013;41:263–306.

85. Fraser GL, Devlin JW, Worby CP, et al. Benzodiazepine versus nonbenzodiazepine-based sedation for mechanically ventilated, critically ill adults: a systematic review and meta-analysis of randomized trials. Crit Care Med 2013;41(9S1):S30–8.

86. Hopkins RO, Suchyta MR, Farrer TJ, et al. Improving post-intensive care unit neuropsychiatric outcomes: understanding cognitive effects of physical activity. Am J Respir Crit Care Med 2012;186(12):1220–8.

87. Morris PE, Griffin L, Berry M, et al. Receiving early mobility during an ICU admission is a predictor of improved outcomes in acute respiratory failure. Am J Med Sci 2011;341(5):373–7.

88. Chao PW, Shih CJ, Lee YJ, et al. Association of post-discharge rehabilitation with mortality in intensive care unit survivors of sepsis. Am J Respir Crit Care Med 2014;190(9):1003–11.

89. Jackson J, Ely EW, Morey MC, et al. Cognitive and physical rehabilitation of ICU survivors: results of the RETURN randomized, controlled pilot investigation. Crit Care Med 2012;40(4):1088–97.

90. Mehlhorn J, Freytag A, Schmidt K, et al. Rehabilitation interventions for postintensive care

syndrome: a systematic review. Crit Care Med 2014;42(5):1263–71.

91. Cuthbertson BH, Rattray J, Campbell MK, et al. The PRaCTICaL study of nurse led, intensive care follow-up programmes for improving long term outcomes from critical illness: a pragmatic randomised controlled trial. BMJ 2009;339:b3723.

92. Mikkelsen ME, Iwashyna TJ, Thompson C. Why ICU clinicians need to care about post-intensive care syndrome. Critical Connections, in press. Available at: http://www.sccm.org/Communications/Critical-Connections/Archives/Pages/Why-ICU-Clinicians-Need-to-Care-about-Post-Intensive-Care-Syndrome.aspx. Accessed February 26, 2016.

# Index

*Note:* Page numbers of article titles are in **boldface** type.

## A

Acid-base balance
  in AKI management in septic patient, 283–284
Acute kidney injury (AKI)
  crystalloids In fluid resuscitation in sepsis and, 245
  defined, 277
  epidemiology of, 277–278
  introduction, 277–279
  pathophysiology of, 279–280
  RIFLE criteria for, 277
  risk factors for, 279
  in septic patient, **277–288**
    management of, 279–284
      acid-base balance in, 283–284
      "euvolemia"-related, 279–280
      future directions in, 284
      goals in, 279–282
      mean arterial pressure–related, 280–281
      nephrotoxins-related, 281–282
      nonpharmacologic strategies, 282–284
      pharmacologic, 282
      renal replacement therapy in, 282–283
Adrenergic nervous system
  activation of
    in sepsis, 322
Age
  as factor in increased incidence of sepsis, 170
Agitation
  in septic patients after initial resuscitation
    management of, 348–352 (*See also* Pain,
      agitation, and delirium (PAD))
AKI. *See* Acute kidney injury (AKI)
Albumin
  in fluid resuscitation in sepsis, 247
Alert fatigue
  as barrier to development and implementation of
    sepsis alert systems, 221
Algorithm alert performance
  as barrier to development and implementation of
    sepsis alert systems, 221
Amygdala
  functional anatomy of
    during sepsis, 340–341
Antibiotics
  empiric
    in goal-directed resuscitation in septic
      shock, 233

  in sepsis management, 182
Antibodies
  anti–LPS
    in sepsis management, 183–184
Anti–LPS antibodies
  in sepsis management, 183–184
Antimicrobial Stewardship Programs (ASPs)
    potential economic impact of rapid molecular
      diagnostic methods and benefits for
        in early identification and treatment of
          sepsis-related pathogens, 201–204
Apoptosis
  cardiac dysfunction in sepsis related to, 292
Arterial pressure
  measurement of
    hypotension, shock, and, 251–252
  for septic shock
    target mean, 252–253
ASPs. *See* Antimicrobial Stewardship Programs
  (ASPs)
Astrocyte(s)
  in SAE, 336, 338

## B

Bacteremia
  sepsis-related
    detection of
      molecular methods in, 192
Biomarkers
  in sepsis
    metabolic changes as, 324–327
Blood transfusion
  in PAD management in septic patients after initial
    resuscitation, 354–355
Brain dysfunction
  in sepsis, **333–345** (*See also* Sepsis-associated
    encephalopathy (SAE))
    clinical presentation of, 333–335
    introduction, 333
    neuroimaging procedures in, 334–335
    neurophysiologic tests in, 334–335
    short- and long-term outcomes of, 335
Brain response
  acute
    during sepsis, 333–334
Brainstem

Brainstem (*continued*)
  functional anatomy of
    during sepsis, 339

**C**

Cardiac dysfunction
  in sepsis, **289–298** (*See also* Sepsis, cardiac
    dysfunction in)
Cardiac failure
  echocardiography in detection of, 303–304
Cardiomyopathy
  septic
    echocardiography in detection of, 303–304
Cardiovascular risk factors
  in sepsis survivors, 371
CCE. *See* Critical care echocardiography (CCE)
Cellular metabolism
  in SAE, 338
Central nervous system (CNS)
  functional anatomy of
    during sepsis, 339–341
CNS. *See* Central nervous system (CNS)
Coagulation
  infection and, 264
Cognitive impairment
  in sepsis survivors, 368–369
Colloids
  in fluid resuscitation in sepsis, 247–248
    albumin, 247
    semisynthetic colloids, 247–248
Comorbid conditions
  as factor in increased incidence of sepsis, 171
Contractile dysfunction
  in sepsis, 292–293
Critical care echocardiography (CCE)
  advanced, 300–301
  basic, 300
  in hemodynamic evaluation
    main views, 301–302
  learning and understanding, 300–302
Crystalloids
  in fluid resuscitation in sepsis, 245–247
    AKI related to, 245
    hyperchloremic metabolic acidosis related to,
      245
    isotonic crystalloids, 245
Cytokine(s)
  in sepsis management, 183
Cytokine release
  metabolic effects of
    sepsis and, 322–323

**D**

Delirium

in septic patients after initial resuscitation
  management of, 348–352 (*See also* Pain,
    agitation, and delirium (PAD))
Dexmedetomidine
  in PAD management in septic patients after initial
    resuscitation, 349
Diabetes
  chronic hyperglycemia effects on, 311–313
  unrecognized, 313
Dobutamine
  in goal-directed resuscitation in septic shock,
    235–236
Dysglycemia
  in septic patients, **309–319**
    glucose targets, 314–315
    interpretation, 316
    introduction, 309
    pathogenesis of, 309–314
    prevalence of, 309–314
    terminology related to, 309–314

**E**

Echocardiography
  critical care (*See* Critical care echocardiography
    (CCE))
  in sepsis, **299–309**
    hemodynamic profiles detected by, 302–304
      cardiac failure, 303–304
      hypovolemia or fluid responsiveness status,
        302–303
      left ventricular diastolic dysfunction, 303
      left ventricular systolic dysfunction, 303
      right ventricular dysfunction, 304
    introduction, 299–300
    in practice, 304–305
Edema
  tissue
    infection and, 264
Electronic medical records (EMRs)
  clinical diagnostic cue not available in
    as barrier to development and implementation
      of sepsis alert systems, 220–221
EMRs. *See* Electronic medical records (EMRs)
Encephalopathy
  sepsis-associated, **333–345** (*See also* Sepsis-
    associated encephalopathy (SAE))
Endothelial glycocalyx
  septic microcirculation and, 267–268
Environment(s)
  hospital
    reengineering of
      in development and implementation of
        sepsis alert systems, 226
"Euvolemia"
  as management goal in AKI, 279–280

# F

Fatigue
  alert
    as barrier to development and implementation
      of sepsis alert systems, 221
Fluid(s)
  IV
    in goal-directed resuscitation in septic shock,
      232–233
    in PAD management in septic patients after initial
      resuscitation, 353–354
  responsiveness to
    echocardiography in detection of, 302–303
  in sepsis management, 182
Frontal cortex
  functional anatomy of
    during sepsis, 340–341
Functional disability
  in sepsis survivors, 369–370

# G

Gender
  as factor in increased incidence of sepsis, 170
Gene expression profiling
  sepsis-related
    considerations for future studies, 216
Genetics
  as factor in cardiac dysfunction in sepsis, 290
Geography
  as factor in increased incidence of sepsis, 171
Gliovascular unit
  in SAE, 338
Glucose control
  during sepsis, **309–319** (See also Dysglycemia, in
    septic patients)
Glycemic variability
  defined, 314
Glycocalyx
  endothelial
    septic microcirculation and, 267–268
Goal-directed resuscitation
  history of, 231–232
  in septic shock, **231–239** (See also Septic shock,
    goal-directed resuscitation in)
Goal-directed therapies
  for septic shock, 254–257

# H

Haloperidol
  in PAD management in septic patients after initial
    resuscitation, 349, 352
Health care delivery
  variability in systems of
    as barrier to development and implementation
      of sepsis alert systems, 221–224

# Heart

Heart
  sepsis effects on, **289–298** (See also Sepsis,
    cardiac dysfunction in)
Hemodynamic management
  of PAD in septic patients after initial resuscitation,
    353–354
Hippocampus
  functional anatomy of
    during sepsis, 340–341
Hospital environment
  reengineering of
    in development and implementation of sepsis
      alert systems, 226
Hyperchloremic metabolic acidosis
  crystalloids in fluid resuscitation in sepsis and, 245
Hyperglycemia
  chronic
    diabetes effects of, 311–313
  defined, 309
  harm secondary to, 310–311
  stress-induced, 309–310
    mechanism of, 310
Hypoglycemia, 313–314
Hypotension
  sepsis-mediated, 251–252
Hypothalamus
  functional anatomy of
    during sepsis, 339–340
Hypovolemia
  echocardiography in detection of, 302–303

# I

Immune paralysis
  in sepsis, 212–214
Immunosuppression
  in sepsis survivors, 371
Infection(s)
  normal microvasculature response to, 263–264
Information overload
  development and implementation of, 221
Inotropic agents
  vasopressors with
    during sepsis, 258
Intravenous (IV) fluids
  in goal-directed resuscitation in septic shock,
    232–233
IRIDICA BAC-BSI assay
  in early identification of sepsis pathogens, 201
Ischemic process
  in SAE, 338

# L

Lactate
  as biomarker in sepsis, 324–325
Left ventricular diastolic dysfunction

Left (*continued*)
    echocardiography in detection of, 303
Left ventricular systolic dysfunction
    echocardiography in detection of, 303
Leukocyte adhesion
    infection and, 264
Levosimendan
    vasopressors with
        during sepsis, 259
Lipopolysaccharide(s) (LPS)
    blocking of
        in sepsis management, 183–184
LPS. *See* Lipopolysaccharide(s) (LPS)


**M**

Machine learning
    mathematical modeling and
        in development and implementation of sepsis
            alert systems, 224
Macronutrients
    metabolism of
        sepsis effects on, 323–324
    in septic patients
        replacement of, 328
Mathematical modeling and machine learning
    in development and implementation of sepsis alert
        systems, 224
Mechanical ventilation
    in PAD management in septic patients after initial
        resuscitation, 352–353
Melatonin receptor agonists
    in PAD management in septic patients after initial
        resuscitation, 352
Metabolic acidosis
    hyperchloremic
        crystalloids in fluid resuscitation in sepsis
            and, 245
Metabolic factors
    cardiac dysfunction in sepsis related to, 290
Metabolism
    sepsis effects on, **321–331**
Metabolomics, **321–331**
Microcirculation
    in sepsis
        therapeutic targeting of, 268–270
    septic
        endothelial glycocalyx and, 267–268
Microglia
    in SAE, 336
Micronutrients
    metabolism of
        sepsis effects on, 324
    in septic patients
        replacement of, 328
Microvasculature
    normal response to infection, 263–264

    in sepsis, **263–275** (*See also* Sepsis,
        microcirculatory dysfunction in)
Milrinone
    vasopressors with
        during sepsis, 259
Molecular factors
    cardiac dysfunction in sepsis related to, 290
Myocardial infiltration
    cardiac dysfunction in sepsis related to, 292


**N**

Necrosis
    cardiac dysfunction in sepsis related to, 292
Neuronal dysfunction
    in SAE, 339
Neurovascular coupling
    in SAE, 338
Nutritional support
    in septic patients, **321–331**
        enteral *vs.* parenteral nutrition, 328
        macronutrient and micronutrient replacement,
            328
        in PAD management after initial resuscitation,
            355–356
        timing of, 327–328


**O**

Oxygen delivery
    in goal-directed resuscitation in septic shock
        assessment of, 235–236


**P**

Packed red blood cells
    in goal-directed resuscitation in septic shock,
        235–236
PAD. *See* Pain, agitation, and delirium (PAD)
Pain
    in septic patients after initial resuscitation
        management of, 348–352 (*See also* Pain,
            agitation, and delirium (PAD))
Pain, agitation, and delirium (PAD)
    in septic patients after initial resuscitation
        management of, 348–352
            blood transfusion in, 354–355
            early mobilization and exercise in, 349
            hemodynamic, 353–354
            mechanical ventilation in, 352–353
            medications in, 349, 352
            nutritional support in, 355–356
            spontaneous breathing trials and
                decreased sedation in, 349
Pituitary gland
    functional anatomy of
        during sepsis, 339–340

Preload
    optimizing
        in goal-directed resuscitation in septic
            shock, 234
Propofol
    in PAD management in septic patients after initial
        resuscitation, 349
Psychological morbidity
    in sepsis survivors, 369

**Q**

Quality of life
    in sepsis survivors, 374–375
Quantitative resuscitation
    in sepsis management, 184

**R**

Race
    as factor in increased incidence of sepsis,
        170–171
Ramelteon
    in PAD management in septic patients after initial
        resuscitation, 352
Red blood cells
    packed
        in goal-directed resuscitation in septic shock,
            235–236
Renal replacement therapy
    in AKI management in septic patient, 282–283
Resuscitation
    fluid
        in sepsis, **241–250** (See also Sepsis, fluid
            resuscitation in)
    goal-directed
        history of, 231–232
        in septic shock, **231–239** (See also Septic
            shock, goal-directed resuscitation in)
    initial
        caring for septic patients after, **347–365** (See
            also Septic patient(s), caring for, after initial
            resuscitation)
    quantitative
        in sepsis management, 184
RIFLE criteria
    for AKI, 277
Right ventricular dysfunction
    echocardiography in detection of, 304

**S**

SAE. See Sepsis-associated encephalopathy (SAE)
Seasonality
    as factor in increased incidence of sepsis, 171
Sepsis
    activation of adrenergic nervous system in, 322
    acute brain response during, 333–334
    AKI and, **277–288** (See also Acute kidney injury
        (AKI))
    altered cellular metabolism in
        mechanisms of, 323
    altered endocrine physiology in, 322
    brain dysfunction in, **333–345** (See also Brain
        dysfunction, in sepsis; Sepsis-associated
        encephalopathy (SAE))
    broader metabolic profiling in, 325–327
    cardiac dysfunction in, **289–298**
        contractile dysfunction, 292–293
        imaging studies of, 295
        impact of chronic heart disease on acute
            hemodynamics, 293
        introduction, 289
        laboratory studies of, 293–295
        mechanisms of, 293
        pathophysiology of, 289–293
            functional abnormalities in, 289–290
            hemodynamic abnormalities in, 292–293
            structural abnormalities in, 290–292
        treatment of, 295–296
    CNS during
        functional anatomy of, 339–341
    defined, **165–179,** 191, 367
    described, 209–210, 367–368
    echocardiography in, **299–309** (See also
        Echocardiography, in sepsis)
    epidemiology of
        changing, **165–179**
        clinical correlations and, 171–177
        future of, 171–177
        global, 170
        U.S. trends in, 165–170
    fluid resuscitation in, **241–250**
        dose for, 242–245
            administration in sepsis resuscitation,
                242–243
            in sepsis management after resuscitation,
                244–245
        fluid choice in, 245–248
            colloids, 247–248
            crystalloids, 245–247
        physiology of, 241–242
    gene expression at onset of, 210–212
    gene expression profiling in
        considerations for future studies, 216
    glucose control during, **309–319** (See also
        Dysglycemia, in septic patients)
    hospital-acquired
        prediction of
            longitudinal studies of, 212
    immune paralysis in, 212–214
    improved outcomes of, 257–258
    incidence of
        increased

Sepsis (*continued*)
    factors associated with, 170–171
    U.S. trends in, 165–170
  introduction, 165, 191–192, 209–210, 241
  metabolic changes in, 322–324
    as biomarkers, 324–327
    mediators of, 322–323
  metabolic effects of cytokine release in, 322–323
  metabolism in, **321–331**
    introduction, 321
    macronutrients effects of, 323–324
    micronutrients effects of, 324
  microcirculatory dysfunction in, **263–275**
    evidence of, 264
    measurement of, 264–266
    novel microcirculation-protective therapies for, 270–271
    pathogenesis of, 266–267
    therapeutic targeting for, 268–270
  mortality data, 209, 367
    prognostication at admission effects on, 210–212
    U.S. trends in, 165–170
  nutritional support for, **321–331**
  organ-specific outcomes in peripheral blood related to
  markers of, 214–215
  pathogens in
    early identification and treatment of, **191–207**
      amplified methods–growth required, 197–198
      broad-based methods, 196–197
      broad-based technologies directly from whole blood, 198–201
      IRIDICA BAC-BSI assay, 201
      molecular methods for bacteremia detection, 192
      nonamplified, growth-dependent methods, 192–197
      pathogen-specific methods, 192–196
      rapid molecular diagnostic methods and benefits for ASPs, 201–204
      T2 Candida magnetic resonance assay, 200–201
  prognosis in, **209–218**
    future directions in, 216–217
    importance of time in studies of, 212
  risk stratification in, **209–218**
  septic shock related to
    described, 251
  subtypes of
    unsupervised learning of, 215–216
  survivors of, **367–380** (*See also* Sepsis survivors)
  terminology related to, **165–179**
  treatment of
    antibiotics in, 182
    anti-LPS antibodies in, 183–184

    clinical trials, 183–184
      optimizing trial design, 186–187
    cytokines in, 183
    evolution of, 182
    fluids in, 182
    future targets in, 184–186
    healing injured epithelium in, 184–185
    large-scale screens of compounds safe for human use in, 185–186
    late mediators of septic organ injury in, 185
    quantitative resuscitation in, 184
    supporting injured organs in, 182
    therapeutic targets in, **181–189**
  ultrasound in, **299–309** (*See also* Ultrasound, in sepsis)
  vasopressors during, **251–262** (*See also* Vasopressor(s), during sepsis)
Sepsis alert systems
  development and implementation of, **219–229**
    barriers to, 220–224
      alert fatigue, 221
      algorithm alert performance, 221
      clinical diagnostic cue not available in EMRs, 220–221
      information overload, 221
      variability in systems of health care delivery, 221–224
    described, 220
    potential solutions to, 224–226
      alert delivery and integration into workflow, 224, 226
      improved alert system: mathematical modeling and machine learning, 224
      reengineering hospital environment, 226
  introduction, 219–220
Sepsis-associated encephalopathy (SAE), **333–345**. *See also* Brain dysfunction, in sepsis
  clinical presentation of, 333–335
  described, 333
  introduction, 333
  neuroimaging procedures in, 334–335
  neurophysiologic tests in, 334–335
  pathophysiology of, 335–339
    ischemic process in, 338
    neuroinflammation in, 335–338
    neuronal dysfunction in, 339
  short- and long-term outcomes of, 335
Sepsis survivors, **367–380**
  health care resource use by, 371–375
    ED visits, 372
    hospital-based acute care use, 372
    hospital readmissions, 372–374
    post–acute care use, 372
  long-term consequences in, **367–380**
    health-related quality of life and mortality, 374–375
    immunosuppression, 371

improving, 375–376
inflammation and cardiovascular risk, 371
neuropsychological and physical impairments,
    368–371
    cognitive impairment, 368–369
    functional disability, 369–370
    psychological morbidity, 369
qualitative experience of, 370–371
Septic cardiomyopathy
echocardiography in detection of, 303–304
Septic patient(s)
caring for
    after initial resuscitation, **347–365**
        introduction, 347–348
        PAD management, 348–352 (*See also* Pain,
            agitation, and delirium (PAD), in septic
            patients after initial resuscitation)
        viral reactivation, 356–358
Septic shock
defined, 252
described, 251–252
goal-directed resuscitation in, **231–239**
    dobutamine in, 235–236
    early identification in, 232
    empiric antibiotics in, 233
    future directions in, 237
    history of, 231–232
    IV fluid resuscitation, 232–233
    optimizing preload in, 234
    oxygen delivery assessment in, 235–236
    packed red blood cells in, 235–236
    vasopressor support in, 234–235
goal-directed therapies for, 254–257
improved outcomes of, 257–258
sepsis and
    described, 251
target mean arterial pressure for, 252–253
vasopressors for, **251–262** (*See also*
    Vasopressor(s), during sepsis)
Sex
as factor in increased incidence of sepsis, 170
Shock

septic (*See* Septic shock)
Stress hyperglycemia, 309–310
    mechanism of, 310

T

T2 Candida magnetic resonance assay
    in early identification of sepsis pathogens,
        200–201
Time
    in studies of acute critical illness
        importance of, 212
Tissue edema
    infection and, 264

U

Ultrasound. *See also* Echocardiography
    critical care
        learning and understanding, 300–302
    in sepsis, **299–309**
        introduction, 299–300
        in practice, 304–305

V

Vasopressor(s)
    in goal-directed resuscitation in septic shock,
        234–235
    in PAD management in septic patients after initial
        resuscitation, 353–354
    during sepsis, **251–262**
        comparisons among, 253–254
        inotropic agents with, 258
        introduction, 251
        monitoring patients on, 258–259
        supplements for
            levosimendan, 259
            milrinone, 259
Viral reactivation
    in PAD management in septic patients after initial
        resuscitation, 356–358

Printed and bound by CPI Group (UK) Ltd, Croydon, CR0 4YY

12/05/2025

01866934-0001